CLARK'S
POSITIONING IN
RADIOGRAPHY

TENTH EDITION
Volume Two

Edited by Louis Kreel MD FRCP FRCR

A WILLIAM HEINEMANN MEDICAL BOOKS
PUBLICATION

Distributed by
YEAR BOOK MEDICAL PUBLISHERS, INC.
35 East Wacker Drive, Chicago

First edition published in January 1939
Second edition published in January 1941
Third edition published in June 1942
Fourth edition published in April 1945
Fifth edition published in October 1949
Sixth edition published in February 1951
Seventh edition published in December 1956
Eighth edition published in July 1964
Eighth edition (revised) published in May 1967
Ninth edition (Volume 1) published in 1973
Tenth edition (Volume 1) published in 1979
Tenth edition (Volume 2) published in 1981

(ISBN 0–8151–5191–8)

Distributed in Continental North, South and Central America,
Hawaii, Puerto Rico and The Philippines by
Year Book Medical Publishers, Inc.

by Arrangement with
William Heinemann Medical Books, Ltd.

Filmset and printed in Great Britain

INTRODUCTION
to the TENTH EDITION

The last ten years have seen considerable advances in radiography, radiology departments and hospital practice. Rare-earth screens are now widely used with a marked reduction in radiation exposure making short exposure times possible without recourse to high kilovoltage or high output generators.

Many old procedures have been modified and new procedures introduced, now being an integral part of normal practice. Angiography is available in all but the smallest departments, double contrast barium meals and enemas performed routinely as well as arthography, renal cyst puncture, antegrade pyelography, mammography and endoscopic retrograde cholangio-pancreotography (ERCP).

Automatic processing is currently so widespread that 'wet processing' is not only unknown in many departments but can hardly be remembered while radiographic equipment with automatic exposure control is gaining wider acceptance. Radiography has consequently become easier and pleasanter with cleaner and more efficient dark rooms, fewer repeat examinations and a saving in cost and radiation.

Fluoroscopy has also become simpler and pleasanter with the universal introduction of image intensification and television viewing. Gone are the old days of red goggles, dark adaptation and barium examinations in the dark. Moreover, the new caesium iodide intensifier tubes produce images of very high quality. Even the films are in the process of change with the acceptance of 70 and 100 mm films, storage by miniaturisation and the use of Xerography.

Central sterilisation departments provide sterile angiographic, aspiration, myelographic and hystersalpingography packs. Emergency examinations are now readily organized with a minimum of fuss and bother, and have consequently become safer and more tolerable for the patient. A more important reason for the increased safety is that the newer contrast agents for these invasive procedures are less toxic and more easily managed.

Intensive Care and Coronary Care units (ITU/CCU) are an accepted part of general hospital practice and many more hospitals move patients to radiology departments in their beds. Mobile examinations are therefore more confined and are of much better quality especially with the new higher output units.

There has also been a greater awareness of the potential hazard from radiation in the early months of pregnancy and the almost universal implementation of the 10 day rule is especially gratifying. The most dramatic change however is the introduction of ultrasonography in obstetrics which has completely displaced conventional radiography. But it is not only in obstetrics that the new scanning methods are revolutionizing diagnostic radiology. Non-invasive methods including isotope imaging, computed tomography and nuclear magnetic resonance scanning are being applied to all areas of the body and every organ. The new generation of radiographers are likely to be as familiar and unimpressed by these innovations as the present generation are with automatic processors and image intensifiers.

Thus radiology departments have changed radically in the last decade, making exact diagnoses more readily available to larger numbers with less discomfort to the patient and easier for the radiographer. However, radiographers now need a far greater knowledge to cover the increasing scope of the subject. With the new scanning methods being introduced computers and computer technology may yet also find a place in radiographic practice. However, there can be no progress in radiography without the basic skills in patient positioning based on an accurate knowledge of basic anatomy. "Positioning in Radiography" will therefore continue as an essential guide to good radiographic practice.

ACKNOWLEDGEMENTS
to the NINTH EDITION

Miss K C Clark was principal of the ILFORD Department of Radiography and Medical Photography, Tavistock House, from 1935 to 1958. Her intense interest in teaching and radiographic projections led to an invitation by Ilford Limited to produce 'Positioning in Radiography' which has now reached its 10th edition. Her infectious enthusiasm was most gratifying to all visitors. She was ably assisted by her colleagues, leading to many innovations in radiography, especially in developing mass miniature radiography.

She accepted Honorary Fellowship of the British Society of Radiographers after being President of the Society and in 1959 was made an Honorary member of the Faculty of Radiologists and an Honorary Fellow of the Australian Institute of Radiography.

Miss Clark died in 1968 and the Kathleen Clark Memorial Library established by the Society of Radiographers at Upper Wimpole Street in fitting respect of her contribution.

The ninth edition was produced in two volumes being edited and revised by James McInnes FSR, TE, FRPS, having been involved with Positioning in Radiography from 1946 when he joined the team at Tavistock House. He originated many aspects in radiography and contributed numerous articles to radiographic journals, becoming Principal of Lecture and Technical Services at Tavistock House and lecturing widely to X-ray Societies in Britain, Canada, America, South and West Africa.

Over two hundred new photographic illustrations have been incorporated in this new edition. Renewal of considerable previous illustrations has taken place, to both up-date and improve the accuracy of presentation. Photographic illustration of all additional techniques has also been included.

In the production of these we are indebted to the photographic artistry and skill of Mr Michael Barrington-Martin.

Acknowledgement is also made to the considerable assistance given by GEC Medical Equipment Limited (Wembley) who, on two occasions, installed the necessary X-ray equipment in the photographic studios and to Sierex Limited and Philips Medical Systems Ltd on further occasions. The accuracy and convenience required, to present photographs of radiographic positioning technique, is largely a function of having good X-ray equipment, and on each occasion We were well served in this respect.

In connection with the above we are also indebted to Leslies Limited (Polyfoam Division) for the use of their Polyfoam positioning aids and foam table mattress, these proved a major factor in comfort, convenience and positional accuracy.

Thanks are also due to Miss H M Fowles MSR, Westminster Hospital X-ray Department for providing the facilities for photographing the tomographic positioning techniques. Thanks are also due to Miss D M Chesney, Hon FSR, TE, Coventry and Warwickshire Hospital for permission to adapt her article, "Acute Abdomen Emergency" within the format of Positioning In Radiography.

Consultation is a very necessary feature in the preparation of descriptive and accurate text, in this respect we are indebted to the following:
Miss S J Smith FSR and Mr J Causton FSR, Salford College of Technology. Mr E Higginbottom MSR, Lodge Moor Hospital, Sheffield. Mr W J Stripp, Royal National Orthopaedic Hospital, London. Miss M England FSR, and Mr Norman Baldock FSR, Royal Northern Hospital, London. Thanks are due to Mr J Coote for making available the X-ray room facilities at Tavistock House, in order to clarify many of the problems associated with positioning technique.
Mr Kenneth Lawley and Mr Michael Smith have been responsible for the design and production of the 9th edition in the new two volume form. We are most grateful for their valued co-operation.

Our thanks are due to the directors of CIBA-GEIGY Limited for making this edition possible and allowing us to be associated with this acknowledged world-wide authoritative work on radiographic positioning.

In preparing the ninth edition of Positioning In Radiography we wish to acknowledge the radiographic illustration content from the following sources:

Albert Einstein Medical Center, Philadelphia, USA
Dr J Gershon-Cohen and Miss Barbara M Curcio

Bradford Royal Infirmary, Yorkshire
Dr R J Carr

Bristol Royal Hospital, Royal Infirmary Branch
Dr J H Middlemiss

Brompton Hospital, London
Dr L G Blair and Miss V G Jones

Child Study Centre, University of London, Institute of Education and Child Health
Dr J M Tanner, group investigations

Children's Hospital Medical Center, Boston, USA
Dr E B D Neuhauser and Dr M H Wittenborg, Mr Eric Hammond

Chorley and District Hospital, Lancashire
Dr G Sullivan

Cuckfield Hospital, Sussex
Miss H E M Noller

Dublin
Dr T Garratt Hardman

Halifax, Yorkshire
Dr R I Lewis

Harefield Hospital, Middlesex
Dr L G Blair, Mr V C Snell and Mr A W Holder

Hospital for Sick Children, London
Dr L G Blair, Dr G N Weber, also Miss H Nicol and Miss M Riocreux

Hospital for Sick Children, Toronto, Canada
Dr J D Munn, Mr Richard Harmes, Mr Walter Johns, also Mr L J Cartwright

Ipswich and East Suffolk Hospital
Miss S M Stockley

Johnson and Johnson (Great Britain) Limited, Slough, Buckinghamshire

Lodge Moor Hospital, Sheffield, Yorkshire
Dr T Lodge and Mr E Higginbottom

London Hospital
Dr J J Rae and Miss F M A Vaughan

Department for Research in Industrial Medicine
Dr L J Rae, Dr A I G McLaughlin and Miss F M A Vaughan

Maidenhead Hospital, Berkshire
Dr A W Simmins, Mr David W Bain and Miss A Crofton

Manchester Royal Infirmary, Lancashire
Dr E D Gray, Dr R G Reid

Medical Arts X-ray Department, Niagra Falls, Canada
Mr Lewis Edwards

Melrose-Wakefield Hospital, Massachusetts, USA
Dr William E Davis and Mr Clarence W Coupe

Memorial Hospital, Cirencester, Gloucestershire
Dr G C Griffiths

Memorial Hospital, New York City, USA
Dr Robert S Sherman and Dr George Schwarz

Middlesex Hospital, London
Dr F Campbell Golding and Miss H J Weller,
Dr M J McLoughlin and Miss Marion Frank

Mulago Hospital, Kampala, Uganda
Dr A G M Davies

National Hospital, Queen Square, London
Dr Hugh W Davies, Dr J W D Bull, Mr
Harvey Jackson and Mr Peter Gortvai,
Dr J Marryat, Mr A M Hastin Bennett,
Mr A E Prickett, Miss A M Hamilton,
Mr L S Walsh

National Heart Hospital, London
Dr Peter Kerley, CVO, CBE and Miss K M A
Pritchard

New Britain Hospital, Connecticut, USA
Dr John C Larkin and Mr Nicholas R Barraco

Newcastle General Hospital, Newcastle-
Upon-Tyne
Dr S Josephs

New England Center Hospital, Pratt Diagnostic
Clinic, Boston, USA
Dr Alice Ettinger

Nuffield Orthopaedic Centre, Oxford
(Wingfield Morris Orthopaedic Hospital)
Dr F H Kemp, Dr J L Boldero,
Mr J Agerholm, Miss B Robbins

NV Optische Industrie 'De Oude Delft',
Holland

Prince of Wales's General Hospital, London
Dr A Elkeles

Queen Victoria Hospital, Plastic Surgery and
Jaw Injuries Centre, East Grinstead, Sussex
Dr William Campbell

Radcliffe Infirmary, Oxford
Dr F H Kemp

Robert Jones and Agnes Hunt Orthopaedic
Hospital, Oswestry, Shropshire
Dr J W Foy, Mr J Rowland Hughes, Mr F B
Thomas, Mr R Roaf and Mr W G Davies

Royal Cornwall Infirmary, Truro
Dr H S Bennett, Mr J G Kendall,
Mrs V Wheaton

Royal Dental Hospital, London
Dr Sydney Blackman, Miss D O Gibb and
Mrs D White

Royal Hospital, Sheffield, Yorkshire
Dr T Lodge and Mr G W Delahaye

Royal Marsden Hospital, London
Dr J J Stevenson, Dr J S McDonald,
Dr E J Pick

Royal National Orthopaedic Hospital, London
Dr F Campbell Golding, Mr J N Wilson,
Mr C W S F Manning, Mr J I P James,
Mr W J Stripp

Royal National Orthopaedic Hospital,
Brockley Hill, Stanmore, Middlesex
Dr F Campbell Golding, Mr J N Wilson,
Mr C V S F Manning

Royal Northern Hospital, London
Dr L S Carstairs, Mr A M Hastin Bennett,
and Miss M J England, Mr N Baldock

Royal Portsmouth Hospital, Hampshire
Dr R S MacHardy

St Anthony's Hospital, Cheam, Surrey
Mr Aubrey York Mason

St Mary's Hospitals for Women and Children,
Manchester
Dr J Blair Hartley and Miss A Stirling Fisher

St Thomas's Hospital, London
Dr J W McLaren

St Vincent's Hospital, New York City, USA
Dr Francis F Ruzicka Jnr, and Dr M M
Schechter

St Vincent's Orthopaedic Hospital, Eastcote,
Pinner, Middlesex
Dr L G Blair, Mr V C Snell and Sister Francis

Salford Royal Hospital, Lancashire
Dr A H McCallum

Stuttgart, Germany
Dr Georg Thieme Verlag

Sydney, Australia
Dr Majorie Dalgarno

Temple University Hospital, Philadelphia,
USA
Professor Herbert M Stauffer and Miss
Margaret J McGann

The Hague, Holland
Dr V Fiorani

Universiteit Van Amsterdam, Holland
Professor Dr B G Ziedses des Plantes

University College Hospital, London
Dr David Edwards, Dr M E Grossmann,
Dr M E Sidaway and Mrs S Gordon and
Sister H Quirke

War Memorial Children's Hospital, London
Ontario, Canada
Dr D S Rajic and Mr Bryan Fisher

Westminster Hospital, London
Dr B Strickland, Dr Roger Pyle and Dr S
Holesh

Weston-Super-Mare General Hospital, Somerset
Dr H B Howell and Mr E J Quick,
Mrs S S Duncan

Women's College Hospital, Toronto, Canada
Dr M E Forbes, Dr Jean Toews and Mrs
Elizabeth Mills

ACKNOWLEDGEMENTS to the TENTH EDITION

We gratefully acknowledge the rôle of the Clinical Research Centre and Northwick Park Hospital. In producing a new Edition to "Kitty" Clark's book; a modern department is obviously essential. The farsighted policy of the Department of Health and Social Security (DHSS) in combining with the Medical Research Council (MRC) under the auspices of the North West Regional Board, helped to conceive and build the institution. Modern equipment and adequate staffing is obviously needed for good radiography.

Our thanks are therefore due to the Staff of the Radiology Department who have developed and maintained high standards since its opening in 1970.

Since July 1980 I have been associated with Mrs Morrison-Jack and her staff at Queen Mary's Hospital of the East End and gratefully acknowledge her enthusiasm for undertaking new procedures and her meticulous attention to detail with routine radiography. The staff at St James' Hospital, Leeds, especially Drs Margaret Bark and Philip Robinson and Mr Steve Henman have been extremely helpful with advice on Ultrasonography, Isotope Scanning and in Management of the CT Machine. Similarly the staff at the Hospital of the University of Pennsylvania, Philadelphia, including Dr Stanley Baum, Dr Ernie Ring, Dr Abbas Alavi, Dr Peter Arger and Dr Igor Laufer were of great assistance. Especial thanks are due to Dr Hans Herlinger who bridges both institutions. I should also like to thank Dr Sam Mindel of the Ashford Hospital, Middlesex for his very valuable contributions to the Ultrasound section, and Mr Malcolm Merrick of the Edinburgh Royal Infirmary for the high resolution isotope bone scan.

I am particularly grateful to my two registrars Dr Jenny Ellert and Dr Grahame Bydder who were a tower of strength, together and individually, during a difficult period.

REVIEW OF EXPOSURE TABLES

Exposure tables

The exposures given in this book are to be used only as a general guide. For any particular region they will vary with different types of equipment and from subject to subject, but are sufficiently similar to obtain acceptable results, provided the technical factors are taken into account. These factors include kilovoltage, milliampere-seconds, focus-film distance, film/screen speed and whether or not a grid is used.

Modern equipment has become more versatile, often more powerful and is frequently designed for particular examinations or regions of the body. Thus equipment is now available with 1000 mA output and a kilovoltage range up to 200 kVp, with automatic exposure selection and phototiming greatly assisting routine examinations. However, to produce films of high diagnostic quality without using automatic exposure equipment the radiographer must have a thorough understanding of the many factors responsible for a diagnostic film. With experience changes in kilovoltage or milliampere seconds can be readily calculated taking into account the size of the patient. For larger patients and great radiodensity higher kilovoltage settings are used, which produces greater penetration and less contrast. For children, restless patients or organs with inherent movement, short exposure times are essential. Low kilovoltages are needed for maximum contrast. Furthermore the radiographic appearance is also markedly affected by screen/film combinations, X-ray beam collimation, the use of grids and the use of contrast medium.

The preference of individual radiologists and departments and the prevailing policies at any particular time are other variables but above all patient radiation must be kept to a minimum compatible with good diagnostic practice, which can only be achieved with radiographic techniques of the highest standards eliminating unnecessary repeat examinations.

Kilovoltage (kVp)

Kilovoltage refers to the electrical tension or the difference in electrical potential across the X-ray tube. A homogenous X-ray beam of constant wavelength giving a high efficiency of emerging photons can only be produced if the kilovoltage from the transformer remains constant. Fortunately most radiographic circuitry today is capable of producing a homogenous wavelength.

Increasing the kilovoltage results in an X-ray beam of a shorter wavelength which is more penetrating and is used for regions of greater radio-density either because of increased thickness or higher atomic numbers. Increased penetration is needed especially for the lower thoracic and upper abdominal paravertebral regions and for large collections of contrast medium particularly in the bladder. For soft tissues and double contrast examinations low kilovoltage and low penetration is needed.

Initially the best method for learning exposure factors for each examination is to choose an appropriate kilovoltage based on the thickness of the part associated with the size of the patient. With experience the exposure factors can subsequently be varied. If the kilovoltage is too low the under-penetration will result in loss of detail, the parts having greater radiodensity not being shown and the radiograph having excessive contrast.

Conversely, with the kilovoltage too high there is over-penetration and loss of radiographic contrast. It becomes more difficult to see small lesions because of the loss of adjacent contrast.

There is thus an optimum kilovoltage for each part which allows for adequate penetration, minimising scatter but producing adequate radiographic contrast. These principles apply particularly to regions of inherently low contrast such as soft tissues where low kilovoltages become imperative, mammography being the outstanding example where kilovoltages down to 25–30 kVp are used. At low kilovoltages collimation becomes extremely important to avoid excessive scatter.

Once the general principle of the relationship between kilovoltage, radiodensity of the region, photon scatter and radiographic contrast is appreciated, further modifications become possible related to

(a) Average thickness of the part
(b) Variations in thickness of adjacent areas
(c) Steep variations of adjacent radio-density.

When there is a wide variation in regional photon absorption differences, the kilovoltages based only on the average thickness of the part would produce excessive contrast and an increase of 20–30 kVp is needed to reduce too steep absorption differences, producing a more uniform exposure of the part being examined.

Other important factors are

(d) Increase radiodensity due to pathological conditions such as a pleural effusion or consolidation obscuring or replacing normal lung, requiring greater penetration.
(e) Decrease in radiodensity due to excessive gas or fatty tissue requiring less penetration.
(f) "Double contrast examinations" when maximum radiographic contrast is highly desirable.

Excessive heat loading of the target area of the X-ray tube becomes a factor in examinations with repetitive exposures such as angiography, cineradiography and tomography. If however the kilovoltage is increased to produce the required radiographic density on films, a greater range of investigations within the rating of small foci becomes possible and a greater accuracy in focal spot size is maintained thereby improving definition.

The use of higher kilovoltages markedly decreases exposure

times and is particularly relevant if the blurring effects of subject movement must be eliminated.

The following table provides a guide as to the increase in kilovoltage required to reduce the milliamperage seconds (mAs) by half.

Range	Increase in kVp for 50% reduction in mAs
40–60	7 kVp
60–80	10 kVp
85–100	15 kVp
100–120	20 kVp
120–150	25 kVp

Milliampere seconds (mAs)

The product of a high tension current in milliamperes and the duration of the exposure in seconds produces milliampere seconds (mAs) (or $mA \times s = mAs$). In many departments only the milliampere seconds is quoted and not milliamperes separately from the time in seconds. Thus to obtain the exposure time in seconds, the value for milliampere seconds is divided by the milliamperes.

The system used by most modern X-ray units has the kilovoltage tied to the milliampere seconds, thereby operating at maximum tube load. The appropriate milliampere seconds chosen for the kilovoltage setting automatically uses the highest mA and the shortest possible time.

The milliampere seconds value is the most important factor in controlling the exposure (radiographic density) on the film. The correct exposure is therefore the most appropriate kilovoltage for the required penetration together with the appropriate milliampere seconds for the correct radiographic density.

If the film is underexposed it will be too white and lack contrast and if overexposed, too black with low contrast.

Most films have considerable tolerance for errors in exposure (milliampere seconds) but exposures become much more critical when using a high kilovoltage technique which requires maximum possible contrast because of its inherently low contrast.

When a short exposure time is critical to eliminate movement blurring, a higher kilovoltage will decrease the exposure time. However if the exposure time is not so critical using lower mA values helps to extend the life of the tube.

The following milliamperes are therefore suggested:

Limbs—with or without intensifying screens—100–120 mA
Skull, Vertebral column, Pelvis—highest mA within rating of smallest foci

Heart and Lungs—300–800 mA
Alimentary Tract—300–500 mA
Gall Bladder—300–500 mA
Urinary Tract—300–500 mA
Dental—8–10 mA

Fluoroscopy with image intensifier—0·3–0·5 mA at 70–80 kVp but without image intensification 3 mA is required.

A free control adjustment is particularly useful for the 100 milliampere setting to obtain low values of mA for long exposure techniques done during quiet breathing and for the long exposure times used with tomography.

Focal-Film Distance (FFD)

When a grid is used the FFD is usually dictated by the radial focus of the grid to obtain a uniform exposure over the entire subject, particularly for large areas as with an AP view of the pelvis, and should not be less than 90 cm (36 ins). The recommended distance is 100–105 cm (40–42 ins). However, where the subject is central to the grid (as in a lateral view of the spine) the FFD may be increased to 120 cm (108 ins) to improve the focus—object to object—film ratio, thereby reducing unsharpness of the image due to displacement of the subject from the film.

When it is important to obtain a true indication of size, as in chest films for the heart, an extended FFD of 150–180 cm (5–6 ft) is needed (teleradiography).

The introduction of small focal spot sizes of 0·3 and 0·6 mm has reduced the need for changing the FFD in general Bucky radiography. The improved sharpness is directly related to the focal spot size, whereas when extending the focal film distance the improved sharpness is related to the square of the distance. Furthermore, by increasing the FFD an increased exposure is required with the attendant possibility of subject movement.

Change in exposure by increasing the FFD can be calculated by

$$\text{New exposure} = \frac{(\text{new distance})^2}{(\text{original distance})^2} \times \text{original exposure}$$

Collimation and Filtration

Collimation by the use of a diaphragm, cone or both limits the X-ray beam to the size and shape of the area to be covered, and is imperative to improve definition and control man-made radiation to the patient.

For further reduction of patient radiation each X-ray tube is fitted with a conventional 2 mm filter placed over the tube aperture. However, filtration will effect both exposure and contrast.

Adequate filtration in the form of a 2 mm thickness aluminium cover over the portal of the X-ray tube in the 60–100 kVp range ensures absorption of the shorter wavelengths. The photons from the shorter wavelengths would otherwise only be absorbed in the patient, adding to the radiation dose, without contributing to the radiographic density.

Filtration can also be used to produce a more uniform radiographic density for areas of the body where there are large adjacent absorption differences, for example, between the upper and lower dorsal spine regions in the antero-posterior projection. Depending on the shape of the part this can take the form of either a wedge shaped filter over the X-ray tube portal with its thickest part over the area of least absorption, or alternatively by increasing the thickness of the conventional tube filter or replacing it by an appropriate thickness of copper.

However, X-ray tube filtration should also be compared with selective under-grid filtration using sheet tin. Under-grid sheet tin filtration also prevents unsuspected scatter from the grid itself reaching the film which of course cannot be done with filtration at the X-ray tube portal.

Radiographic Grids

Radiographic grids are either stationary or moving. Stationary grids require an increase of approximately $\times 3$ exposure relative to a non-grid exposure and a moving grid approximately an increase of $\times 4$.

Grid efficiency is dependent on and can be judged by two essential features namely primary transmission and secondary elimination, which are determined by the composition of the grid and the grid ratio. Satisfactory performance in both respects can be obtained with a 7:1 metal or a 10:1 plastic grid with kilovoltages up to 100 kVp and produce similar results.

For kilovoltages over 100 kVp grid ratios of 12:1 with metal and 16:1 with plastic are available but the higher primary absorption creates a problem particularly with short exposure times not coinciding with the uniform de-centralised grid excursion. In these circumstances, conventional grids complemented by selective filtration behind the grid is often more favourable.

Fineline Stationary Grids

The construction of the modern fineline grid makes the gridlines almost invisible on the film thus overcoming the difficulties associated with movement at ultrashort exposure times and giving an efficiency comparable to a 7:1 metal moving grid.

Film

The manufacture of the modern film is largely dictated by the speed of automatic processing usually 90 secs or $3\frac{1}{2}$ minutes. The film characteristics must be suited both to the high activity in developing, fixing and drying as well as to the rapid transport. As a result there is now an almost "universal" type of film suited to the extreme conditions associated with rapid processing producing a standard result and virtually eliminating high definition non-screen films. Non-screen films were formally used for hands and feet. Modern film can still be used without screens and are then suitable for 90 sec processing. Alternatively slow speed, high definition screens are available particularly for increased contrast giving a reduced exposure time and radiation dosage when compared with non-screen film.

Choice of Film and Screen

The choice of film is determined by its quality, cost and availability and must obviously be compatible with the processing technique as well as the screens but is undergoing change due to the recent introduction of rare earth screens; one manufacturer's films are not necessarily compatible with another's screens.

Intensifying Screens

Only about 10% of the radiographic film density comes from direct radiation, the remainder is from fluorescence from the intensifying screens, which is why a much smaller exposure is required and why the speed of film/screen combinations are much greater when compared with non-screen film.

The general purpose screen is a screen of high quality and efficiency, but the fast tungstate screen requires only half the exposure to obtain improved definition, while with the high definition screens 50% greater exposure is needed.

The latest rare-earth screens are some 4–5 times faster than conventional screens without significant loss of definition. Short exposure times have thus become possible with low output equipment in the 100–300 milliampere range, less radiation to the patient and less wear-and-tear on the equipment especially the X-ray tube. Improved results are particularly noticeable in double contrast barium examinations and with cholecystography.

Subject

The extreme variation in size from babies to adults is the most important single factor determining exposure factors. However, even considering adults only there is a marked variation from one individual to another especially with sex and age. The elderly are often much thinner and their bones have a lower radiodensity due to oesteoporosis. Heavy set and muscular individuals require more exposure than those of similar size due to adiposity and similarly if there is marked enlargement of liver and spleen the exposure will need to be increased. A much greater exposure is needed when radiographs are taken through plaster casts or splints.

The suggested exposure factors for adult subjects of average physique will therefore be varied by as much as 25 to 50 percent in mAs or 5–10 kVp depending on the size of the individual.

Radiographic Quality Control

The quality of a radiographic examination is judged entirely on the film produced as related to the clinical problem. The main factors responsible for downgrading the image are incorrect exposure and unsharpness, and the major factor in producing unsharpness of the image is subject movement. However, unsharpness can also be due to geometrical projection, the physical properties of the screens and the type of X-ray film used. The highest quality radiograph is produced when all the factors involved are optimised.

Subject Movement Unsharpness

Movements causing blurring occur especially in restless patients or children unable to co-operate but also from breathing and pulsation of the cardiovascular system. During breathing there is movement of the thorax, diaphragm and upper abdominal organs. Unless these movements stop or the exposure time is sufficiently short to nullify the effects of cardiovascular pulsation, even the most modern and expensive equipment, the finest quality film and screen combination and the optimum geometric factors will not produce a diagnostically acceptable radiograph. An absolute essential for good radiography is therefore the elimination of all the patient's voluntary movement and the use of short exposure times to obviate involuntary movements.

Short exposure times can be obtained in different ways. High output units with three-phrase generators giving milliamperes of 500–1000 produce exposure times in the millisecond range. Short times can also be produced with single phase units using rare-earth screens which have made a major contribution to obtaining good radiographic quality by reducing exposures by about a factor of four. Not only can short exposure times be used with rare earth screens but there is correspondingly less radiation to the patient. Shorter exposure times can also be obtained, again with diminished radiation dose, by increasing the kilovoltage but this produces a loss of radiographic contrast.

Geometric Unsharpness

Most radiographic units now have X-ray tubes with 0·6 and 0·3 mm foci greatly reducing geometric unsharpness which is directly proportional to focal spot size. However, the rating of the focal spot must not reduce the energy of the output below the requirement for a particular examination.

The balance between focal spot size and energy output is well illustrated by the requirements for a lateral view of the lumbar spine which inevitably increases the subject-film distance to about 25 cm requiring an increase in the focal-film distance to 100 cm to compensate for geometric unsharpness. With a FFD of 100 cm and a focal spot size of 2 mm the geometric unsharpness is 0·6 mm which is unacceptable. A 1 mm focus would reduce the unsharpness to 0·3 mm in keeping with the degree of unsharpness of standard type screens. However, the unsharpness could be reduced to 0·15 by a 0·5 mm focus to match the full improvement gained by using high definition screens.

Contrast

The difference in radiographic density between adjacent areas constitutes contrast and is a function of the X-ray film contrast associated with its processing as well as the degree of radiographic density due to secondary radiation.

Secondary radiation lessens radiographic contrast and must therefore be reduced as much as possible, by effective collimation which limits the area from which scattered radiation can occur, by effective soft tissue compression allowing a lower kilovoltage to be used, by use of effective grids and by preventing backscatter. Higher kilovoltages produce less radiographic contrast than low kilovoltages.

Sharpness

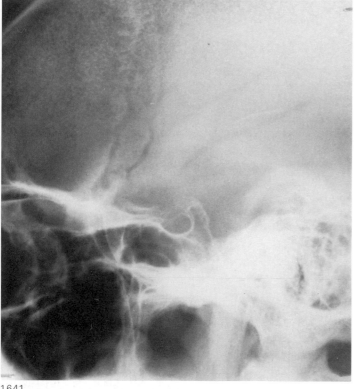

1641

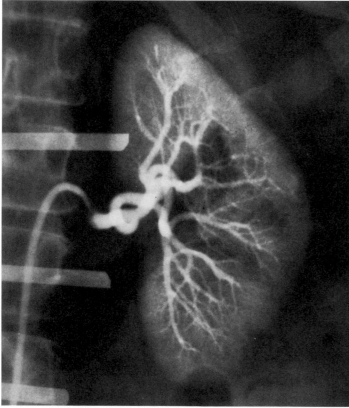

1642

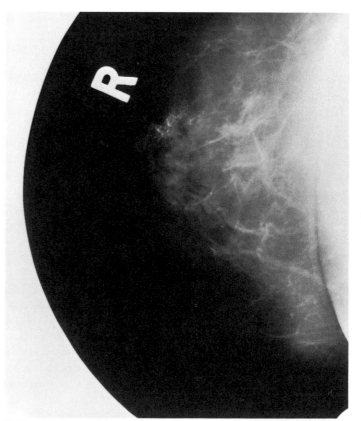

1643

Radiographs

1641 The lamina dura of the pituitary fossa appears as a fine white line.

1642 Selective left renal arteriogram showing small vessels.

1643 Mammography with minimal flecks of calcification in a localised area.

1644 Lateral lumbar spine with narrowing of the disc space at L3/4.

1645 With greater contrast the vertebral end plates appear whiter and the small anterior osteophyte on L4 is more obvious.

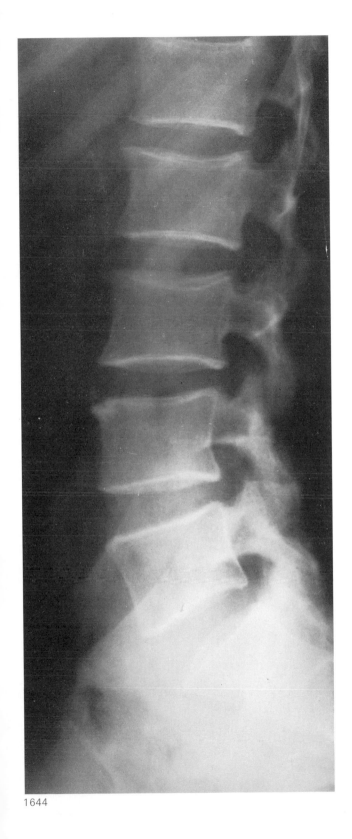

1644

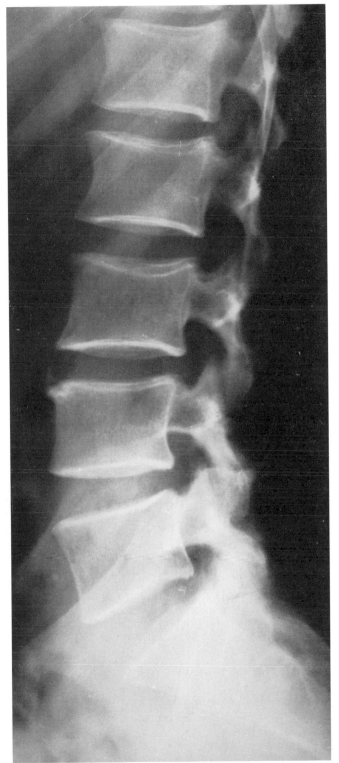

1645

Sharpness

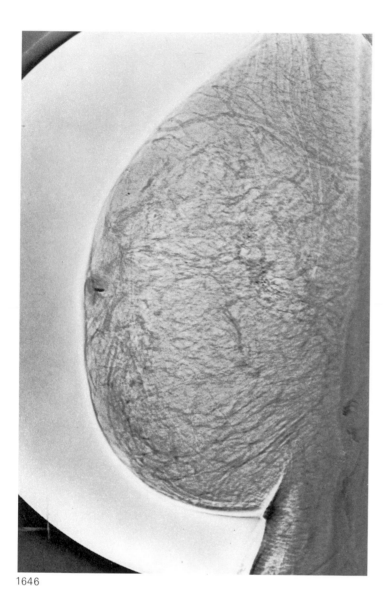

1646

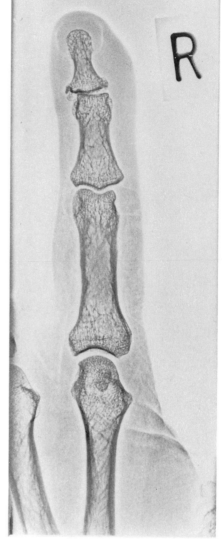

1647

1646 Xeroradiograph of the breast showing marked edge enhancement which accentuates the small flecks of calcification.

1647 Xeroradiograph of an index finger. The bone trabeculae are markedly accentuated by edge enhancement.

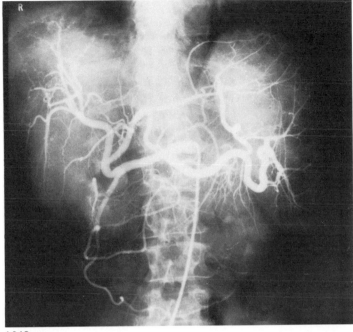

1648

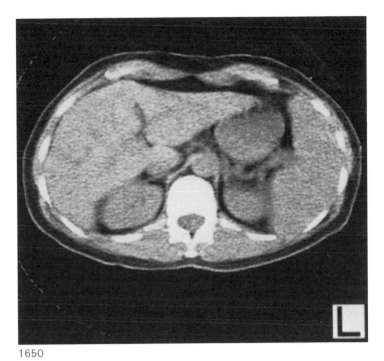

1650

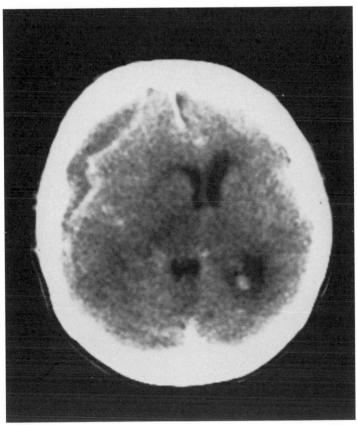

1649

1648 Selective coeliac axis arteriogram showing small vascular pattern.

1649 Subdural haematoma seen on a computed tomography brain scan with contrast enhancement of the margin after an intravenous injection of contrast medium.

1650 Computed tomography section through the liver, spleen and kidneys. The fat planes of the body act as natural contrast demarcating the abdominal organs.

CONTENTS
VOLUME TWO

SECTION 35
Contrast and Opaque Media
Barium preparations. Organic iodine compounds.

SECTION 36
Medical Imaging
Scanning images. Scanning modalities.

SECTION 37
Isotope Scanning
The apparatus. Organ imaging. Isotopes. Projections.

SECTION 38
Ultrasonography
History. Theory, physics. Images. Summary of preliminary adjustments. Indications for ultrasound. Techniques for various abdominal regions.

SECTION 39
Computed Tomography
History. General principles. The apparatus. Preparation for CT examinations. Preparations for different regions. Machine management.

SECTION 40
Nuclear Magnetic Resonance
Scanning.
History. General principles. The apparatus. Positioning.

SUPPLEMENT ONE
The Effects of Radiation, and Protection Methods in Diagnostic Radiology

SUPPLEMENT TWO
Working Metric Equivalents of Dimensions and Quantities.

The Tenth Edition of Positioning in Radiography has been produced in two volumes. An outline of the contents of volume one is shown below:

CONTENTS
VOLUME ONE

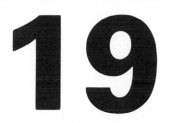

19

DENTAL
PANAGRAPHY
ROTOGRAPHY

19 SECTION 19

DENTAL

Radiographic terms for positioning in the mouth differ from other regions, particularly because antero-posterior and lateral cannot be used for the teeth or dental arches.

The Dental arches

Radiographs of the mouth show the upper and lower dental arches with the upper teeth rooted in the maxilla above (1651) and the lower teeth in the mandible below (1652). The term "mesial" is used for the anterior parts of the arches near the canines and incisors and "distal" describes the posterior parts of the arches at the molars. Labial or buccal refers to the outer or cheek side of the dental arch and lingual or palatal to the inner side within the month (1651, 1652) which would be described in other regions of the body as external and internal.

Dentitions

Humans (homo sapiens) have two successive sets of teeth known as dentitions. There are twenty, temporary or deciduous teeth, the "milk teeth" of childhood (1662) which appear between six months and two years of age. The deciduous teeth are followed by permanent teeth and are 32 in number when complete (1663) erupting from the sixth year onwards with the last four distal molars or "wisdom" teeth normally emerging at 18 years of age. However, the wisdom teeth may not erupt until the twenty-sixth year and is the reason for always including this region in a complete examination even if the wisdom teeth are not visible within the mouth. Impaction of wisdom teeth are a common cause for non-appearance and clearly shown on radiographs. However wisdom teeth may be entirely absent.

In the extra-oral films of a child of eight (1653, 1654) both deciduous and permanent teeth are shown. In (1659) a panoramic projection shows the arrangement of the permanent teeth in an adult.

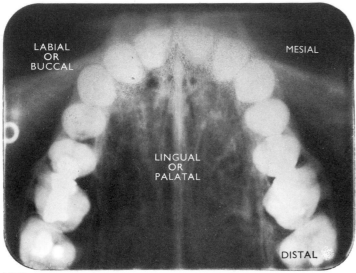

1651

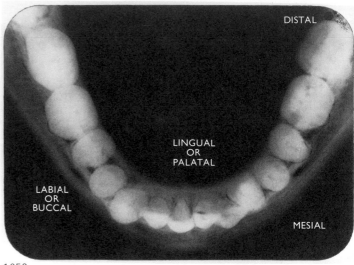

1652

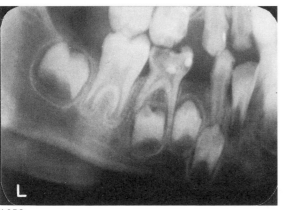

1653

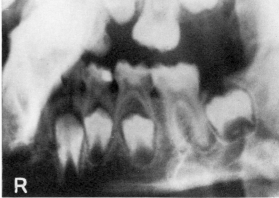

1654

Anatomy

Each tooth is divided into crown, neck and root(s) with each root ending at its apex and being set in the jaw. Normally only the crown is visible and the rest of the tooth is embedded in the alveolar part of the jaw which is covered with soft tissue forming the gum (1655).

An intra-oral film placed in contact with the crown and gum is separated from the root of the tooth by a variable amount of tissue. The angle between the tooth and film will therefore vary from patient to patient and with the region being examined, being greatest with the upper incisors and negligible with the lower molars where the film is almost parallel to the tooth (1656).

An antomical diagram of two adjacent teeth are shown within their individual tooth sockets in (1657) and a radiograph of the lower three molars in (1658). In the centre of the neck and root is the pulp cavity surrounded by dentine which is capped by enamel of the crown. The cement layer lies between the dentine and dental periosteum reaching up to the neck of the tooth just below the crown. On the radiograph the pulp cavity appears as a darker area lying within each tooth and the interdental table of alveolar bone lies between adjacent teeth with a marginal white line known as the lamina dura. The periodontal membrane lies between the tooth root and the lamina dura (1657, 1658).

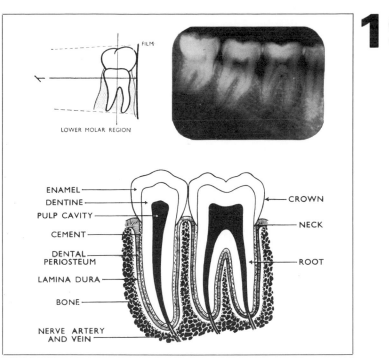

1656/1657

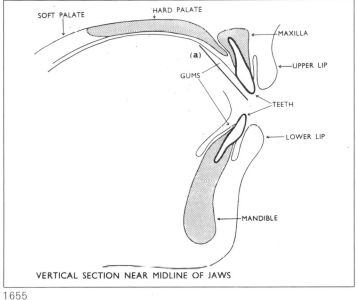

1655

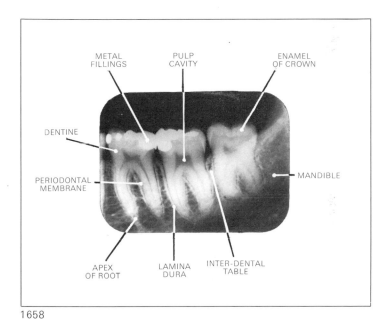

1658

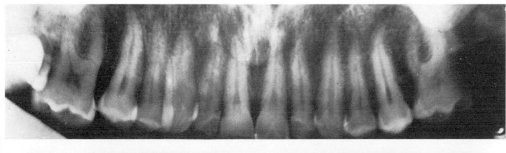

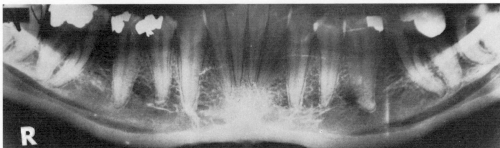

1659

The Dental Formula

For a deciduous set the teeth are represented as four groups of five to correspond to left and right and upper and lower (1660) being represented by the letters 'a' to 'e' from mesial to distal. The permanent teeth are similarly divided into four groups of eight but numbered 1 to 8 from mesial to distal (1661a). Requests for dental examinations are specified accordingly. Even in the case of missing teeth or an edentulous patient, either retained roots or the alveolar margin can similarly be requested. In children a radiograph of "milk" teeth will also show unerupted permanent teeth (1653, 1654)

Films

There are two types of dental film—Standard and Fast, the speed of the fast film being twice that of the standard film and packed singly or in pairs. The use of the latter pack allows one set to be retained for record purposes. The film-pack contains a lead foil between film and label to absorb secondary radiation thereby enhancing definition and each film is embossed with a dot for correct alignment with the tube. The film packs are damp proof.

Intra-oral films come in a standard size of 3×4.5 cm ($1\frac{1}{4} \times 1\frac{5}{8}$ ins) and a substandard size of 2.5×3 cm ($1 \times 1\frac{1}{4}$ ins). The smaller films are more suitable for the incisors and canines in shallow mouths and particularly for children.

The occlusal film is larger, measuring 5.5×7.5 cm ($2\frac{1}{4} \times 3$ ins)

and is positioned for an exposure in the occlusal plane between the jaws. It is supplied in packs similar to those of the smaller intra-oral films.

Whole plate and half-plate films are also used for the investigation of the mandible and maxilla but of course for extra-oral examination.

Equipment

Patients almost invariably have their examination in the sitting position but occasionally such an examination on an ill patient needs to be done with the patient horizontal. Once the angulation for dental technique is understood this should present no problem.

Dental units are shock free and the special bakelite or plastic cone is placed in contact with the skin. The technique employed will be governed by the type of equipment in use and the length of the cone. The tube head of dental units move freely around the patient when seated in a dental chair or chair with a modified head support. The tube can thus be moved into any required position.

However, with a general purpose X-ray unit and the patient supine the head must be moved into the various positions in relation to the X-ray tube. A focus-film distance of 50–72 cm (20–24 ins) with a small localising cone is used and a small aperture to cover only a small area beyond the size of the intra-oral dental film.

Diagrams

Diagram (1660) is the dental formula of a set of deciduous teeth which are labelled 'a' to 'e' from mesial first incisor to distal second milk molar showing upper and lower and right and left teeth.

The formula for a set of permanent teeth (1661a) is numbered sequentially from 1 to 8 from mesial first incisor to distal third molar.

Examples of requests for dental examinations in (1661b) are for

(a) upper right 1–8 i.e. all the right upper teeth
(b) lower left 7 and 8 or left lower 2nd and 3rd molars
(c) upper left 4, 5, 6 and lower right 6, 7, 8.

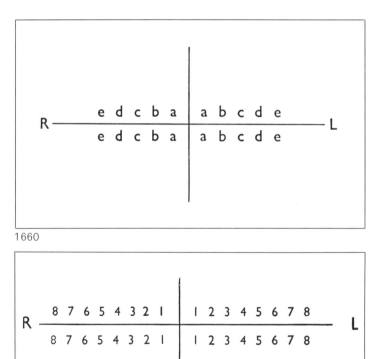

1660

R ——— e d c b a | a b c d e ——— L
      e d c b a | a b c d e

R ——— 8 7 6 5 4 3 2 1 | 1 2 3 4 5 6 7 8 ——— L
      8 7 6 5 4 3 2 1 | 1 2 3 4 5 6 7 8

1661a

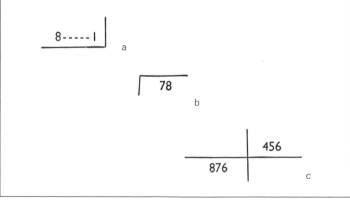

1661b

In (1662) the arrangement of a set of deciduous teeth is shown consisting of two incisors, a canine and two molars in each of the four quadrants and the teeth are designated by letters 'a' to 'e'. The upper molars have three roots and the lower molars only two.

The arrangement of a set of permanent teeth (1663) designated by numbers 1 to 8, consists of two incisors, one canine, two premolars and three molars in each quadrant. Again the upper molars have three roots each and the lower molars two roots.

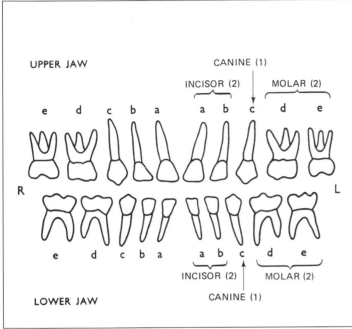

1662

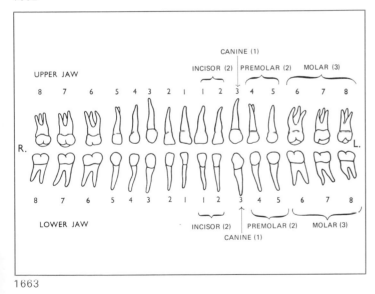

1663

Placing the film in position
Film-holders

Film holders can be used to maintain the film in position but more commonly the patient holds the film on the lingual aspect of the teeth to be examined after it has been correctly placed. The patient's thumb is used for the incisors with the fingers hyperextended and moved out of the way of the X-ray beam. For the other teeth the patient's contralateral index finger holds the film in position, thus for the patient's right teeth the left index finger is used and vice versa.

The radiographer must not in any circumstances hold the film because this may result in radiation burns of the fingers from exposure to the direct X-ray beam.

When the patient cannot co-operate film holders are used to avoid displacement of the film. However, "bite" film holders can only be used if there are sufficient teeth to grip the film holder, otherwise a holder with a handle is required or it must be gripped by a forceps.

Colyer's dental film holders consist of a group of four stainless steel holders (1664) each having a metal film support on a suitable handle and a hard rubber bite block.

The number 1 holder carries the film with the long edge vertically for the upper incisors and canines. With the number 2 holder the film is suspended downwards in the centre of the lower arch for the incisors.

The number 3 holds a film for both the upper left premolars and molars and lower right premolars and molars.

The number 4 is reversed to hold the film for the upper right premolars and molars and lower left premolars and molars.

The number 3 and 4 holders are somewhat large, being uncomfortable far back in the mouth. The film should therefore be placed to extend well beyond the holder for the molars (5).

Forceps holders have a locking mechanism to grip the film edge and includes a bite block. The light weight forceps (6) are easily manipulated and adjusted to cover the various positions but the radiographer must not continue holding the forceps during the exposure.

Balsa wood or plastic bite blocks are also light weight and easily held in the mouth. They can be suitably shaped with an appropriate slot for the film and an adjustable handle simplifies positioning in the mouth. These disposable blocks are inexpensive and are thrown away after use, which saves the bother and expense of resterilisation.

For all types of film holders the film must of course always be loaded with the tube-side surface of the film towards the bite block.

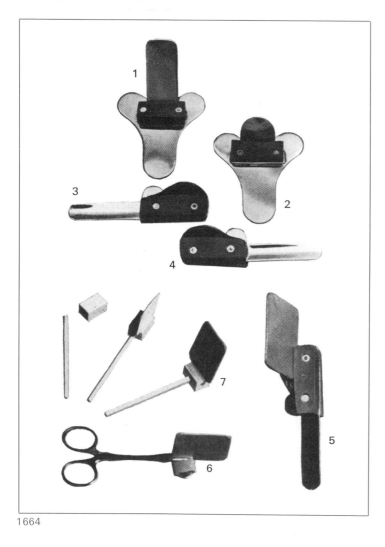

1664

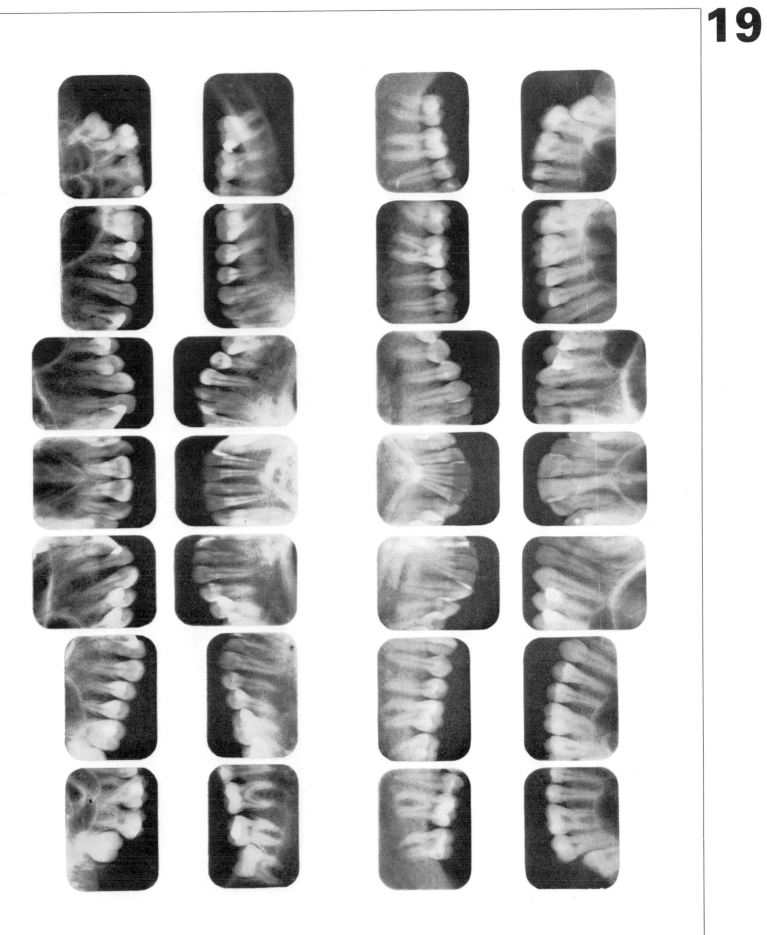

Technique

The size and number of films used for a complete set of teeth will depend on the size and shape of the mouth and can be as little as ten or as many as fourteen. Centring for both the ten-film and fourteen-film series are therefore shown.

The examination is usually done with the patient sitting in a dental chair and for both the upper and lower jaw the head is supported and immobilised against the head rest with the median-sagittal plane vertical. The occlusal plane is horizontal for each jaw in turn (1666, 1667) and this position must be maintained throughout the examination. However, when the patient is being examined in the horizontal position some movement of the head as well as movement of the tube is necessary.

The head is positioned for the upper jaw with its occlusal plane horizontal (1666) and the mouth open. For the lower jaw the head is extended to bring the occlusal plane of the lower jaw horizontal (1667) again with an open mouth. The positioning line for the upper jaw which is used for the centring points for the upper teeth (1666) extends from the tragus of the ear to the ala of the nose, and is 4 cm (1½ ins) above the occlusal plane. For the level of the lower occlusal plane, with the mouth open, a line is drawn from the tragus of the ear to the angle of the mouth which is 2 cm (¾ in) above the lower occlusal plane (1667). The centring points for the lower teeth are just above the level of the low border of the mandible and spaced similarly for both upper and lower teeth (1669) hence perpendicular lines can be drawn between the centring points for the upper and lower teeth.

The angles in relation to both the upper and lower occlusal planes are shown in profile (1668) and enface (1669) but will of course vary somewhat from individual to individual and must only be used as a guide.

Two full sets of films of adult teeth (p. 491) show how they may be grouped for an adequate examination.

The correct projection

The correct projection for dental radiography is particularly important because of the short focus-film distance.

To obtain as little distortion as possible of the length of the

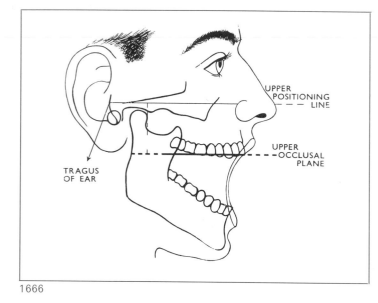

1666

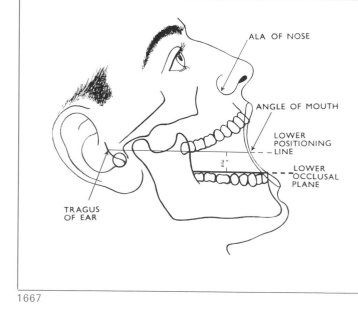

1667

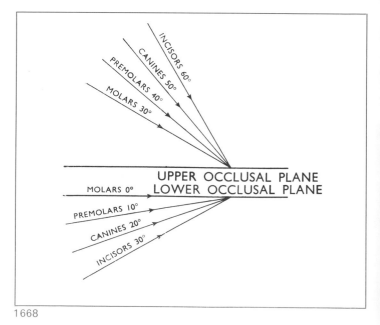

1668

tooth on the radiograph the X-ray beam must be directed at right angles to a line bisecting the angle between the tooth and the film (1670). Angling the tube more vertically towards the crown produces fore-shortening (1671) and more horizontally towards the root produces elongation of the tooth shadow (1672). Some foreshortening is permissible but elongation must be avoided and for the best results the central ray should be directed towards the apical half-section of each tooth.

In the diagrams (1670–1672) the effects of varying the tube angulation in the incisor region are shown together with the corresponding radiographs. The foreshortening in (1671) and elongation in (1672) are compared with correct tube angulation (1670).

Similarly lateral distortion which causes overlapping of tooth shadows must be avoided (1673a) by correct centring in the axial plane to the long axis. Sometimes overlapping is unavoidable because of malposition of the teeth or the shape of the mouth but careful centring will minimise distortion due to projection (1673b).

The shape of the mouth and the direction of the teeth must therefore be noted before starting the examination. The broad

mouth with a large, regular, anterior curve is most easily examined but for the narrow mouth with a tight anterior curve the small sub-standard sized films must be used, centring to each of the front teeth in turn. Furthermore for a shallow palate greater tube angulation will be needed than for a high arched palate.

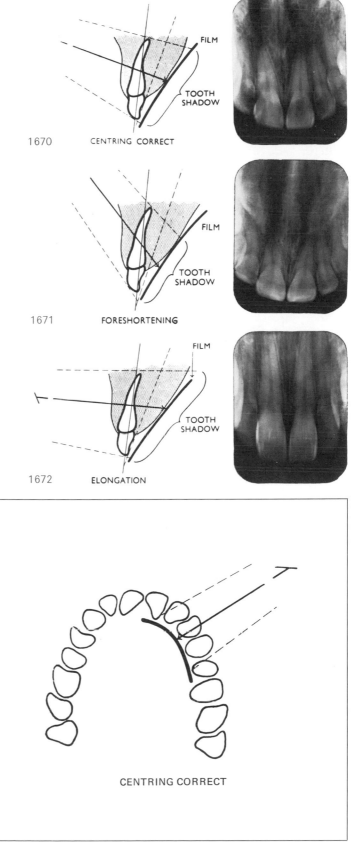

1670   CENTRING CORRECT

1671   FORESHORTENING

1672   ELONGATION

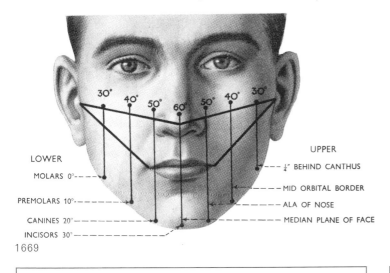

1669

LOWER

MOLARS 0°

PREMOLARS 10°

CANINES 20°

INCISORS 30°

UPPER

¼″ BEHIND CANTHUS

MID ORBITAL BORDER

ALA OF NOSE

MEDIAN PLANE OF FACE

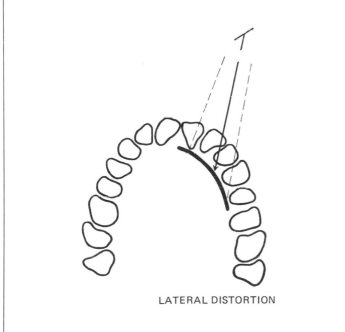

LATERAL DISTORTION

1673a

CENTRING CORRECT

1673b

Radiation protection

Radiation protection for both patient and operator is important in dental radiography because of the short focal-film distance and the number of overlap exposures necessary to cover a full set of teeth. A 2-millimetre aluminium filter at the tube-aperture usually built into the unit by the manufacturer, is essential to stop unwanted soft radiation. Protective lead rubber aprons extending from the neck to the lap (1674a) are available in suitable sizes for the patient especially during pregnancy.

However, the special localising dental cone with its small angled aperture (1674b) limits the X-ray beam to little more than the size of the dental films employed for intra-oral examinations with minimal overlap beyond the 3 or 4 teeth being radiographed and furthermore the use of fast film reduces the radiation to a minimum. Nevertheless the most important way of limiting radiation is to undertake only essential examinations, using accurate positioning, centring and exposures to avoid repeating films.

The operator must never hold the film in the patient's mouth during an exposure even though each film pack incorporates a backing of protective lead foil. Suitable film holders are available or the patient must hold the film in position, and the operator must be at the maximum working distance from the X-ray unit. Wherever possible radiography of a full set of teeth should be done with pantomography which requires considerably less radiation.

Exposure factors

Most dental radiography is done by dental surgeons or assistants but some examinations continue in general radiology departments. Apparatus thus varies from the small specially designed dental unit to the large general purpose unit.

An output with a small range between 55 to 65 kVp is adequate for dental radiography but there are units with lower or higher ratings, or both, from 45 to 70 kVp.

The small units generally with a rating from 45 to 60 kVp have a fixed current of 8–10 milliamperes. There is however a smaller unit rated at 45 kVp and 5 milliamperes which is used at a very short focus-film distance of 10 cm (4 ins). All units are fitted with a 2-mm aluminium filter to stop soft radiation as recommended by the Code of Practice.

A unit with a long cone for a 40 cm (16 ins) focus-film distance has a special film holder to keep the film vertically in the mouth and therefore uses less tube angulation. Most units however have specially fitted dental cones for set distances of 14–23 cm (5½ to 9 ins) with small apertures which restrict the X-ray beam to little more than the intra-oral dental film.

Dental units are usually fitted with clockwork timers which need periodic checking for accuracy. The more recent models have a range of 0·1 to 10 seconds.

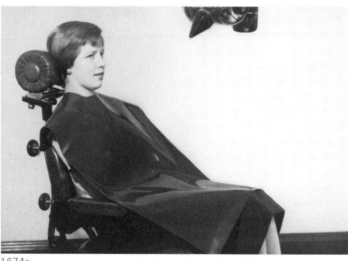

1674a

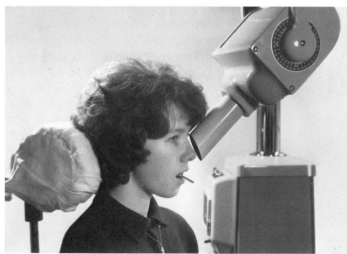

1674b

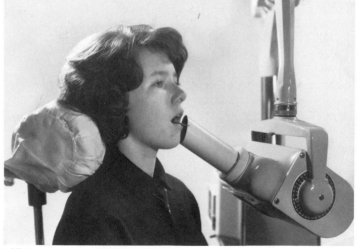

1674c

Exposure table for dental films

As with other regions of the body the correct exposure varies with the area being examined, the subject, the output of the X-ray tube, the focus-film distance and the processing.

In the table below the recommended exposures are for an adult of average physique. Using a 23 cm (9 ins) focus-film distance, at 60 kVp and 10 mA with 2 mm aluminium filtration. Exposure times are given for standard and for fast film.

	Exposure time	
Region	Standard	Fast
Upper Incisors	1 sec	$\frac{1}{2}$ sec
Upper Canines	1 sec	$\frac{1}{2}$ sec
Upper Premolars	1 sec	$\frac{1}{2}$ sec
Upper Molars	$1\frac{1}{2}$ sec	$\frac{3}{4}$ sec
Lower Incisors	$\frac{1}{2}$ sec	$\frac{1}{4}$ sec
Lower Canines	1 sec	$\frac{1}{2}$ sec
Lower Premolars	1 sec	$\frac{1}{2}$ sec
Lower Molars	1 sec	$\frac{1}{2}$ sec
Upper Occlusal	$2\frac{1}{2}$ sec	$1\frac{1}{4}$ sec at 12 in FFD
Lower Occlusal	$1\frac{1}{2}$ sec	$\frac{3}{4}$ sec at 10 in FFD

For the general purpose unit the focus-film distance should be doubled and the milliampere seconds changed accordingly, i.e. increased by 4 times.

Processing

Most general departments use automatic processing for large films and therefore dental films must be processed separately. Small automatic processing units for dental films are now also available but for departments doing only the occasional examination manual processing in small dental units will still be needed. For satisfactory dental radiographs, processing must be meticulous using a fixed time temperature technique, usually 4 minutes at 68°F with the regular renewal of developing and fixing solutions.

A complete set of dental films can be processed simultaneously by hand using the special developing hanger, with the films in the conventional positions (1675) for final mounting. The patient's identification must be noted on a small celluloid tab fitted for the purpose (1675).

Identification

Individual films must not be marked with a pencil before being processed as it inevitably obscures part of the radiograph. A small embossed 'pip' in similar positions on the front of the pink paper covered pack and on the film marks the position of each film. The pink surface is positioned in the mouth to face the tube with the embossed 'pip' lying nearest the crown and also avoids the possibility of obscuring the apices.

Films should be mounted to correspond to a view of the teeth from the labial aspect, that is with the patient's right to the left of the mount and with the embossed convexity toward the observer.

In handling dental films great care is needed to avoid finger marks. If this becomes a problem the film should be handled between tissue paper or by using celluloid dental film loaders for the cardboard mounts.

Viewing

In a complete series the films should be arranged for each tooth to appear free from distortion on at least one film (1665, p. 491). The films should be viewed and checked before the patient leaves the department to establish whether a faulty examination needs to be repeated or to elucidate an unusual variation.

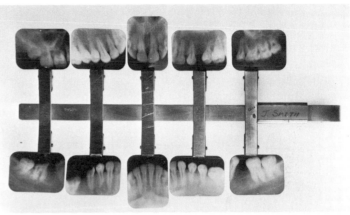

1675

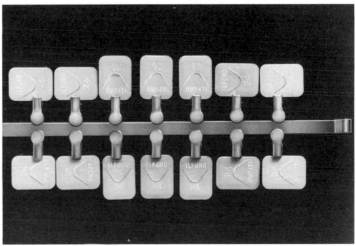

1676

Upper jaw

Tube angulation for teeth of the upper jaw
Incisors: tube-occlusal plane angle 60°
Canines: tube-occlusal plane angle 50°
Premolars: tube-occlusal plane angle 40°
Molars: tube-occlusal plane angle 30°

For the shallow, low arched maxilla with prominent incisors, the tube-occlusal plane angle needs to be increased up to 70° and for receding teeth or a high palate the angle must be decreased.

Centring the tube for the upper teeth
Incisors. The film is placed with the long edge upright in the mouth behind the incisors and the tube, angled 60° to the occlusal line, is centred in the midline on the occlusal line projected onto the face. This is usually at the tip of the nose but may be above or below depending on the shape and height of the palate. The radiograph should show both the central and lateral incisors (1678, 1679, 1680a, 1680b).

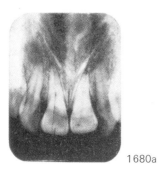

1680a

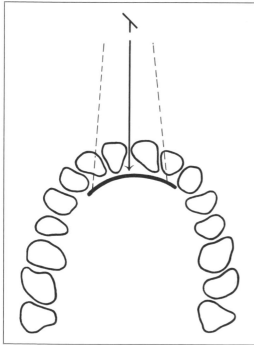

496
1680b

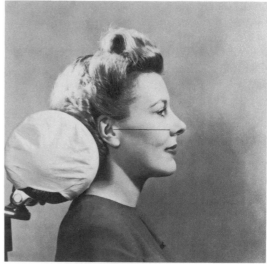

1677

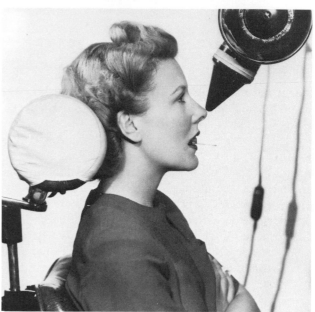

1678

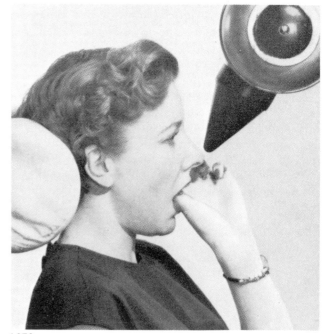

1679

Canines. The film is inserted with the long edge upright behind the canine and the tube is centred to the canine at an angle of 50° to the occlusal plane. Centring is usually over the ala of the nose (1681, 1682) but the canine may be more distal; it is thus best to see the position of the canine by lifting the upper lip.

In a narrow mouth there may be difficulty in placing the film because the canines lie on the curve of the arch. A smaller, substandard sized film should then be used to obtain a satisfactory view of just the one tooth. These films are large enough if used vertically to include even the long root of a canine and probably the lateral incisor will also be included on the radiograph.

However in wide mouthed patients films are much more easily positioned and a larger standard film should be placed long edge horizontally with its medial edge in the midline between the central incisors. The tube should then be centred more mesially between the lateral incisor and the canine giving a good view of both teeth (1683). In these subjects, with a wide mouth, the lateral incisor is often not completely shown on the first film taken.

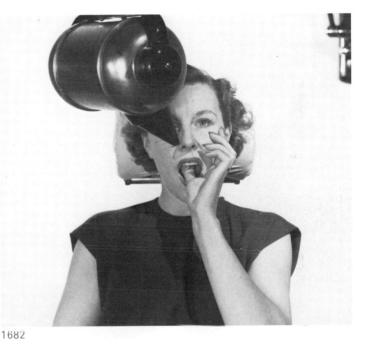

1682

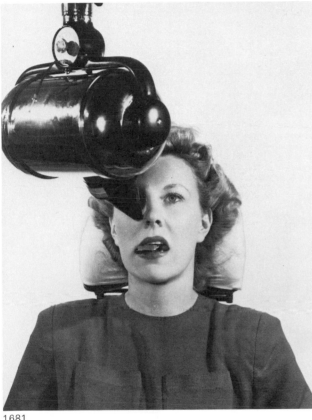

1681

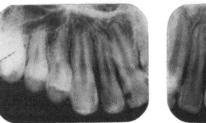
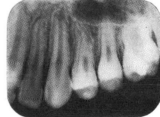

1683

Premolars. A standard sized film is placed behind the pre-molars long edge transversely with the tube angled 40° to the occlusal plane. Centre on a point along a line midway between the inner and outer canthus of the eye by swinging the tube around the curve of the cheek. The tube is centred just above the occlusal line along the mid inter-canthus line (1684, 1685).

The two premolars should appear evenly spaced on the film (1686). The image of the buccal cusp is projected below the palatal cusp due to its distance from the film and the angle of the tube (1684, 1685, 1686, 1687).

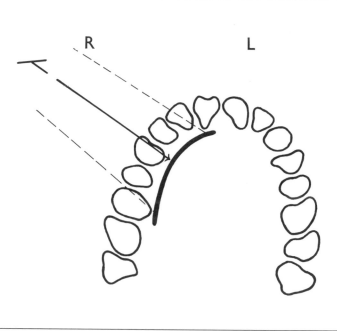

1687

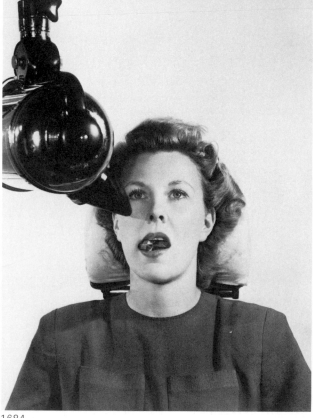

1684

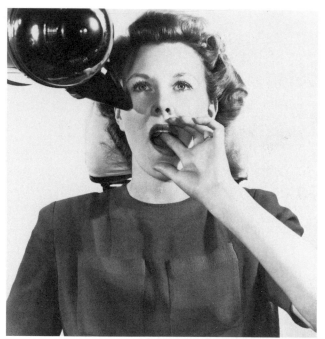

1685

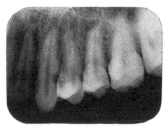

1686

Molars. In this region the patient may have difficulty in tolerating the film placed far back in the mouth and there is also the problem of not projecting the protruding zygomatic bone over the molar roots. The film is better tolerated if the upper inner corner is slightly bent over a finger prior to positioning to prevent too close a contact with the soft palate. To avoid the zygomatic bone the tube should be centred where a line running perpendicularly downwards from a point 0·5 cm ($\frac{1}{4}$ ins) behind the outer canthus of the eye intersects the occlusal line or slightly below. When positioning the tube place a finger on the zygomatic bone and to avoid projecting its shadow onto the film, direct the tip of the tube cone under its lower border (1688, 1689).

In the diagram (1690), (a) is of the lateral view of the zygoma and (b) shows the X-ray beam in the frontal view directed 30° to the occlusal plane to avoid overshadowing of the molar. An alternative method (c) uses a horizontal beam with a film holder having a wide bite block by placing a dental roll between the teeth and the film to bring their general line parallel to the film and at right angles to the X-ray beam. With this method a longer focus film distance is needed to compensate for the greater object-film distance and the exposure time must be correspondingly adjusted.

All three molars should be shown on this film with the floor of the maxillary antrum projected across the apices of the roots (1691a), nevertheless showing the teeth clearly, whereas in (1691b) the roots are obscured by overshadowing of the zygomatic bone.

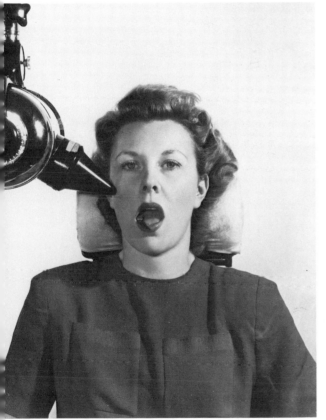

1688

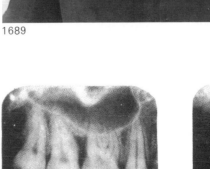

1689

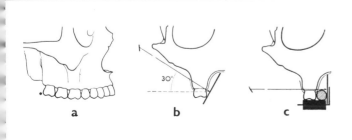

1690

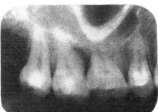

1691a   1691b   499

Lower jaw

Tube centring for the lower teeth

Incisors. The arch of the lower jaw is smaller than the upper and as a general rule the smaller sub-standard sized films placed long edge vertically are preferable to the larger standard film, long edge horizontally. The larger horizontally placed films will need bending before insertion into the apex of the lower jaw arch which usually causes crimp marks and will be painful if the patient has tender gums. The smaller film placed vertically will thus be more comfortable, free of crimp marks and distortion of the root image.

The head is tilted back to bring the lower occlusal line horizontal (1692), the tube is angled upwards 25°–30° to the occlusal plane and centred to the symphysis menti (1693, 1694). Both the medial and lateral incisors should appear evenly spaced on the film (1695, 1696).

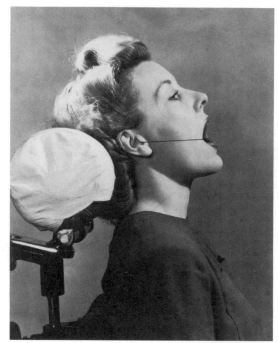

1692

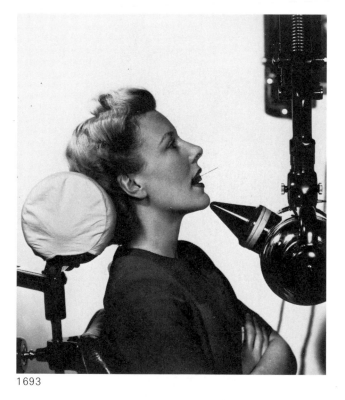

1693

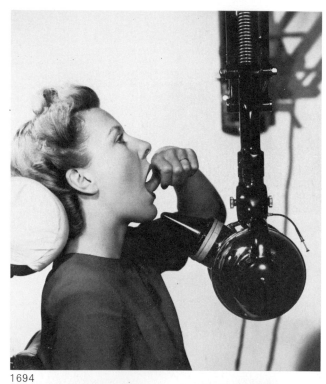

1694

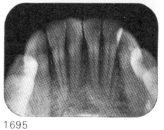

1695   1696

Canines. In narrow arched lower jaws better radiographs may again be obtained by using smaller films, long edge vertically and examining only the canine. However, standard films, long edge horizontally or vertically can also be used with wide arched lower jaws. The tube is angled 20° to the occlusal plane and centred at the lower border of the mandible on a vertical line from the outer edge of the ala of the nose. (1697, 1698)

If a standard film can be used horizontally the premolars may be included in this view (1699) and so complete the examination of the lower jaw with five films rather than seven (1697, 1698, 1700, 1701).

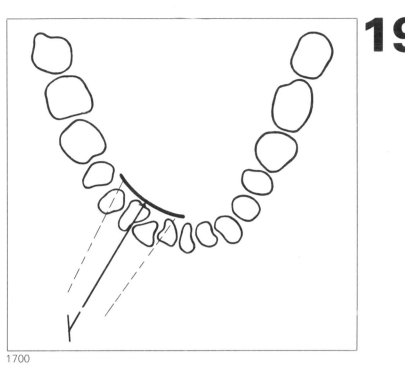

1700

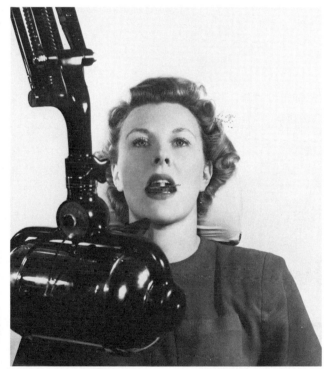

1697

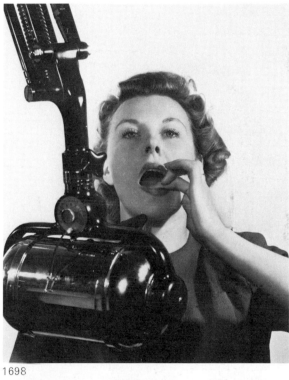

1698

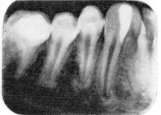

1699

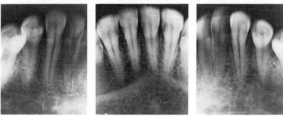

1701

Premolars. A standard film, long edge transversely is recommended, with the tube swung round to direct the X-ray beam squarely to the film plane from the lateral angle (1705). The tube is angled 10° to the occlusal plane and centred on the intersection of the vertical line midway between the angle of the canthus of the eye and the lower border of the mandible (1702, 1703, 1704).

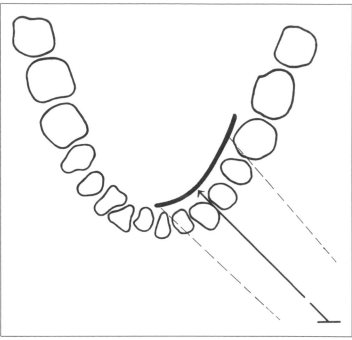

1705

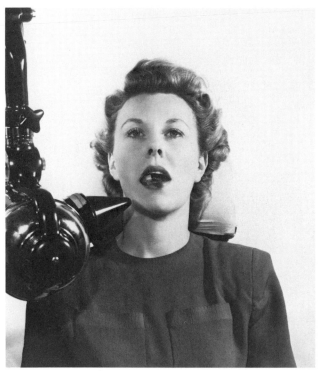

1702

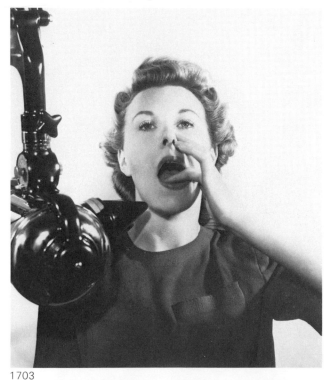

1703

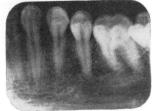

1704

Molars. A standard film is placed long edge horizontally behind the molars and a vertical centring line similar to the upper molars is used which lies 0·5 cm ($\frac{1}{4}$ ins) behind the outer canthus of the eye. Because the X-ray beam is parallel to the occlusal plane which is horizontal and the film parallel to the plane of the molars, the centring point must be higher than for the other lower jaw teeth namely above the lower border of the mandible (1706, 1707). In (1708), the 3rd molar is fully erupted and (1709) shows impacted 3rd molar or wisdom tooth.

The molar teeth are well in front of the angle of the mandible which serves as a guide to their position.

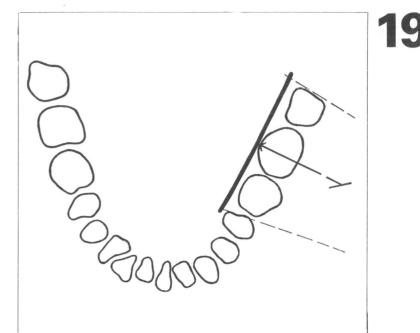

1710

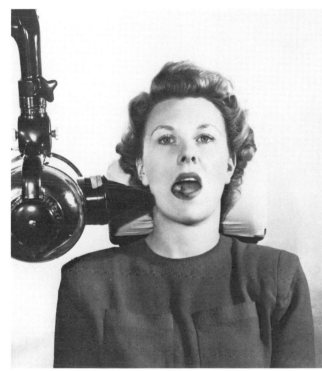

1706

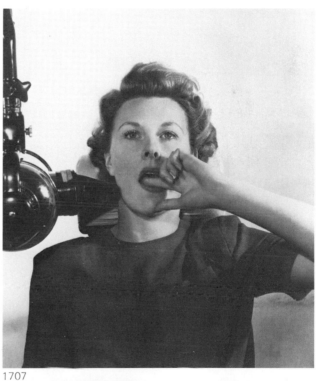

1707

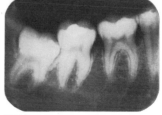

1708

1709

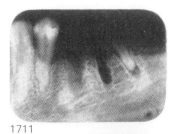

1711

Edentulous subjects

Following the recent extraction of teeth the tooth sockets and lamina dura are still clearly visible (1711) with a normal height of alveolar margin at the dental table. However, with time the alveolar margin is absorbed, the tooth sockets are no longer visible and all trace of the lamina dura lost. It is difficult to keep the intraoral film parallel to the long standing edentulous jaw because the film tends to lean to the buccal or palatal aspects unless a film holder with a dental roll can be used.

When no film holder is being used the angulation of the tube must be increased to correspond to the position of the film. If the denture for the jaw not being examined is replaced a better grip on the film holder can be obtained.

Good quality films are essential to show the trabecular pattern of the bone and because no teeth are present the exposure time must be reduced. The dental canals should be clearly visible (1712).

A general extra-oral or occlusal film will show the position of a buried or unextracted root (1713) should there be any difficulty in locating it on the intra-oral film.

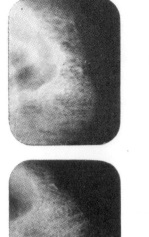
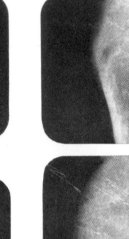

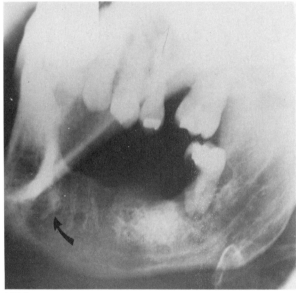

1713

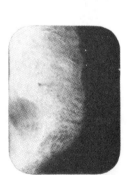
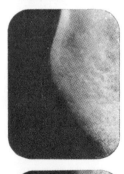

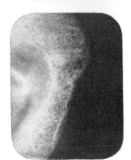
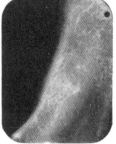

1712

Investigation of crowns

Both upper and lower crowns can be shown on one film if special holders are used which support the film midway between the teeth by a special bite-block. Two different designs are shown in (1714). It is thus possible to examine the crowns of a complete set of teeth with only 4 or 5 films.

Disposable film holders can be made of tasteless tubular plastic which is supplied in 1 foot lengths from which a suitable sized piece for holding the film, can be cut (1715). The method for folding the tubular plastic into a T-shape is shown in (1715) to insert the film central to the bite block. The tube side faces the support, with the teeth over the bite block to maintain its position.

The tube is centred at right angles to the film (1716) with the central ray parallel to the occlusal plane. In the molar region a 5° downward angulation is needed. The radiographs show both upper and lower crowns. When the bite block is made of metal it appears as a thin radio-opaque strip between the crowns (1717).

If special film holders are not available a tab of adhesive tape can be attached to the centre of the tube side of the film. The patient bites on the adhesive tape which holds the film against the crowns. Only radiolucent tape must be used and not zinc oxide plaster which is radio-opaque. If there is any doubt the tape should first be tested.

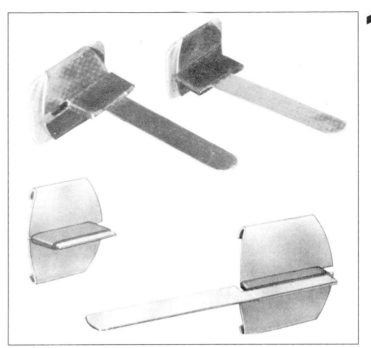

19

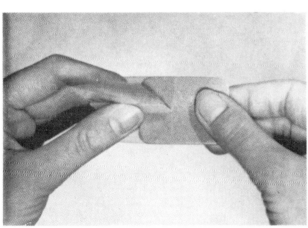

1714

1715

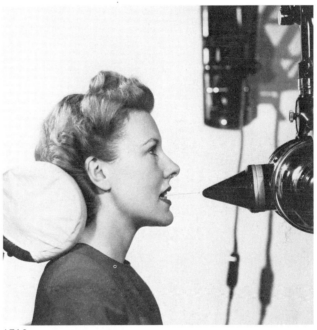

1716

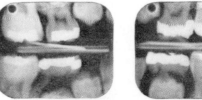

1717

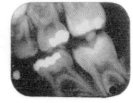

1718

505

Occlusal

Occlusal view of upper incisor region

With the narrow end of a number 3 occlusal film in the mouth, the tube is centred as for the standard view of the upper incisors just above the level of the occlusal line (1719). Because the film is horizontal the tube-occlusal plane angle must be increased to 70° with the pink side of the wrapped film facing the tube.

The radiograph shows foreshortened incisor teeth (1720) but in addition the incisive fossa, possibly the canals, the central area of the palate and the overlying air-filled nasal cavity (1720).

Oblique occlusal views of the upper teeth

With the same type of film but placed transversely with the pink surface uppermost, the tube angle is increased to 65° to the occlusal plane (1721) again because of the horizontal position of the film. Centre halfway along the lower orbital margin for the lateral incisors and canine and just below the outer canthus of the eye for the premolars and molars (1721, 1722).

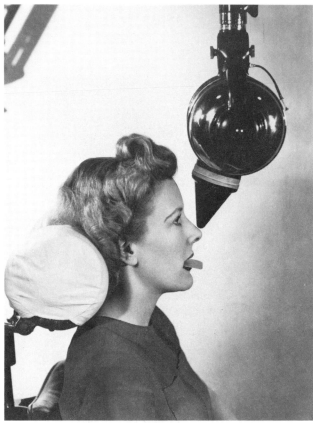

1719

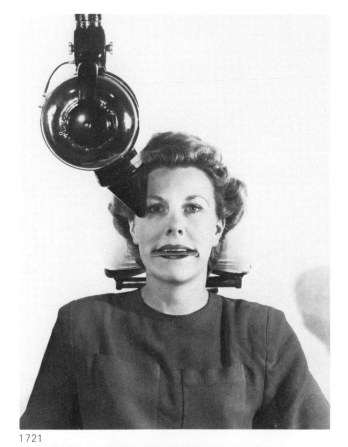

1721

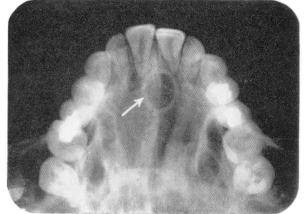

1720

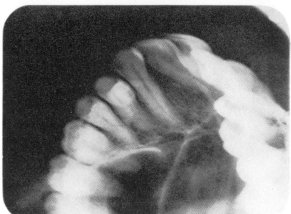

1722

Occlusal view of the lower incisors

The patient's head is tilted back to bring the lower occlusal plane horizontal and with the narrow end of a number 3 occlusal film in the mouth the tube is centred in the midline to the lower jaw as for the intra-oral radiograph of the incisors. The tube angulation is however increased to 35°–40° to the lower occlusal plane because the film is horizontal. The radiograph includes the whole length of the symphysis menti down to the lower border of the jaw because a larger film is used, but the incisors appear foreshortened because the film is horizontal (1723, 1724).

Occlusal view of the lower jaw

The film is placed in the mouth as for the previous view but the neck is more fully extended for the tube to be centred between the angles of the mandible perpendicular to the film (1725). For this view the head must be sufficiently far back to place the tube well down almost onto the patient's chest. In males a prominent thyroid cartilage (Adam's apple) may make it impossible to centre the tube quite so far back but marked neck extension will usually produce the necessary clearance.

These radiographs provide a plan view of the lower mandible to show fracture displacements (1726), unerupted teeth (1727) or the direction of displaced roots (1724).

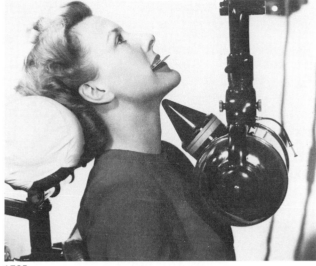
1725

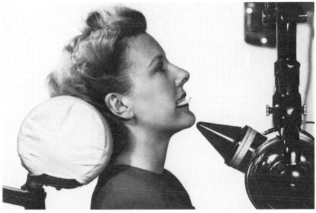
1723

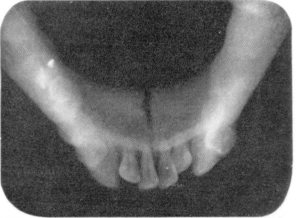
1726

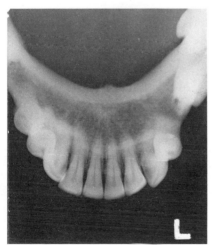
1724

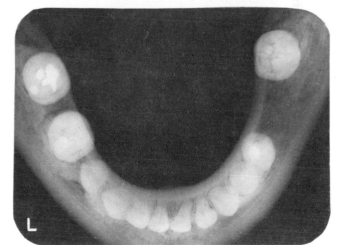
1727

507

Extra-Oral

The Mandible to show the ramus

A small cassette film preferably with rare earth screens, 18 × 13 cm (7 × 5 ins) or 26 × 20 cm (10 × 8 ins) is used.

The patient may stand with the head bent over an angled board (1728), be seated in a dental chair (1729) or at a table (1730). In each case the median line of the face is parallel and the inter-orbital line at right angles to the cassette with the tube tilted 20°–25° towards the head, centring 5 cm (2 ins) below the angle of the jaw remote from the film. The sub-mental triangle forming the floor of the mouth (1731) should be visible from the position of the X-ray tube. The radiograph shows the ramus and posterior half of the body of the mandible (1732).

The Mandible to show the body

If the angle board is used for this view it is set at 25° and the patient's head is turned towards the cassette to bring the body of the mandible close to the film. Centre the tube 5 cm (2 ins) below the angle of the jaw remote from the film with a tube tilt of 110°–120° towards the head. (1733, 1734, 1735)

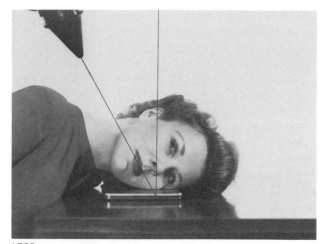
1730

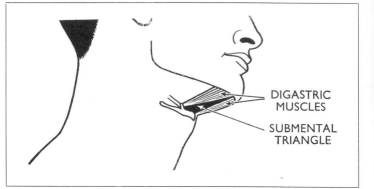

DIGASTRIC MUSCLES

SUBMENTAL TRIANGLE

1731

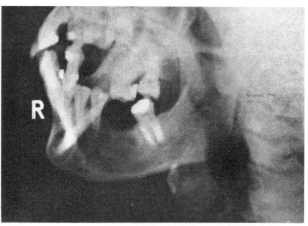
R

1732

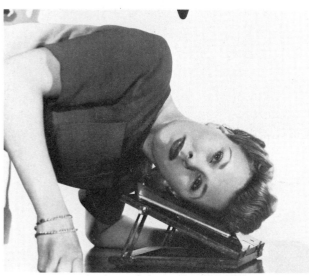
1728

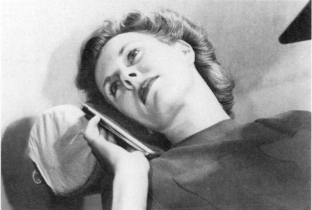
1729

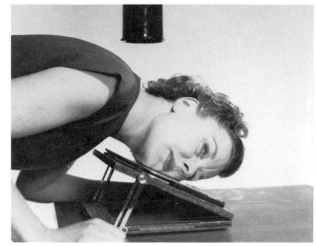
1733

Superior-inferior, "Collar" radiography

For the patient with a fracture of the mandible the occlusal axial view (p. 507) may not be possible. A specially designed cassette, with half an elipse cut out, fits around the neck and under the mandible from the chin to the rami (1737).

The cassette can be used with any table although a skull unit is most convenient (1737) and produces a plan projection of the mandible including the condyles.

Centre in the median sagittal plane at the level of the molars with the tube tilted 15° towards the chin and the orbito-meatal base line at 15° to the horizontal (1736, 1737, 1738).

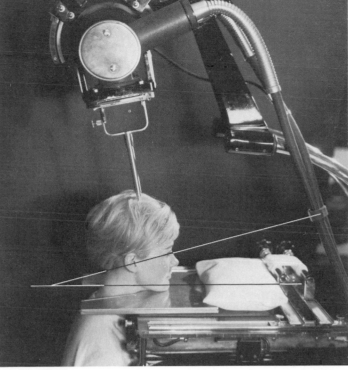
1737

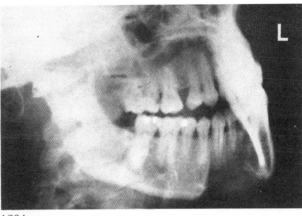
1734

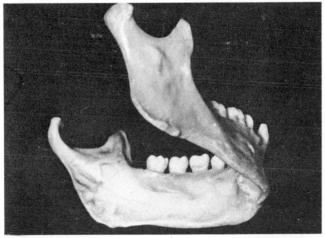
1735

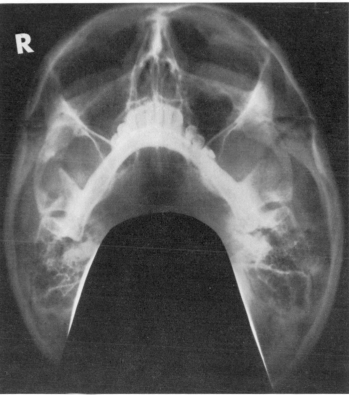
1738

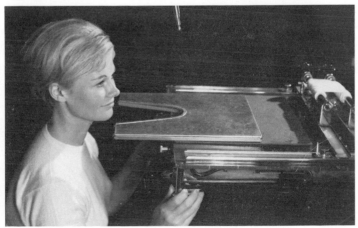
1736

Panagraphy

Pan-oral radiography or panagraphy uses an X-ray source within the mouth to examine the upper and lower dental arches and has become possible with the introduction of a special X-ray tube (1740). The main part of the oil-immersed tube containing the filament and magnetic focussing of the cathode stream is outside the mouth and only the anode, at the end of a narrow metal tube, is inside the mouth. The tube has a low rating of 60 kVp, 0·5 milliamperes and 0·1 second and therefore the exposures are limited to one per second. Lead protection in the anode stem and 2 mm aluminium filtration of the target area reduces radiation to a minimum. Only two exposures are needed for a complete examination of upper and lower jaws as against 10–14 intra-oral views.

The focal spot is 0·1 mm (1/120th ins) and at the tip of the pyramidal shaped anode. The pin-point focus ensures maximum definition and the low kVp good contrast while the short film-focus distance has the added benefit of ×2 magnification. The tube output is low due to the small focal spot but ample for a focus-film distance of 4 cm. Maximum effective radiation is produced by a constant potential and the anode is earthed to eliminate the danger of electric shock.

A 10 × 25 cm (4 × 10 ins) flexible cassette lined with calcium tungstate or rare earth screens is used with rapid-R or other suitable film and the outer side is lead-lined to absorb scattered radiation and for radiation protection.

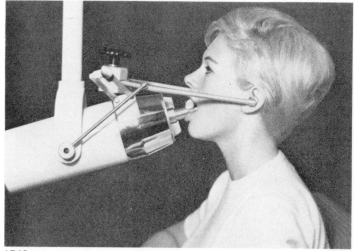

1740

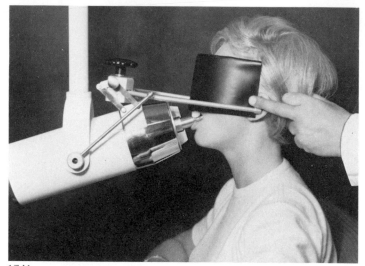

1741

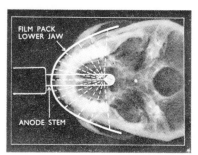

1739

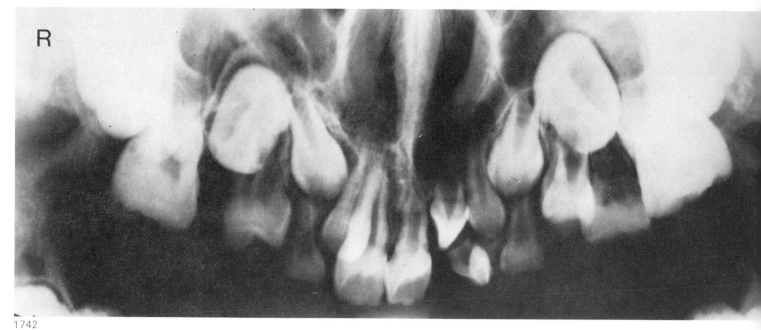

1742

The pin-point tube focus, at the "centre" of the dental arch, produces radiation through a wide angle of 270° (1739). The flexible film cassette is wrapped round the patient's cheeks (1741) or chin (1744) from ear to ear and positioned accordingly for a film of the upper (1745) or lower teeth (1746).

The metal tube leading to the anode is adjustable usually 2·5 cm (1 ins) for adults and 2 cm ($\frac{3}{4}$ ins) for children, and there is also a bite ridge for the incisors to vary the length inside the mouth from about 5 cm (2 ins) in adults to 4 cm ($1\frac{1}{2}$ ins) in children. A sterile disposable polythene cover is used for each patient.

The flexible film pack, placed around the face from ear to ear, has its lower edge touching the anode tube for the upper teeth and is just a little below the level of the occlusal plane. For the lower teeth the wrap around cassette touches the lower aspect of the anode tube reaching just a little above the occlusal plane. Usually the patient can hold the cassette in position otherwise a face board or special chair attachment is needed. In the photographs (1741, 1744) an assistant is holding the cassettes for demonstration purposes only so as not to obscure its position. Under no circumstances must the radiographer hold the cassette in this way during the exposure.

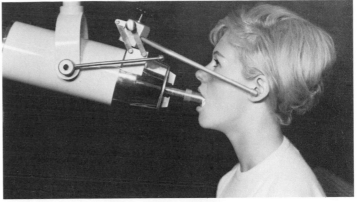

1743

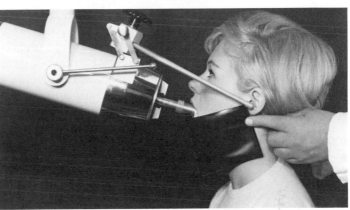

1744

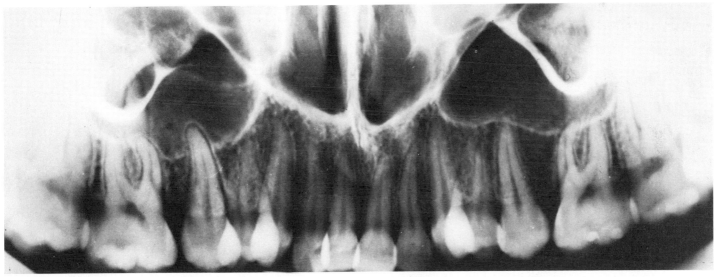

1745

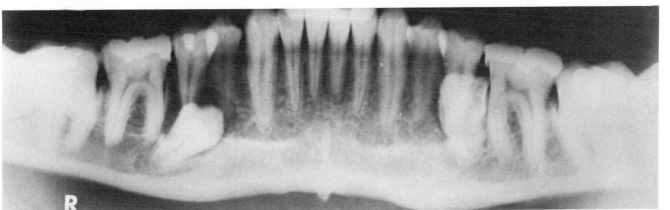

1746

Upper jaw

The seated patient is immobilised against a head and back support with the median sagittal plane vertical and the upper occlusal plane horizontal. A tube attachment (1740) is used to check the position of the occlusal plane. The tube is angled 30° upwards and the bite position adjusted to 5 cm (2 ins) for the adult. The anode head is slowly introduced into the mouth. The patient then bites gently on the padded bite ring and if the tube is correctly positioned will feel no discomfort. (1741, 1745)

Panagraphy of the upper jaw of a child (1742) shows multiple unerupted teeth.

Lower jaw

With the patient seated and immobilised the median sagittal plane is vertical and the *lower* occlusal plane horizontal using the tube attachment as a guide (1743). The tube is angled 20° *downwards*. The tubular anode is placed in the mouth and the flexible-film cassette is positioned with its upper border against the anode tube and extending upwards to the level of the tragus of the ear on both sides (1743, 1744, 1746).

Rotography

Roto-tomography or rotography produces radiographs of curved structures such as the mandible or parts of the skull. Basically the system combines tomography and slit scanography, using a synchronous rotatory movement of both the patient and the film (1747).

In practise the patient and curved film-cassette rotate in opposite directions while a stationary X-ray tube projects a vertical slit beam of X-rays. Because the film and the patient rotate at the same speed only one "plane" is sharply in focus and the other "planes" moving faster or slower are blurred out. To limit the thickness of the section in focus and to avoid too many overlapping shadows, the vertical X-ray beam must be very narrow, a slit beam diaphragm of 0·8 mm (1/32 in) at the tube aperture is used.

There is another vertical slit diaphragm between the patient and cassette to shield the film from scattered radiation.

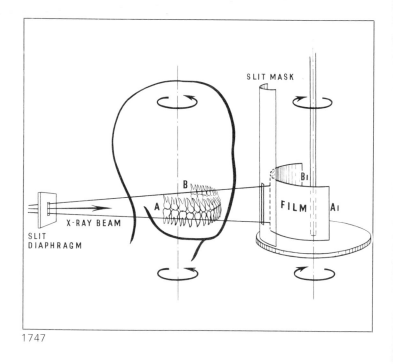

1747

A modified craniostat consisting of a head clamp with adjustable pads, plastic earplugs, a chin rest and a centring device is used for immobilising the patient's head in the correct position (1748). A 10 × 25 cm (4 × 10 ins) flexible film cassette shaped to correspond to the patient's jaw is fixed on a turntable which is geared to rotate synchronously with the patient's chair.

The shape of the jaws can be checked from a bite into a wax block and the hinged cassette holder adjusted accordingly as well as extra holders being provided for unusual features or to examine other regions.

The axis of rotation of the craniostat can be adjusted. If moved backwards along the sagittal plane the temperomanibular joints and whole of the mandible is included while moving the axis of rotation forwards confines the examination to the teeth. There are corresponding scales on the head clamp and film holder for synchronous adjustment. Locating pins on the curved cassette-holder and chin rest establish the correct relationship between the face and film.

Although the apparatus rotates through a full circle the predetermined exposure is made only during 180° to correspond with the region being examined; (1749) shows the position at the beginning of the exposure and (1750) approaching half-way.

In the incisor region the X-ray beam passes through the cervical vertebrae but only through soft tissues in the molar region, hence two density wedges are fitted to produce a more uniform exposure on the film.

The procedure must be explained to the patient before the examination and a practice rotation without radiation also helps to obtain the necessary reassurance and co-operation during the exposure. Other than for patients with vertigo there is no discomfort associated with the procedure.

Exposure factors

There is a long exposure time of 10 secs and with Rapid R film and fast intensifying screens, at 80 kVp 30 milliamperes are needed, giving an exposure of 300 mAs for the fixed focus-film distance of the equipment. The slit diaphragm is 0·8 mm wide (1/32 in). The central axis is irradiated throughout the exposure but the teeth and skin surface for only a fraction of the exposure. The pituitary fossa must thus be above the height of the slit beam of radiation and the central axis of rotation along the sagittal plane must be anterior to the pituitary fossa to minimise the radiation dose to the pituitary gland. A 3 mm aluminium filter at the tube aperture eliminates the unwanted softer radiation.

Rotographs on the following page show in (1751a) a fracture just anterior to the angle of the mandible on the right, in (1751b) the condylar heads taken with the mouth open and in (1752) fracture dislocation of the right condyle in a four year old child with both dentitions visible.

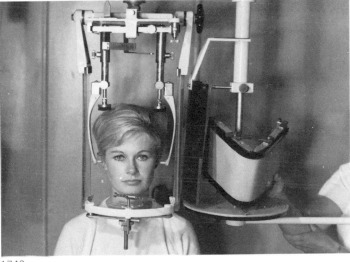

1748

1749

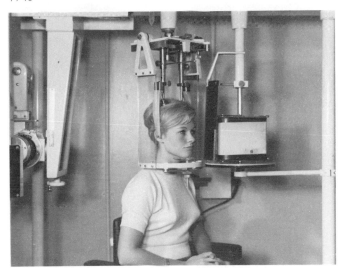

1750

19

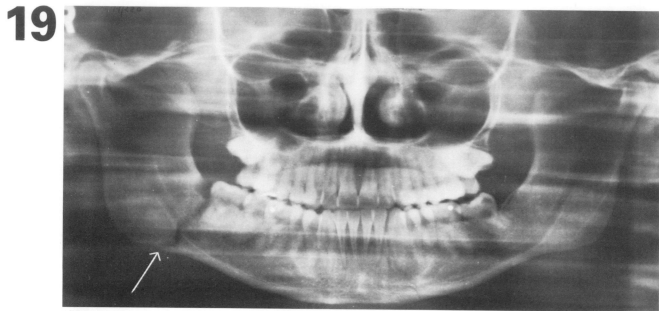

1751a

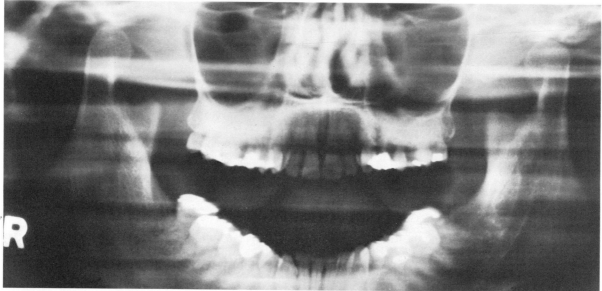

1751b

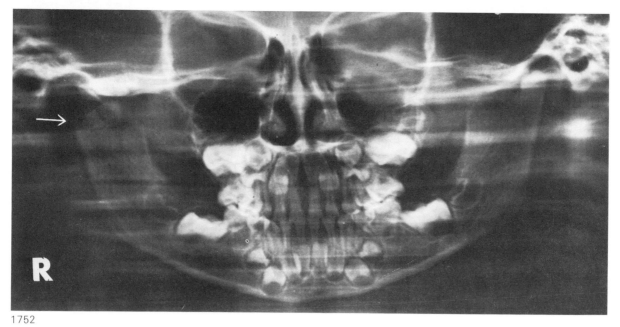

1752

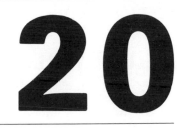

SALIVARY GLANDS
LACRIMAL SYSTEM

SALIVARY GLANDS

Parotid

There are three pairs of salivary glands, the parotid, sub-mandibular and lingual, adjacent to the side and floor of the mouth (1753) which secrete saliva into their respective ducts draining into the mouth to lubricate the mucosa. Saliva contains a digestive enzyme called ptyalase.

Calculi or duct stones may produce obstruction and marked swelling of the gland. If radio-opaque these calculi can be shown on radiographs taken with proper projections.

The main ducts and the intra-glandular branch ducts can be shown by injecting contrast medium, a procedure known as sialography.

The parotids are the largest of the salivary glands, lying just below the zygomatic arch, in front of and below the ear and on the masseter muscles over the ramus of the mandible. The duct from the parotid gland (Stensen's duct) runs along the outer surface of the masseter muscle around its anterior margin to the buccal mucous membrane opposite the upper second molar where it forms a small visible papilla.

Stone formation in Stensen's duct is relatively uncommon compared with the submandibular duct but when present is best shown by an intra-oral film against the inner surface of the cheek on the labial side of the upper molars. A very low dose exposure is needed otherwise the film will be overexposed hiding the calculus on the radiograph.

Radiograph (1754) shows a parotid duct calculus on an intra-oral film barely visible on the fronto-occipital view (1755).

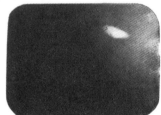

1754

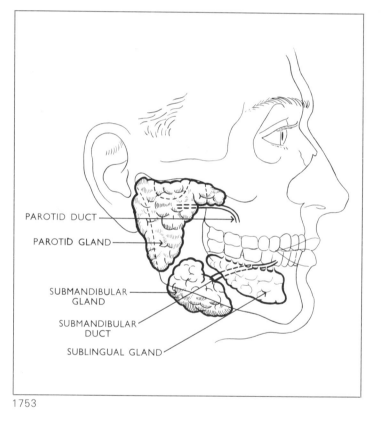

PAROTID DUCT

PAROTID GLAND

SUBMANDIBULAR GLAND

SUBMANDIBULAR DUCT

SUBLINGUAL GLAND

1753

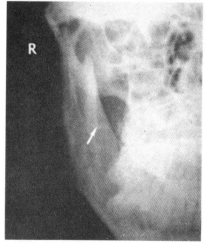

R

1755

Sialography

A cannula tip or fine catheter is inserted into the duct orifice after locating the papilla opposite the upper second molar. A small amount (1–2 ml) of 60% water soluble contrast medium is injected, each gland being examined in turn. The exposure is made as the patient signals a feeling of discomfort from the distension of the duct system. Both lateral and frontal views are needed to show the main duct and its branches.

The projections for the parotid are the same as for the ramus of the mandible and an oblique or lateral view can be done.

Lateral oblique

In the lateral oblique view (1756) the head is straight and the tube angled to separate the right and left sides of the mandible.

The head is in the true lateral position with the median sagittal plane parallel to and the intraorbital line at right angles to the cassette.

■ Centre below and behind the angle of the jaw away from the film with the tube tilted 25° towards the head (1756, 1757)

Lateral

The head is in the true lateral position with the angles of the mandible overshadowing each other. The neck is slightly extended to show as much as possible of the parotid between the mandible and cervical spine.

■ Centre with the tube perpendicular over the angle of the mandible (1758, 1759)

Exposure table

			Oblique view		
kVp	mAs	FFD	Film ILFORD	Screen ILFORD	Grid
Oblique 60	5	105cm(42″)	RAPID R	FT	—
Lateral 70	5	105cm(42″)	RAPID R	FT	—

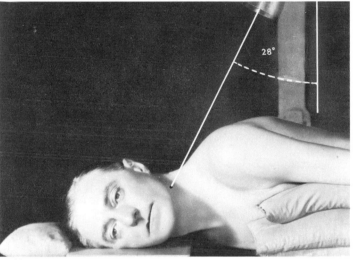

1756

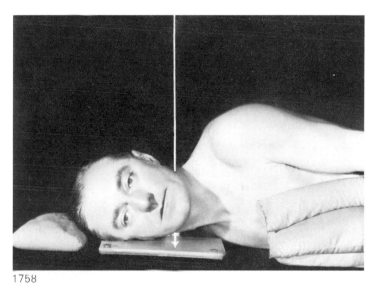

1758

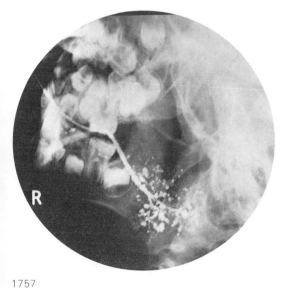

1757

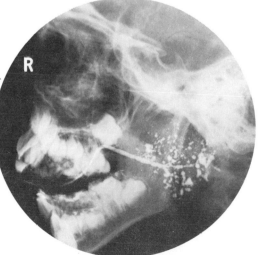

1759

Frontal Projection

Although the parotid region can be shown in both the antero-posterior and postero-anterior positions, the projection for sialography is antero-posterior for the injection of contrast medium. However, the main duct is projected across the mandible while the gland is free of overlying bone; the exposure for the two areas being quite different. When the duct is well shown the gland is overexposed (1762) and when the gland is well shown the film is underpenetrated for the main duct as it crosses the mandible. Both regions can be shown with one exposure if a non-screen film is placed in front of the cassette and an exposure used as for the cassette-film.

Antero-posterior

With the patient supine, the head is raised on a small non-opaque pad and the chin lowered toward the chest bringing the base line perpendicular to the cassette. The median plane is also at right angles to the film.

■ Centre in the midline, immediately below the lower lip (1760, 1761, 1762)

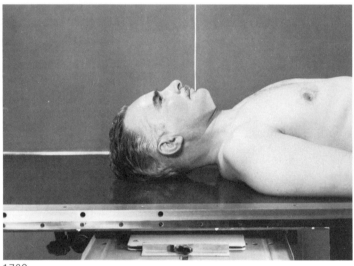

1760

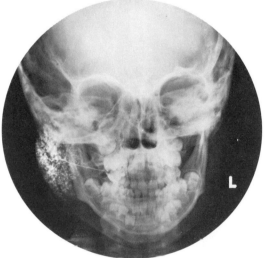

518   1761

Even when only one side is being examined the tube must still be perpendicular and centred to the midline to use the oblique ray to project the gland free of overshadowing by bone. Soft tissue exposures are essential for the gland itself and must be considerably less than that for the view of the mandible (1761).

Radiographs

A normal sialogram is shown in lateral (1763) and in antero-posterior view (1762). The main duct of Stensen is well shown as it crosses the mandible but the gland region is overexposed with the intraglandular ducts largely obliterated.

In (1761) the gland is well demonstrated including the intraglandular or branch ducts.

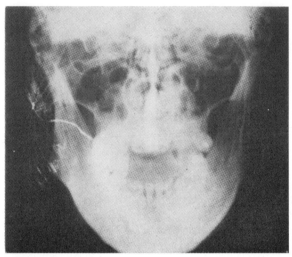

1762

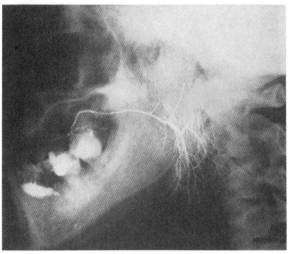

1763

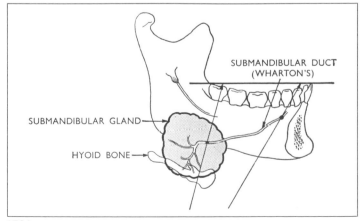

1764

Salivary glands

Submandibular (Submaxillary)

The two submandibular glands lie on either side of the neck forming part of the soft tissues on the medial margin of the body of the mandible and between the mandible and hyoid bone (1764). The submandibular or Wharton's duct runs forwards, upwards and medially crossing the lingual nerve, lying on the medial surface of the sublingual gland along the floor of the mouth to open on a small papilla at the side of the frenulum of the tongue. There are three standard projections for the submandibular duct and gland, the infero-superior (occlusal), the infero-superior (occlusal) with the head tilted and the lateral.

Infero-superior (occlusal) (1)

The patient is seated and the neck well extended supported on a head rest. An occlusal film, well over to the side being examined and well back in the mouth is held lightly between the teeth.

■ Centre to the film from beneath the jaw with the axial ray at right angles to the film (1765)

Infero-superior (2)

A modified occlusal view for calculi lying far posteriorly is done with the patient's head tilted to one side.

The patient is seated, the chin raised and turned away from the affected side. An occlusal film is positioned diagonally in the mouth with the long edge along the jaw of the affected side thus allowing the film to be placed well back in the mouth. The film is held lightly between the teeth.

■ Centre beyond the angle of the jaw at right angles to the film (1766, 1768)

The value of this projection is shown by comparing (1768) which shows two calculi in Wharton's duct with (1767) which shows only the anterior opacity.

Occlusal infero-superior					
kVp	mAs	FFD	Film ILFORD	Screen —	Grid
60	20	75cm(30″)	FAST OCCLUSAL	—	—

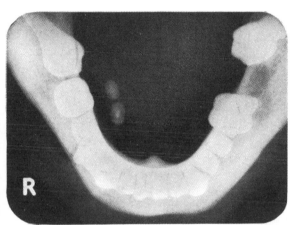

1765

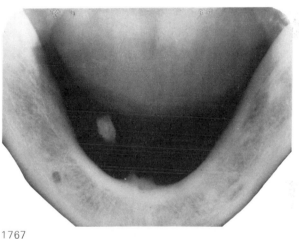

1767

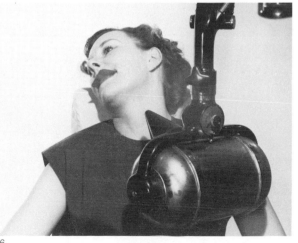

1766

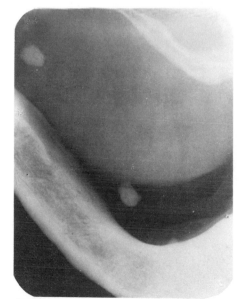

1768

Lateral

The oblique projection is more suitable for the parotid gland while the true lateral with the tongue depressed (1769) is more appropriate for the submandibular gland.

To show calculi on the lateral view the tongue must be well pressed down with a spatula over the affected side to bring the soft tissues of the floor of the mouth below the level of the bone (1769). An opacity in the posterior two thirds of the duct or in the gland will then become visible on the radiograph.

The stone often lies at the bend of the duct just medial to the roots of the third molar.

Sialography

Contrast examinations of the submandibular glands are similar to parotid sialography which show both the main duct and the intraglandular branch ducts. Lateral and oblique views are taken as for parotid sialography and demonstrate the main duct lying over the body of the mandible and the gland lying in the gap below the angle of the mandible and above the hyoid bone (1770, 1771).

Radiograph (1770) was exposed during the injection and (1771) immediately after removal of the cannula.

Sublingual

The two sublingual glands lie in the floor of the anterior part of the mouth below the tongue. Their secretions enter the mouth by several small openings on either side of the frenulum and some may open into the submandibular duct.

The projections are the same as for the submandibular gland with the occlusal projection being the most important which easily covers the glands as they lie anteriorly. (1772)

Occlusal view (sublingual)					
kVp	mAs	FFD	Film ILFORD	Screen —	Grid
60	20	90cm(36″)	FAST OCCLUSAL	—	—

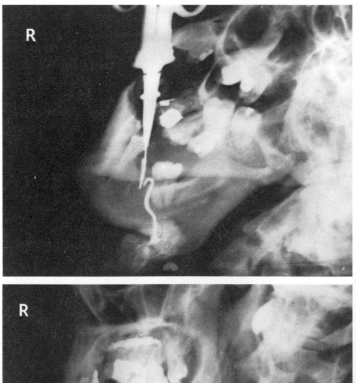
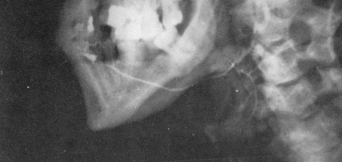

1770 1771

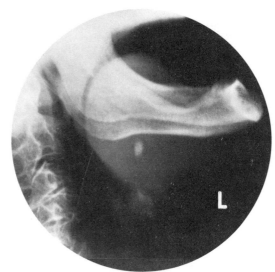

1769

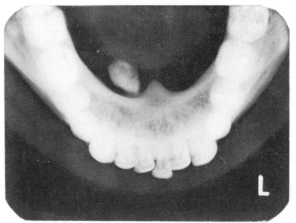

1772

The Lacrimal Apparatus

The lacrimal apparatus includes the lacrimal gland, which secretes the tears, and the lacrimal sac and ducts through which the tears pass into the nose (1773).

The lacrimal gland lies anteriorly in the upper, outer quadrant of the orbit, forming the tears which wash over the eye and drain into the lacrimal sac by two small openings in the medial aspects of the lids—the puncta lacrimalia, which can be seen when the inner aspects of the lids are everted. They communicate with the lacrimal sac by fine lacrimal canaliculi which run horizontally.

The lacrimal sac drains into the naso-lacrimal duct which runs vertically in the lateral nasal wall on the medial aspect of the maxillary antrum. The lengths of the canaliculi are approximately 1 cm, the lacrimal sac 1 cm and the naso-lacrimal duct 2 cm which finally ends below the inferior nasal conchus well back in the nose.

When the lacrimal duct system is blocked a "watering" eye is produced and is investigated radiographically by a contrast examination.

The patient is supine and two drops of local anaesthetic are inserted into the medial aspect of the lower lid. The orifice of the inferior punctum lacrimila is dilated with a blunt dilator. An anionic water soluble contrast medium such as Amipaque is injected through a cannula with a 2 ml syringe.

A film is taken when the fluid enters the nostril or regurgitates through the upper punctum. Antero-posterior and lateral radiographs of the nose and antrum are required (1774, 1775).

When the duct system is patent contrast medium may show its whole length or be seen on the floor of the nasal cavity. With an obstructed duct the contrast medium is held up proximal to the site of obstruction.

The lacrimal duct inclines posteriorly as it runs downwards. To bring the duct parallel to the film in the antero-posterior position the chin must be raised a further 5°–10°.

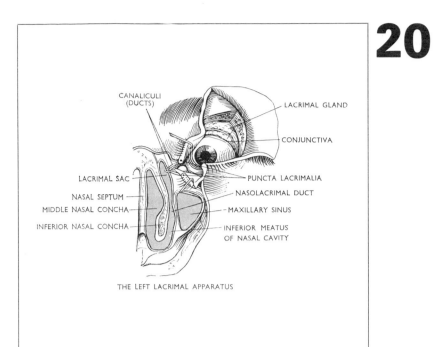

THE LEFT LACRIMAL APPARATUS

1773

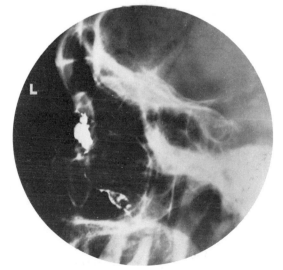

1774

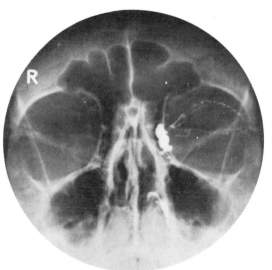

1775

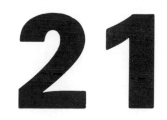

TEMPORAL BONES

TEMPORAL BONES

Anatomy: position and structure

The temporal bones form part of the lateral walls and floor of the cranium and consist of squamous, tympanic, mastoid and petrous portions with zygomatic and styloid processes. This section is mainly concerned with the mastoid and petrous portions.

The squamous part is a flat, thin area of bone lying mainly above and behind the external auditory meatus and giving off the zygomatic process anteriorly (1781a).

The tympanic part forms the antero-inferior aspect of the external auditory meatus lying just behind the articular fossa of the tempero-mandibular joint which lies mainly on the squamous temporal (1781a).

The styloid process is long and thin, lying just behind and medial to the ramus of the mandible and pointing to the anterior part or body of the hyoid (1778).

The mastoid lies behind and below the external auditory meatus containing the mastoid or tympanic antrum and numerous air cells which vary in size, shape and number from one individual to the next (1776, 1781a).

The petrous part or pyramid is the most complex containing the organ of hearing and position sense and being wedged between the sphenoid and occipital bones at the base of the skull (1781b, 1781c). There are three parts to the organ of hearing

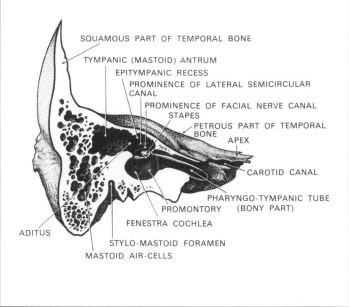

SQUAMOUS PART OF TEMPORAL BONE
TYMPANIC (MASTOID) ANTRUM
EPITYMPANIC RECESS
PROMINENCE OF LATERAL SEMICIRCULAR CANAL
PROMINENCE OF FACIAL NERVE CANAL
STAPES
PETROUS PART OF TEMPORAL BONE
APEX
CAROTID CANAL
PHARYNGO-TYMPANIC TUBE (BONY PART)
PROMONTORY
FENESTRA COCHLEA
STYLO-MASTOID FORAMEN
MASTOID AIR-CELLS
ADITUS

1776

and position sense, the external ear, the middle ear or tympanic cavity and the internal ear or labyrinth (1777).

The external expanded part of the ear is called the auricle, and the external auditory meatus or ear hole, extends from the auricle to the tympanic membrane (1777). The tympanic membrane or ear-drum is a sheet of fibrous tissue between the external and middle ear and is 1 cm in diameter, almost circular and oblique in position (1777, 1779).

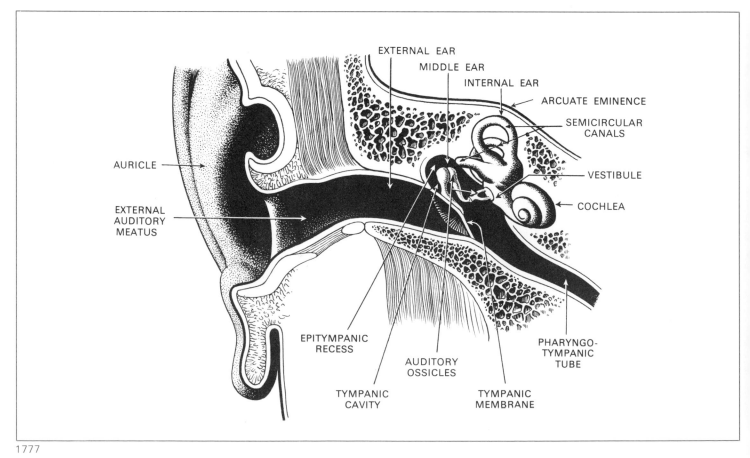

EXTERNAL EAR
MIDDLE EAR
INTERNAL EAR
ARCUATE EMINENCE
SEMICIRCULAR CANALS
VESTIBULE
COCHLEA
AURICLE
EXTERNAL AUDITORY MEATUS
EPITYMPANIC RECESS
TYMPANIC CAVITY
AUDITORY OSSICLES
TYMPANIC MEMBRANE
PHARYNGO-TYMPANIC TUBE

1777

The middle ear is an air space containing the malleus, incus and stapes which are three small interlinked bones, the auditory ossicles, connecting the tympanic membrane and the internal ear; the base of the stapes being attached at the oval window or fenestra vestibuli.

Sound waves causing vibrations at the tympanic membrane are transmitted across the middle ear or tympanic cavity by the auditory ossicles to the internal ear. The auditory ossicles lie in an upward extension of the middle ear air cavity called the epitympanic recess (1779) which has a posterior triangular opening, the aditus, leading to the tympanic or mastoid antrum.

The internal ear is a series of bony channels and chambers lined by delicate membranes forming the labyrinth named the vestibule, semi-circular canals and cochlea. The three semi-circular canals, the superior, posterior and lateral face in three different directions at right angles to each other (1780).

A connecting passage, the pharyngo-tympanic or Eustachian tube between the pharynx and the tympanic cavity allows the air pressure to be equalised on either side of the tympanic membrane (1777).

The internal auditory meatus which is about 1 cm long and

0.5 cm wide is almost opposite the external auditory meatus. The lateral end of the internal auditory meatus, adjacent to the vestibule and cochlea, is the fundus. From it the internal auditory meatus passes medially through the petrous bone, transmitting the facial and auditory nerve and internal auditory artery and vein to open just above the jugular foramen (1778).

Radiographs of the temporal bone, in different projections, can show the features of the middle and internal ear remarkably clearly, but a good understanding of the anatomy of such a complicated structure is needed to produce diagnostic radiographs. Initially the student should practice the various projections on a skull specimen to learn both the radiographic technique and anatomy and then proceed to study the anatomy on radiographs of patients before undertaking these examinations.

The anatomical relations of the temporal bone are shown on the skull specimen from the external (1781a), internal (1781b) and internal basal (1781c) aspects. The main structures are shown on each illustration. The more detailed anatomy on the drawings of the various parts of the temporal bone (1776–1780) should subsequently be used to study radiographs taken with different projections.

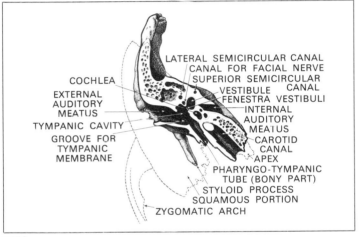

1778

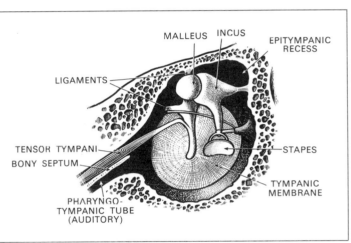

1779

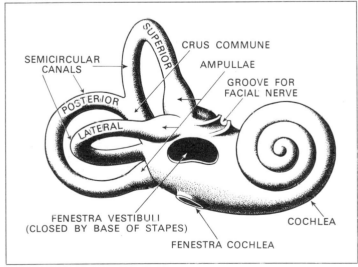

1780

Planes, lines and landmarks

All radiography of the skull whether concerned with a specific region such as the temporal bone or with views of the whole skull uses recognised planes, lines and landmarks as a guide for positioning the patient. The terms used in the illustrations (1782, 1783) follow the recommendations of the Neuro-radiological Commission with the radiographic projections being related to these planes, lines and landmarks.

The view from the lateral aspect is of particular interest as angulation of the X-ray tube, especially in the axial plane, is related to the base line of the skull. Thus positioning of the skull always starts with the base line at right angles to the length of the Bucky top which is adjusted accordingly and then tube angulation to right and left in turn is related to the radiographic base line (orbito-meatal base line—OMBL) of the skull (1783).

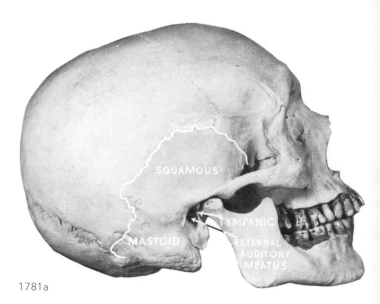

1781a

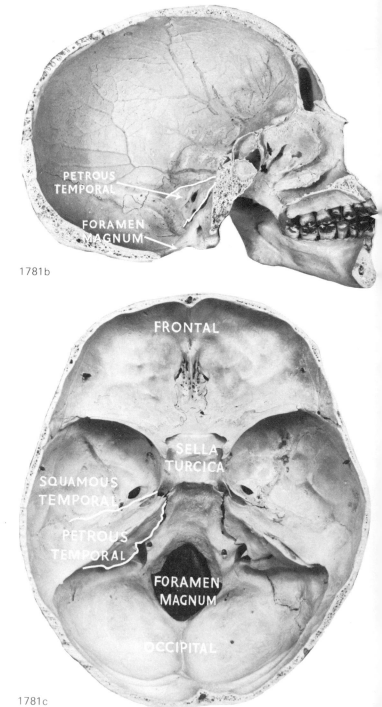

1781b

1781c

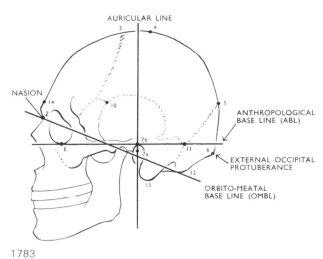

1782

1783

Technique and equipment

Detailed radiography of the temporal bones is only possible because the contained spaces and passages such as the internal and external auditory meatuses, the middle and internal ear and the mastoid air cells are contrasted against bone. The whole purpose of the many projections is to show these spaces and passages, their contents and deformities, to best advantage, free of unnecessary superimposed shadows and away from each other. To show these structures which are so small, so close together and so deeply set within the temporal bones requires precise positioning and finest film definition. To obtain the required film definition a fine-focus tube, a small localising cone and fine grain intensifying screens are essential.

The patient may be either erect or horizontal and the examination may be done with or without grids but in the vast majority of cases both sides are radiographed for comparison and may be supplemented by stereoscopy, macroradiography and tomography.

Basic precepts

As with other sections the exposure factors quoted refer to an adult of average physique and each film should be carefully labelled not only with the patient's identification but also as right or left and for the latter 0·5 cm ($\frac{1}{4}$ ins) lead letters are recommended.

Usually several projections are done for each examination, lateral, oblique and axial but the method used depends very much on whether a special skull unit is available or the patient is being examined on a standard radiographic couch with a vertical stand or ceiling suspended tube.

The skull unit has many advantages. The tube is automatically centred from any angulation or position to the central intersection of the cross-lines on the table top, the required angle of the tube in the correct plane can be located precisely and the position of the head can be seen on the transparent table in a suitably placed mirror by moving the Bucky out of the way. Furthermore, if only routine and easily adjusted positions of the head are used, repeatable projections can be obtained through precise tube angulations. A specialised skull unit is therefore recommended for radiography of the temporal bone.

For other apparatus the tube is centred to the tube-side surface of the head and the cassette is displaced to allow for off-centre projection of the image. But it is then necessary, if the technique described for the skull unit is to be converted for use on a standard couch and vertical stand, to transpose the position of the intersecting lines on the table top to the tube-side surface of the skull. A pointer or frame carrying crossed threads is used to first centre the tube with the necessary angulation to the intersection of the crossed lines on the table top. The head is then interposed, positioned accordingly and the cassette off centred to the tube angulation.

Temporal bone projections

Several methods are given for each projection using both a skull unit and standard equipment and there is a summary of the projections for a skull table on page 535 with radiographs on pages 536 and 537.

Projections using standard equipment are described separately for the mastoids on pages 528–534 and for the petrous temporals on pages 538–540. Although the simplest method for examining the mastoids in profile is with an angle board, the vertical profile projection is more commonly used and set out on pages 530–531.

For lateral projections either the patient's head may be tilted using a vertical X-ray beam or the median sagittal plane is parallel to the table top and the tube tilted as shown on pages 532 and 533.

In both the axial and half-axial projections (35° fronto-occipital and occipito-frontal) both mastoids are shown on one film (page 534).

Two oblique projections are given for the petrous temporal, Stenver's projection (1824) and a similar position using the skull unit, (p. 540). Further views include the axial and half axial and the two lateral projections.

A complete examination of the mastoids and petrous temporals on a skull unit is obtained with four or five projections, often three with the head lateral and two in the frontal plane.

The three projections with the head lateral include two with the tube angled 15° and 35° towards the feet and for the third with a 30°–35° angle to the face, the grid is rotated for the grid slats to be in the same direction as the X-ray beam; on a standard radiographic table a stationary grid must be used.

The axial and half axial projections are similar on both types of equipment but for the basal projection positioning is more comfortable for the patient and more convenient for the operator on the skull unit. Both the axial and half axial projections may be taken with the tube-film positions reversed and narrow rectangular coning eliminates scattered radiation producing better definition.

The base line must be adjusted to the correct angle for all projections including the lateral projections particularly when there is a tube tilt, otherwise the views of right and left sides will not be comparable. In fact this principle applies throughout the whole of skull radiography and not just for projections of the temporal bone.

Mastoid

The mastoid processes are palpable behind and below the ears and best seen on the lateral aspect of the skull (1781a). The mastoids are superimposed on each other on a true lateral radiograph; oblique projections are used to separate the shadows of both sides.

For the profile views the mastoids must be projected clear of the cervical spine. The head is rotated on its axis and at the same time the chin is well tucked in to separate the shadows of the mastoid and occipital bone.

The projections used may be either antero-posterior or postero-anterior, done with or without a grid or angle board and with suitable apparatus the right and left sides can be exactly duplicated. The walls of the air cells must be sharply defined with adequate contrast between the air cells and their walls.

Profile

The profile projections show the less dense mastoid clear of the shadows of the skull base, with the denser shadow of the mastoid antrum included on the film. However, a compromise exposure is used to show both densities with a high kilovoltage suitable for the mastoid antrum and sufficiently high to reduce the difference in contrast between the tip and the antrum. At lower kilovoltages brilliant contrast is produced in the region of the air cells but then either the antrum is over-exposed or the tip under-exposed and will require viewing by a bright light.

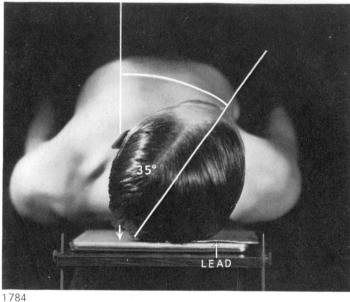

1784

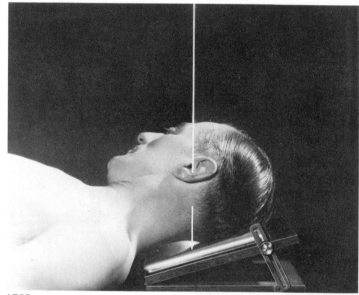

1785

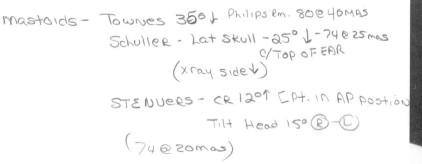

mastoids — Townes 35° ↓ Philips Rm. 80 @ 40MAS
Schuller - Lat Skull -25° ↓ -74 @ 25mas
C/TOP OF EAR
(xray side ↓)
STENUERS - CR 12° ↑ [Pt. IN AP postion
Tilt Head 15° ℞ - ℄
(74 @ 20mas)

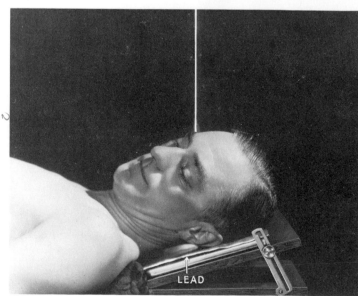

1786

(1) Antero-posterior oblique (basic)
Angle board

With the patient supine, the head is on the cassette which lies on a variable 15°–25° angle board, the radiographic base line being at right angles to the film. From this position the head is turned 35° away from the side being examined and the chin kept well down towards the chest and looking at a side view of the head (1785) the mastoid can be seen lying directly over the cassette without being overlapped by adjacent bone structure.

The two sides can be exposed on a single film by covering each half in turn (1786) or by using a special cassette tunnel.

■ Centre over the base of the mastoid process remote from the film using a small localising cone (1784, 1785, 1786, 1787, 1788).

Radiographs (1787, 1788) of this view should show the mastoid process and antrum clearly. The angle board can be replaced by an angle block or by suitably placed sandbags.

The required angle on the angle board varies with the subject. If the shoulders are thin and the neck long an angle of 15° will be comfortable for positioning the head but for a patient with thick shoulders and a short neck a 25° angle is essential.

The positions of the patient and angle board may be reversed to produce similar results. The patient is then prone with the open end of the angle board toward the neck. The head is rotated 55° toward the cassette and the tube centred over the mastoid nearest the film (1789) to be compared with (1784) shown supine.

Exposure table

Mastoid AP oblique (basic)

kVp	mAs	FFD	Film ILFORD	Screen ILFORD	Grid
65	15	90cm(36")	RAPID R	HD	—

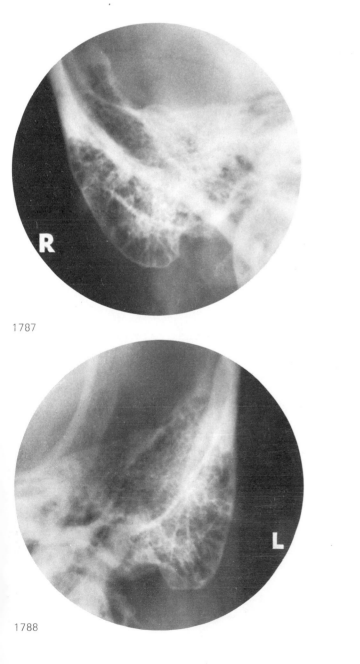

1787

1788

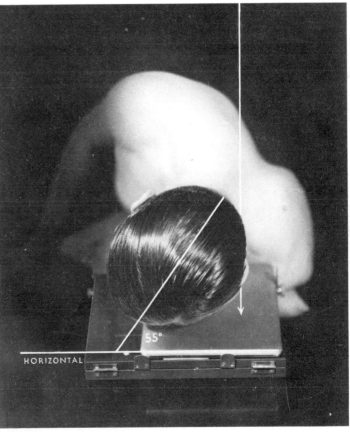

1789

(2) Postero-anterior oblique

The patient may be either erect or horizontal for this projection and usually the Potter-Bucky diaphragm is used.

The head is in the occipito-frontal position, with clamps on the biparietal diameter, and turned through 35° away from the mastoid being radiographed which is brought closer to the film. The base line-film angle is at 85°. With the patient horizontal the protractor is used on the head from the end of the couch to obtain the correct angle (1792).

■ Centre midway between the occipital protuberance and the external auditory meatus of the side nearest the film with the tube angled 12° toward the head (1790, 1791, 1792, 1793, 1794)

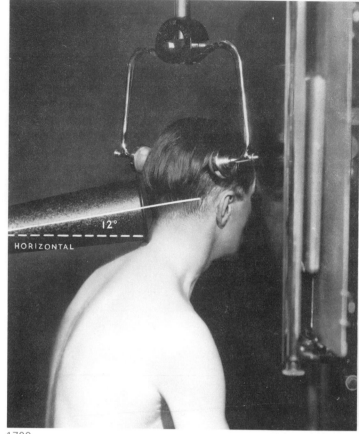

Mastoid postero-anterior oblique

kVp	mAs	FFD	Film ILFORD	Screen ILFORD	Grid
70	40	90cm(36")	RAPID R	HD	Grid

Looking at the head in this position from the tube side (1790) the mastoid is seen in profile free of overlapping bone structures as with the previous positions on the angle board (1785).

The two pairs of films taken postero-anterior (1793, 1794) should be compared with those taken antero-posterior (1795, 1796).

The postero-anterior view has the advantage of producing considerable less radiation to the lens of the eye than the antero-posterior projection.

1790

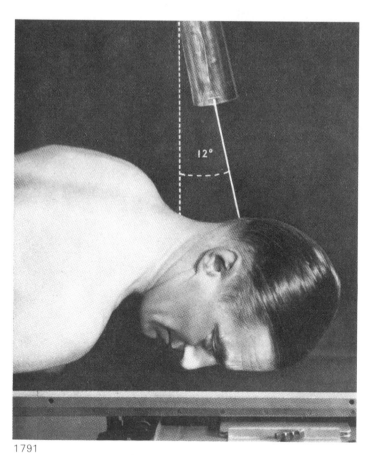

530
1791

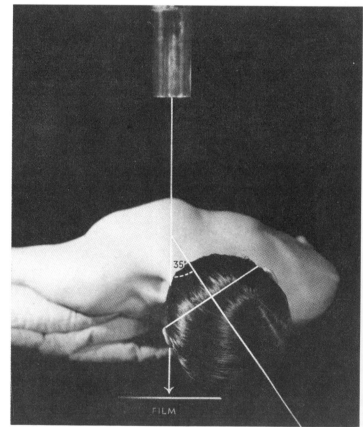

1792

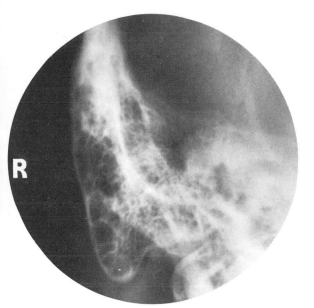

1793

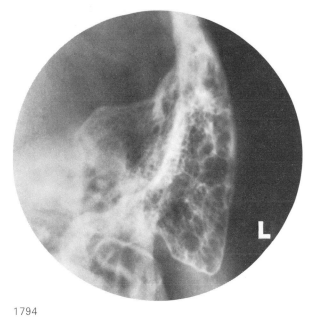

1794

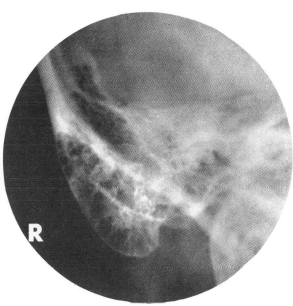

1795

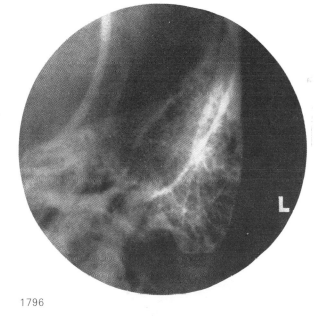

1796

Lateral oblique

To obtain maximum definition the shadows of the two sides are separated on the lateral projection either by tilting the head or by angling the tube thus avoiding superimposition of the mastoid images. The auricle of the ear nearest to the cassette is folded forward. The air cells are shown through the overlying cranial bones.

(1) Angle board

The face is rotated 15° towards the couch top and inclined 15° downward using either an angle table with the patient seated (1797) or an angle block when the patient is prone on a couch or seated (1798, 1802).

The auricle of the ear is folded forward (1802), the median sagittal plane parallel with and the interorbital line at right angles to the angle board.

A diagram of a suitable angle block is shown in (1801).

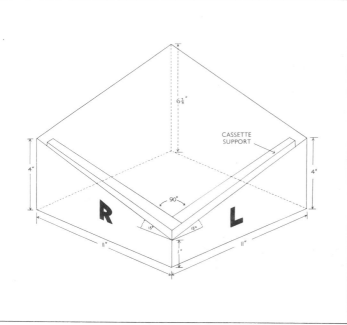

1801

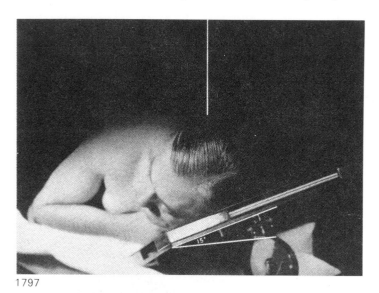

1797

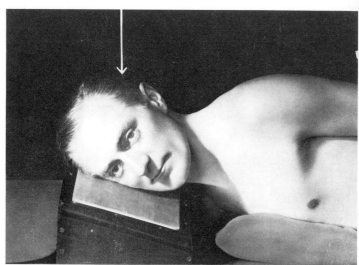

1798

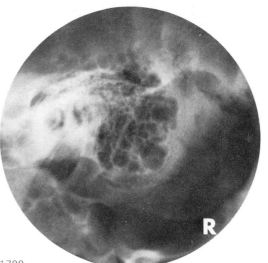

1799

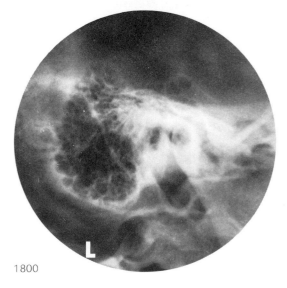

1800

(2) Head tilted

With the head in the true lateral position and the auricle of the ear folded forward away from the mastoid, the face is rotated towards the table top with the chin slightly downward. The chin and cheek should be nestling comfortably on the table top with the median sagittal plane inclined at an angle of 15° to the table (1803).

■ Centre 5 cm (2 ins) above and behind the external auditory meatus remote from the film, with the tube straight and using a small extension cone. Both sides are examined for comparison (1802, 1803, 1799, 1800)

(3) Tube angled

With the head in the true lateral position and the auricle of the ear fold forward away from the mastoid, the tube is angled to separate the shadows of the mastoid. Each side is examined in turn (1804).

The double angulation of the tube makes this projection more difficult and requires at the very least, a centre finder or long extension cone.

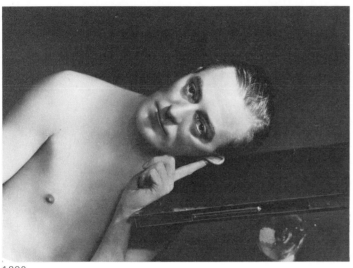

1802

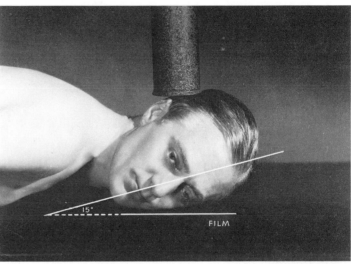

1803

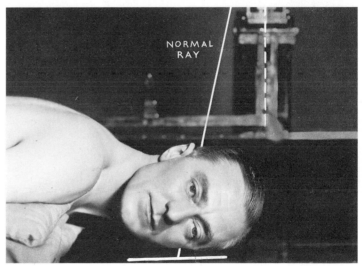

1804

In the following projections both the right and left sides are shown on the one film with a single exposure and may be done with the patient erect or in the horizontal position.

35° Fronto-occipital (half axial)

With the patient facing the tube and the chin well down on the chest, the cervico-occipital region is against the film support. The median sagittal plane and the orbito-meatal line are at right angles to the film.

■ Centre in the midline between the mastoid processes with the tube angled 35° toward the feet (1805, 1806).

Both mastoids are shown symmetrically on the film (1806) with a single exposure.

Occipito-vertical

With the patient facing the film, the head is well flexed to bring the vertex against the film support. The base line-film angle should be at 50° and the median sagittal plane at right angles to the film (1807).

■ Centre midway between the mastoid processes.

kVp	mAs	FFD	Film ILFORD	Screen ILFORD	Grid
80	80	90 cm (36″)	RAPID R	HD	Grid

Both mastoids are shown symmetrically on the one film with a single exposure (1808).

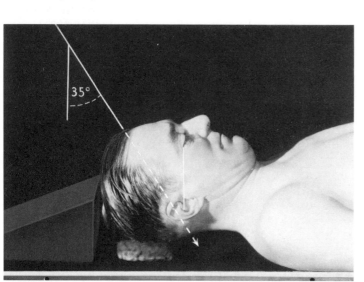

1805

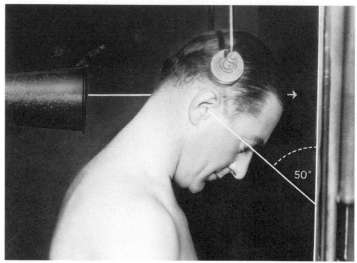

1807

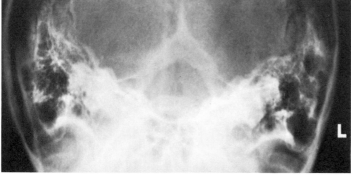

1806

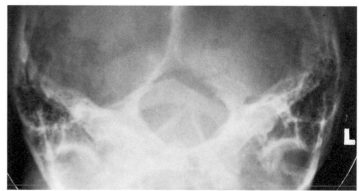

1808

Petrous

Before reading the section on the middle and internal ear or attempting the projections, the illustrations and anatomical descriptions of the region on pages 524–526) should be reviewed. The radiographic and corresponding annotated diagrams on pages 536–537 should also be studied.

Projections are described for use with the general X-ray couch and vertical stand or ceiling suspended tube and for the skull table. For the lateral and oblique views each side is radiographed separately. Two different tube angles are used for the lateral projections and the oblique views are done either from the postero-oblique or lateral oblique aspects. The fronto-occipital and submento-vertical projections show both sides on a single film with a single exposure.

The patient may be erect or horizontal for the examination and a fine focus tube, a small localizing cone and a moving grid are essential for good contrast. High definition films are recommended and owing to the high radio-density of this region a fairly high kilovoltage is used.

Auditory nerve tumour

Auditory (eighth cranial) nerve tumours may enlarge the internal auditory meatus and formerly detailed views of the petrous temporal were considered mandatory but these patients are now investigated by computed tomography. To show the internal auditory meatuses the radiograph must include the petrous portion of the temporal bone, both side being taken either separately or simultaneously for comparison, as shown on pages 536–537 on radiographs and annotated diagrams.

It is of interest to compare the appearances of the axial projection on a stillborn (1842b) with that of an adult (1842a).

The radiographs on pages 536 and 537, each accompanied by an annotated anatomical diagram, were taken as follows:

(1809, 1810)

Head lateral, auricle folded forward with the external auditory meatus centred to the intersection of the cross-lines on the table top, base line parallel to the transverse line, tube angled 15° toward the feet and centred to the cross-lines (1831), page 541. On standard couch (1821), page 538.

(1811, 1812)

Head lateral, auricle folded forward, a point 2 cm (1 ins) below the external auditory meatus placed over the intersection of the cross lines, base line parallel to the transverse line, tube angled 35° toward the feet and centred to the cross lines (1833), page 541. On the standard couch (1821), page 538.

(1813, 1814)

Head lateral but slightly flexed to bring the base line 5° to the transverse line and tube tilt 10° to the head (1835, 1836), page 542. A point 2 cm (1 ins) in front and 1 cm ($\frac{1}{2}$ ins) above the external auditory meatus is placed over the intersection of the cross lines, tube angled 35° toward the face and centred to the cross lines.

(1815, 1816)

Stenver's projection, page 539. Radiographs are very similar to (1813, 1814).

(1817, 1818)

Half axial 35° fronto-occipital with slit diaphragm, patient is supine and nape of neck is over the intersection of the cross lines, with the base line vertical, tube angled 35° toward the feet and centred to the cross lines, page 543.

(1819, 1820)

Axial or base projection, submento-vertical with slit diaphragm, the base line parallel to the film, the tube is centred between the angles of the jaw with the central ray at right angles to the base line (1841) page 543.

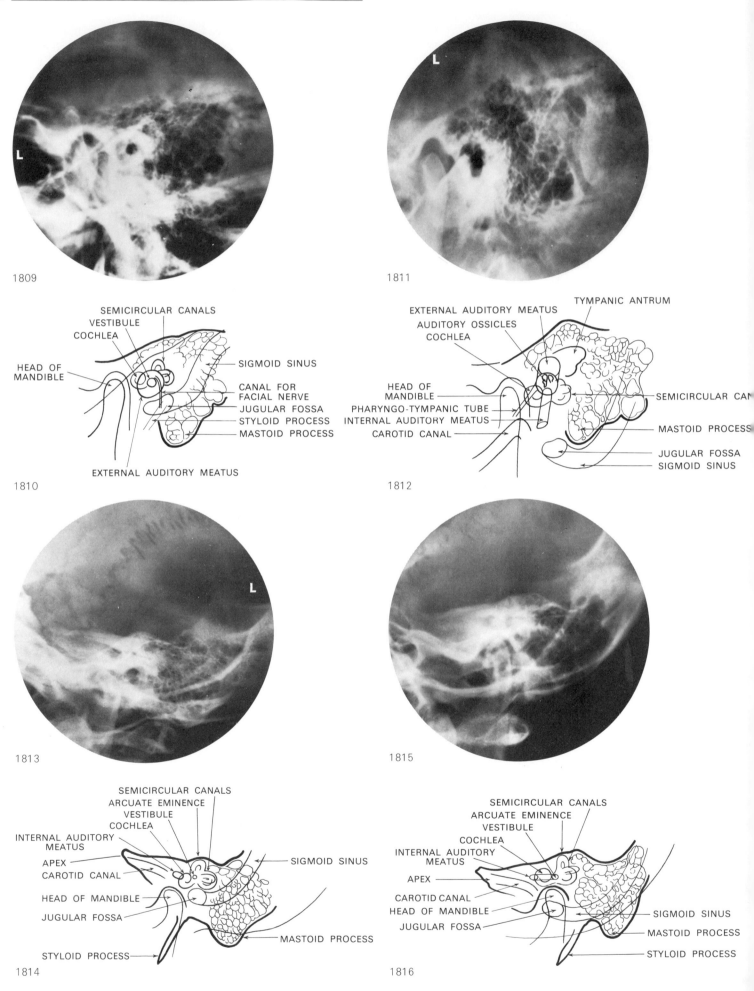

1809

1810

SEMICIRCULAR CANALS
VESTIBULE
COCHLEA

HEAD OF
MANDIBLE

SIGMOID SINUS

CANAL FOR
FACIAL NERVE

JUGULAR FOSSA
STYLOID PROCESS
MASTOID PROCESS

EXTERNAL AUDITORY MEATUS

1811

1812

EXTERNAL AUDITORY MEATUS
AUDITORY OSSICLES
COCHLEA

TYMPANIC ANTRUM

HEAD OF
MANDIBLE
PHARYNGO-TYMPANIC TUBE
INTERNAL AUDITORY MEATUS
CAROTID CANAL

SEMICIRCULAR CAN

MASTOID PROCESS

JUGULAR FOSSA
SIGMOID SINUS

1813

1814

SEMICIRCULAR CANALS
ARCUATE EMINENCE
VESTIBULE
COCHLEA

INTERNAL AUDITORY
MEATUS

APEX
CAROTID CANAL

HEAD OF MANDIBLE

JUGULAR FOSSA

SIGMOID SINUS

MASTOID PROCESS

STYLOID PROCESS

1815

1816

SEMICIRCULAR CANALS
ARCUATE EMINENCE
VESTIBULE
COCHLEA
INTERNAL AUDITORY
MEATUS

APEX

CAROTID CANAL
HEAD OF MANDIBLE
JUGULAR FOSSA

SIGMOID SINUS

MASTOID PROCESS

STYLOID PROCESS

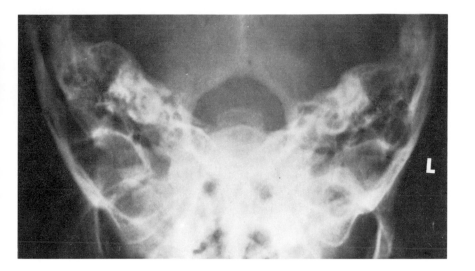

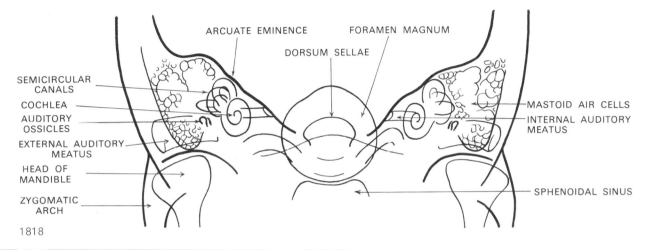

ARCUATE EMINENCE   FORAMEN MAGNUM

DORSUM SELLAE

SEMICIRCULAR
CANALS

COCHLEA

AUDITORY
OSSICLES

EXTERNAL AUDITORY
MEATUS

HEAD OF
MANDIBLE

ZYGOMATIC
ARCH

MASTOID AIR CELLS

INTERNAL AUDITORY
MEATUS

SPHENOIDAL SINUS

1818

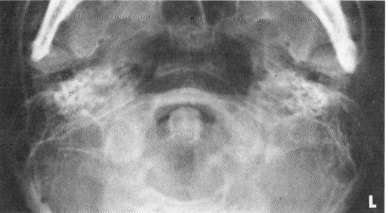

1819

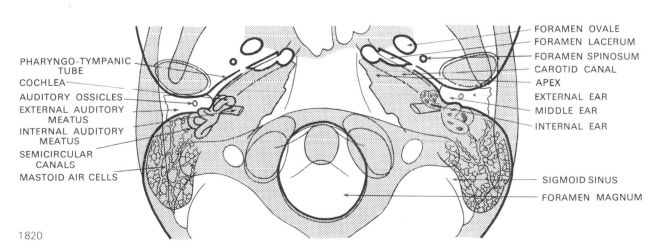

PHARYNGO-TYMPANIC
TUBE

COCHLEA

AUDITORY OSSICLES

EXTERNAL AUDITORY
MEATUS

INTERNAL AUDITORY
MEATUS

SEMICIRCULAR
CANALS

MASTOID AIR CELLS

FORAMEN OVALE

FORAMEN LACERUM

FORAMEN SPINOSUM

CAROTID CANAL

APEX

EXTERNAL EAR

MIDDLE EAR

INTERNAL EAR

SIGMOID SINUS

FORAMEN MAGNUM

1820

kVp	mAs	FFD	Film ILFORD	Screen ILFORD	Grid
70	50	90 cm (36″)	RAPID R	HD	Grid

General purpose couch or stand

Lateral

There are two standard projections for the petrous temporal bone with the head in the true lateral position and the auricle folded forward, but to ensure comparable projections for left and right sides the radiographic base line must be at right angles to the direction of tube angulation. In the first projection the tube is angled 15° toward the feet and centred 2·5 cm (1 ins) above the external auditory meatus (1821, 1822). In the second projection the tube is angled 35° toward the feet, and centred 7·5 cm (3 ins) above the external auditory meatus (1821, 1823). The annotated diagrams (1811, 1812) on page 536 indicate the anatomical features of these radiographs.

A high penetration and close coning is needed to show the labyrinth in these projections and increasing the angulation from 15° to 35° requires an addition of 10 mAs for the latter exposure.

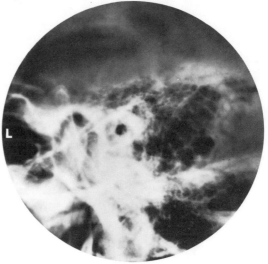

1822

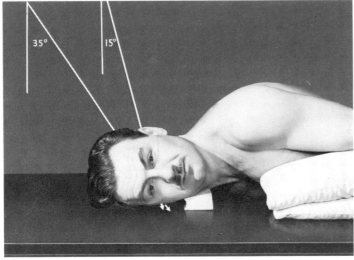

1821

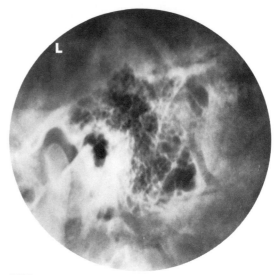

1823

Oblique postero-anterior

With the patient prone and the head in the occipito-frontal position, the central line of the table must be under the middle of the supraorbital margin of the side being examined and the radiographic base line at right angles. Rotate the head 45°, bringing the petrous bone being examined nearer the film so that its superior margin is parallel to the film (1825). The position of the head should be checked with a protractor from the end of the couch (1824).

■ Centre with the tube angled 12° towards the head between the external auditory meatus and the occipital protuberance on the side furthest from the film. A small diaphragm aperture or cone should be used.

This projection is a modified Stenver's view (1826) and is illustrated on a dry skull (1825) which is positioned to show the relationship of the petrous temporal to the film and tube. It clearly demonstrates the importance of correct positioning to bring the superior margin of the petrous parallel to the film for a satisfactory projection.

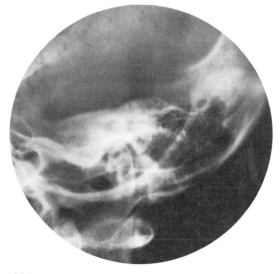

1826

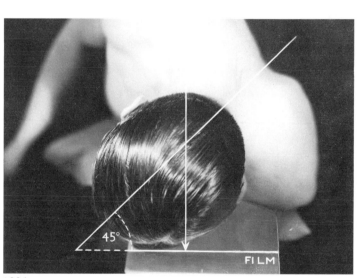

1824

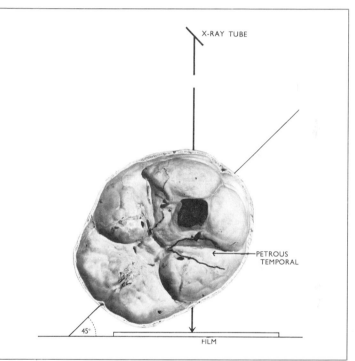

1825

Simultaneous views of petrous for comparison
Fronto-occipital

The patient is supine for the fronto-occipital projection with the base line and median sagittal plane at right angles to the film and centring is in the midline over the vertex to project the petrous directly within the orbits (1827, 1828). Although the orbits are magnified in the fronto-occipital compared with the occipito-frontal view, the radiation dose to the lens of the eye is very much higher in the fronto-occipital view and therefore the occipito-frontal projection is preferred.

Occipito-frontal

For the occipito-frontal view the patient is prone, the base line and median sagittal plane are at right angles to the film and centre in the midline 5 cm (2 ins) below the base line to project the internal auditory meatuses and middle ear through the orbits, page 257 (925, 926, 927, 928).

Modified Stenver's view on the skull table

With the patient prone in the occipito-frontal position, the base line and median sagittal plane are at right angles to the table top with the supraorbital margin of the side being examined over the cross lines. Rotate the head to bring the median sagittal plane 45° to the table top and the superior margin of the petrous temporal nearest the film parallel to the cassette.

■ Centre midway between the external auditory meatus and the occipital protuberance with the tube angled 12° towards the head, using a small diaphragm aperture or cone for greater definition. Both sides are examined in turn for comparison (1829, 1830).

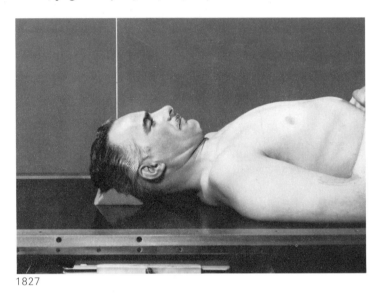

1827

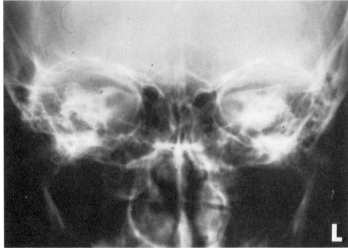

1828

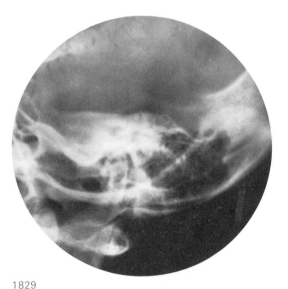

1829

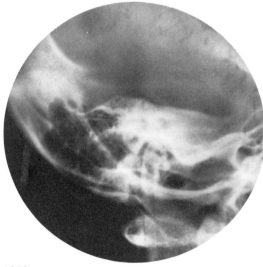

1830

Skull table

Lateral (1)

With the patient prone, the auricle folded forward, the median sagittal plane parallel and the interorbital line at right angles to the table top, the external auditory meatus is positioned just in front of the cross lines as seen in the mirror. The base line must be at right angles to the direction of the tube angulation.

■ Centre with the tube angled 15° toward the feet to the centre of the cross lines, just behind the external auditory meatus on the table top (1831, 1832)

kVp	mAs	FFD	Film ILFORD	Screen ILFORD	Grid
75	150	90 cm (36″)	RAPID	HD	Grid

Lateral (2)

With the patient prone, in the true lateral position with the auricle folded forward as in the previous projection, the external auditory meatus is 1 cm in front of and above the cross lines.

■ Centre with the tube angled 35° toward the feet to the cross lines as seen in the mirror, 1 cm (½ ins) below and behind the external auditory meatus (1833, 1834)

Note—The central ray of the skull unit is automatically centred to the cross lines on the table top.

The annotated diagrams on page 536 indicate the anatomical features of these two basic lateral views as shown on radiographs of the petrous temporal bones (1809, 1810, 1811, 1812)

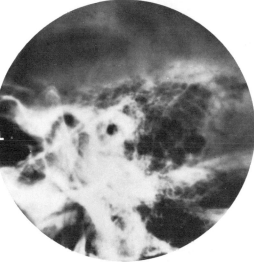

1831

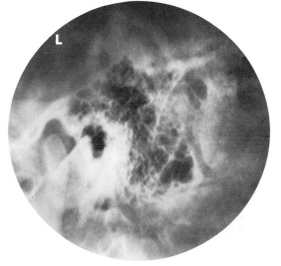

1832

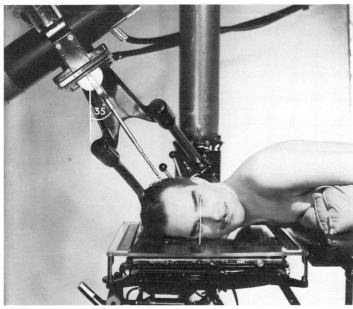

1833

1834

kVp	mAs	FFD	Film ILFORD	Screen ILFORD	Grid
85	100	90 cm (36")	RAPID R	HD	Grid

Oblique-lateral

With the patient prone, in the true lateral position the auricle folded forward, the external auditory meatus is now 2 cm behind and 1 cm below the cross lines as seen in the mirror. The head is flexed to bring the base line 5° to the transverse line.

■ Centre with the tube angled 30° toward the face and 10° toward the head, the central ray passing through the intersection of the cross lines.

The grid is rotated to bring the grid slates parallel to the direction of the angled X-ray beam (1835, 1836, 1837, 1838)

The direction of the beam is at right angles to the long axis of the petrous bone and the radiograph produced is similar to that of the Stenver's projection (1826) which are compared in the radiographs and annotated diagrams (1813, 1814, 1815, 1816) on page 536.

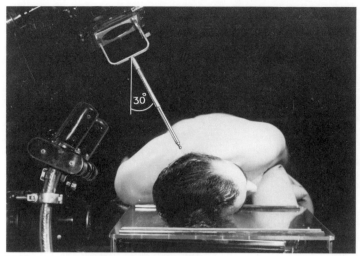

1836

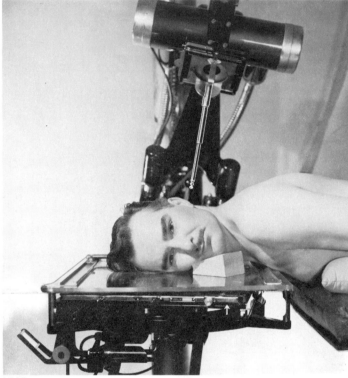

1835

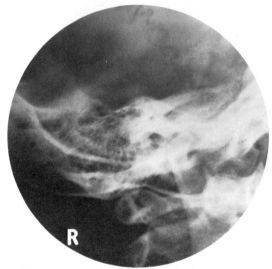

1837

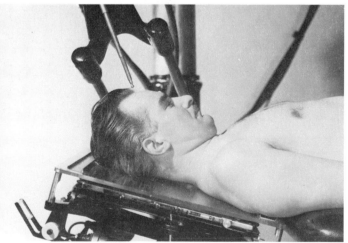

1839

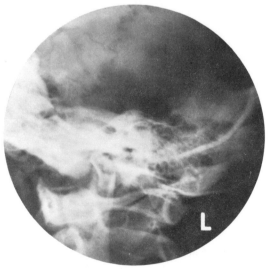

1838

Axial and Half-axial

In the half-axial and axial projections the right and left temporal bones are shown on a single film, both sides examined simultaneously. A narrow rectangular aperture of the diaphragm is used for these exposures.

Radiographs and accompanying annotated diagrams of these projections are shown on page 537 (1817, 1818, 1819, 1820).

35° Fronto-occipital (half axial)

With the patient supine, the skull table is tilted to bring the radiographic base line at right angles to the film. The nape of the neck is centred to the cross lines on the table top as seen in the mirror.

■ Centre in the midline with the tube angle 35° toward the feet (1839, 1840)

kVp	mAs	FFD	Film ILFORD	Screen ILFORD	Grid
80	120	90 cm (36″)	RAPID R	HD	Grid

Submento-vertical (axial)

With the patient supine, the head is extended to bring the vertex of the skull into contact with the skull table which is lowered and angled for the patient's comfort. In the ideal position the base line is parallel to the table top.

■ Centre midway between the external auditory meatus from below the mandible with the tube angled 95° to the base line (1841, 1842a)

kVp	mAs	FFD	Film ILFORD	Screen ILFORD	Grid
85	150	90 cm (36″)	RAPID R	HD	Grid

Axial views of the base of the skull are readily obtained on *computed tomography*. With the patient supine 0·5–1 cm sections are taken in the axial plane and viewing at wider window settings shows bone detail (1842c); fractures (1842d) and bone destruction are clearly demonstrated.

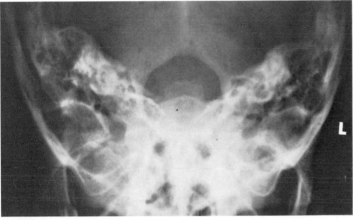

1840

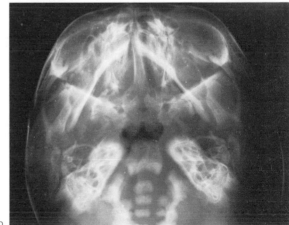

1841

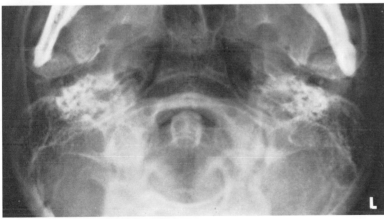

1842a

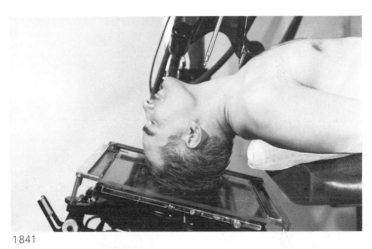

1842b

21 Tomography

While the gross structure of the temporal bone are visible on routine films and even the position of the ossicles can be determined, the intimate details of the middle and inner ears are hidden by the surrounding dense bone and overlapping of the various compartments.

Thin section tomography of 1–2 mm can show each part separately including the cochlea, semicircular canals, ossicles, epitympanic recess and internal auditory meatus. The sections can be done individually or with a multisection technique in which the 1 mm thickness of the card backing of the intensifying screens is used to produce the necessary interval between films. Six to nine exposures may be needed to cover the middle and internal ears and tomography can be performed in the lateral, postero-anterior or Stenver's projections.

Hypocycloidal tube movement on a polytome gives the thinnest sections and is recommended for fine detail. The occipito-frontal position is essential and not the fronto-occipital to minimise radiation to the lens of the eye.

The three pairs of radiographs (1843) of right and left sides were taken at 1 mm apart in the frontal plane.

Technique
Occipito-Frontal

With the patient prone, the forehead resting on a soft pad, the base line and median sagittal plane at right angles to the couch top, the head is immobilised by a head band or clamp.

Spaced diaphragm apertures 15 mm in diameter are used and the tube is centred to the nape of the neck.

The largest possible tomographic "angle" available should be used to produce the thinnest sections and requires either a circular or hypocycloidal tube movement.

The first sections are taken from the table top to the posterior margin of the external auditory meatus and with the trisection multisection cassette the level is lowered 3 mm at a time for each of the two successive exposures.

Lateral

With the patient in the true lateral position, the median sagittal plane parallel to the table top and the base line in the transverse plane, the tube is centred to the external auditory meatus in the centre of the table. The first sections are taken 4–5 cm from the table top, each side being examined in turn.

Tomographic sections of the middle and internal ear can also be done in the Stenver's oblique antero-posterior position.

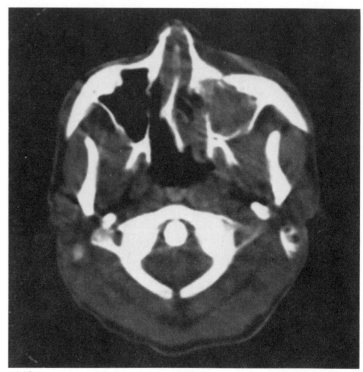

1842c

1842d

CT base of skull.
(1842c)—normal
(1842d)—fracture through walls of antrum

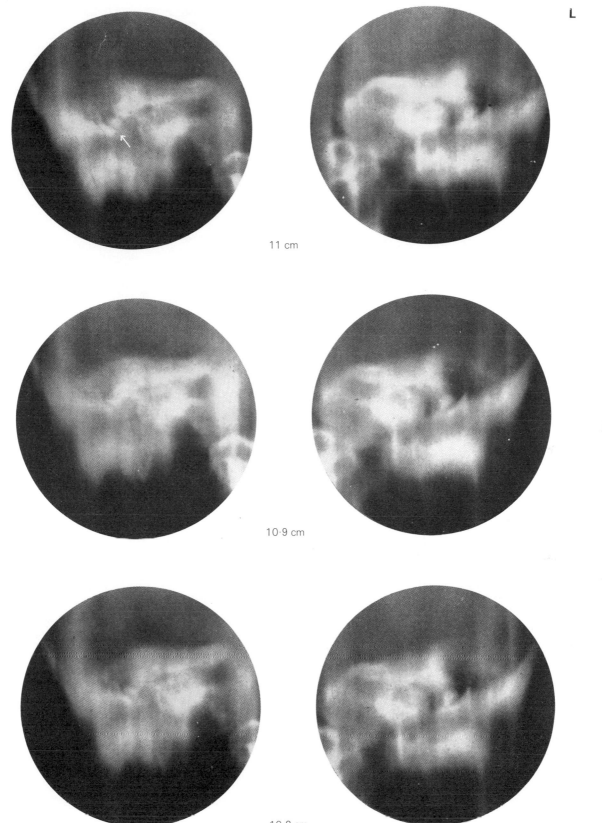

11 cm

10·9 cm

10·8 cm

Macroradiography

Increased detail of the middle and internal ear can be obtained on a skull unit by using an enlargement technique.

With the patient prone and the base line and median sagittal plane at right angles to the table top, the head is immobilised and the tube with a narrow slit diaphragm is centred over the nape of the neck. A 0·1–0·3 mm focal spot is essential to obtain the necessary definition.

The grid is removed from the skull top unit and the cassette is placed in the cassette holder on the far end of the semi-circular arm of the tube support (1844). The air-gap obtained attenuates the scattered radiation improving definition. Standard screens are used and 2× enlargement produced because the petrous temporal is midway between the focus and film.

The skull unit is quite easily adapted for this technique (1844) to produce radiographs of high quality showing the petrous temporal bone with good definition within the orbits (1845).

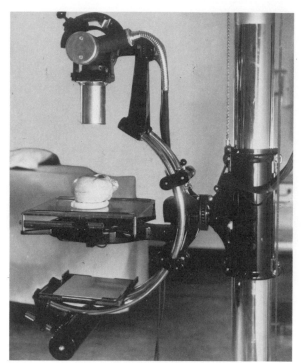

1844

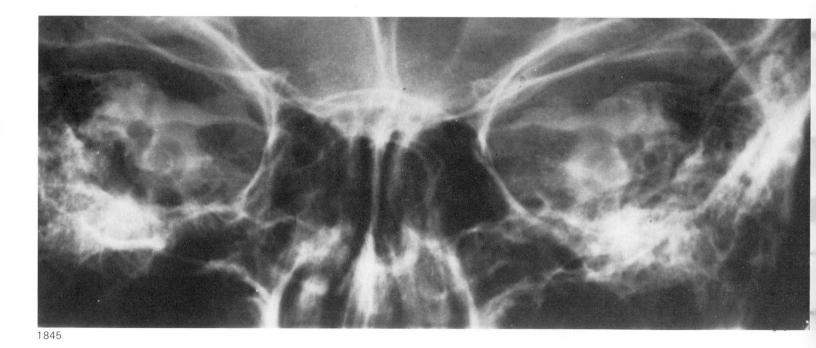

1845

Optic foramen

The optic nerve on each side passes through the optic foramen into the optic canal en route from the eye to the base of the brain.

Radiographs demonstrating an optic canal containing a coil of lead foil on the right side as it runs forward (1846) downward (1847) and outward (1848) to the apex of the orbit from the middle fossa of the cranium show how short the canal is. The position of the right optic canal is thus indicated on the lateral (1846) frontal (1847) and axial (1848) views demonstrating the projections required for the optic foramina.

The views of the orbit to show the optic foramina on a dry skull were taken with different degrees of rotation of the head (1849–1851). With 35° rotation the optic foramen appears circular (1849) but at 25° and at 5° appears oval (1850, 1851) indicating that the projection for the optic foramina should be done at 35°.

Two methods are described, namely for the general couch and the skull table. In the general couch method the head is adjusted in relation to the tube whereas with the skull table the tube is adjusted with the head in the standard symmetrical prone position.

A further series of radiographs of the orbit of a dry skull (1856–1859) show little change in appearance of the optic foramen on centring the tube 2·5 cm (1 ins) forward (1856), backward (1857), upward (1858) and downward (1859) from the recommended centring point, provided the head is positioned correctly.

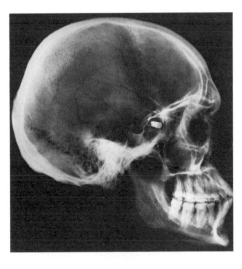

1846

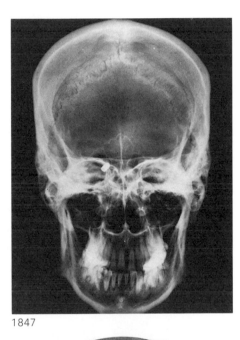

1847

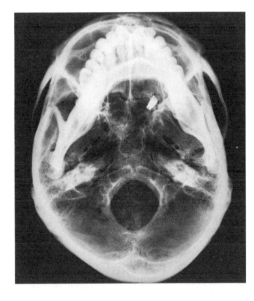

1848

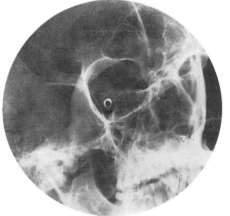

1849

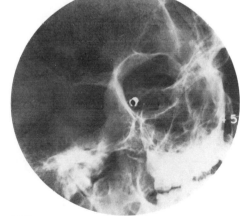

1850

1851

General couch method

With the patient prone and the base line at 35° to the couch (1852), the median sagittal plane is rotated 35° to the vertical (1853) to each side in turn bringing the orbital margin parallel to the film.

■ Centre 7·5 cm above (3 ins) and 6 cm (2½ ins) behind the uppermost external auditory meatus, directly through the orbit being examined (1852, 1853, 1854, 1855)

Optic Foramina

kVp	mAs	FFD	Film ILFORD	Screen ILFORD	Grid
70	100	90 cm (36″)	RAPID R	HD	Grid

Compare radiographs (1855) taken on the general couch with (1862) taken on the skull table using a similar projection.

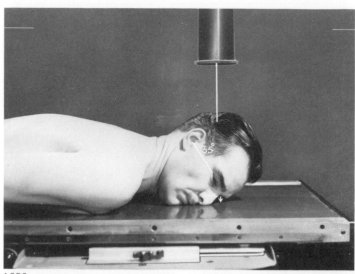

1852

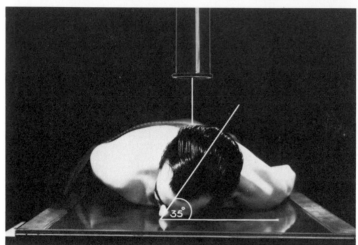

1853

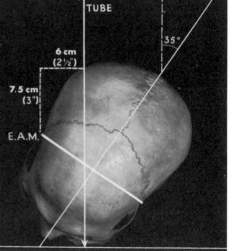

1854

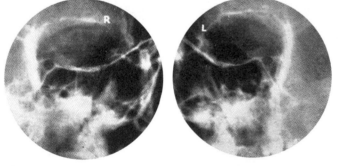

1855

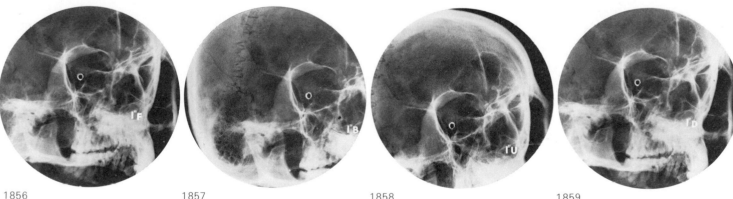

1856   1857   1858   1859

Skull table method

With the patient prone, the median sagittal plane and base line are at right angles to the film and the inner canthus of the orbit being examined is positioned over the cross on the table top as seen in the mirror. Position the cassette 2·5 cm (1 in) toward the side being examined and 2·5 cm (1 in) toward the feet. Rotate the grid to bring the slats parallel to the direction of the X-ray beam and use an eccentric diaphragm to confine the X-ray beam to the side being examined.

■ On the skull table the tube is automatically centred to the centre of the table top. Angle the tube 20° to the feet and 20° to the centred orbit from the opposite side (1861). Both orbits are examined for comparison.

For the examination of the other side the grid, eccentric diaphragm and cassette must all be repositioned accordingly.

Compare radiographs (1863) taken on the skull table with (1862) on the general couch.

In radiographs (1863) of the optic foramina the right side is larger than the left as occurs with an optic nerve glioma.

Tomography

The optic formina can be well defined by tomography if not clearly visible on the standard projections by using a multi-section technique with a backing thickness of 1–2 mm on the intensifying screens. (1864)

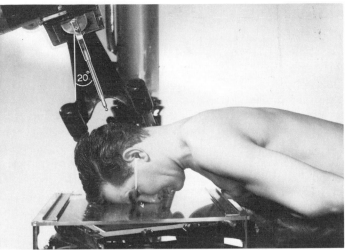
1860

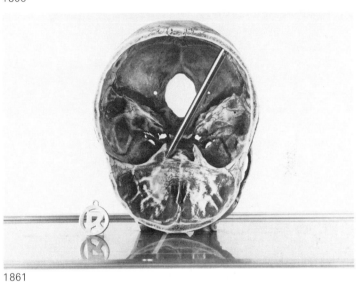
1861

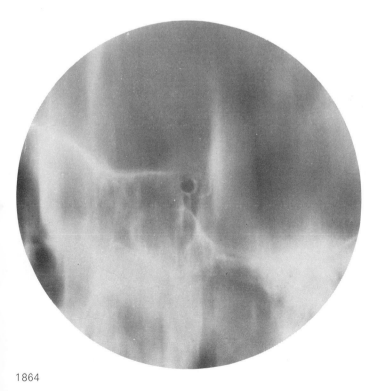
1864

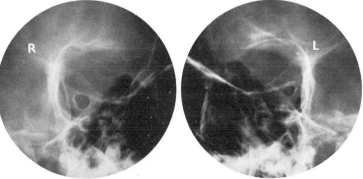
1862

1863

Alternative position for optic foramen

The optic foramina are examined in the postero-anterior position in preference to the antero-posterior position because the object film distance is smaller and radiation to the lens of the eye is considerably less in the postero-anterior position. Very occasionally however, the patient cannot be examined prone and an alternative projection in the supine position is required. Good definition is possible in the antero-posterior projection with the extended ratings of the tubes of 0·3–0·6 mm focal spot size. The orbit and optic foramina are correspondingly enlarged on the radiographs without loss of definition.

Reversed optic foramina technique

The head is antero-posterior and displaced 2·5 cm (1 ins) from the midline towards the side being examined. The chin is raised to bring the base line 35° to the table top and rotate the median sagittal plane 35° away from the orbit being radiographed. The superior and inferior orbital margins are then parallel to the table top.

■ Centre directly over the eye with the central ray perpendicular to the film (1865, a, b)

Both orbits are examined for comparison. By displacing the head 2·5 cm (1 ins) towards the side being examined, the orbit is positioned over the centre of the table top (1865b).

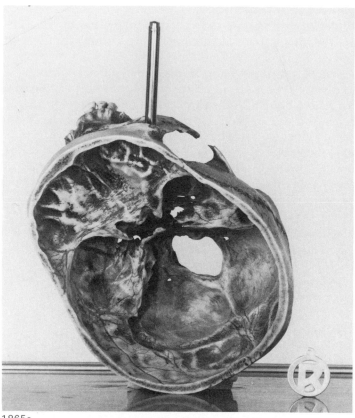

1865a

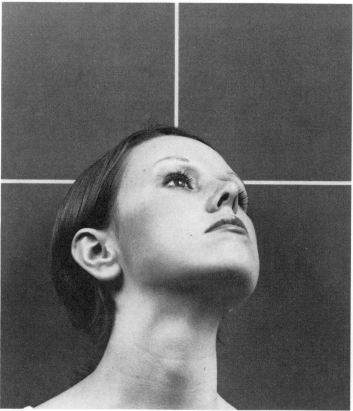

1865b

Temporal bone
Petrous

The petrous temporal may also be examined in the antero-posterior position but the postero-anterior is preferred because of the lower radiation dose to the lens of the eye.

Antero-posterior oblique
With the head in the antero-posterior position and the base line perpendicular to the film rotate the median sagittal plane 45° *away* from the side being examined.
■ Centre 2·5 cm (1 ins) anterior and above the external auditory meatus with the central ray angled 10° toward the feet (1866, 1867)

45° Antero-posterior oblique
With the head in the antero-posterior position and the base line perpendicular to the film, rotate the median sagittal plane 45° toward the side being examined.
■ Centre 5 cm (2 ins) above the outer angle of the eye closest to the tube with the central ray angled 45° toward the feet (1868, 1869)

The photographs of the inner aspect of the base of a dry skull show how the petrous on the side towards which the skull is turned lies vertically (1869) providing a view at right angles to the previous projection (1866).

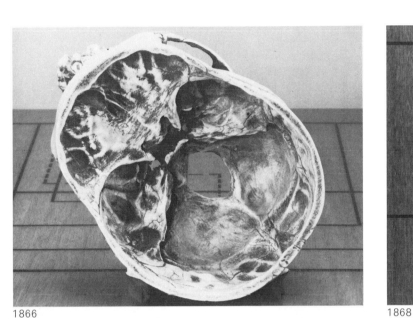

1866

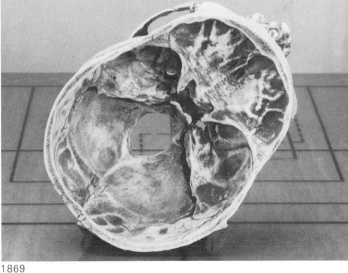

1868

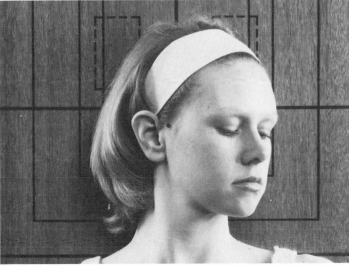

1867

1869

25° Occipito-frontal

With the patient horizontal or sitting in the postero-anterior position, the radiographic base line and median sagittal plane are at right angles to the film.

■ Centre to the nasion with the tube angle 25° toward the head (1870)

This view is useful for demonstrating the palate, styloid processes, orbital floor and intra-orbital fissure.

Ethmoidal bone

Cribriform plate

From the true postero-anterior position with the baseline and median sagittal plane at right angles to the film rotate the head 45° to the side being examined and raise the chin to bring the radiographic base line 35° to the horizontal (1871).

■ Centre to the orbit in contact with the Bucky top with the tube angled 10° toward the feet

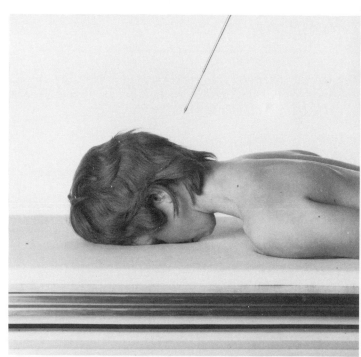

1870

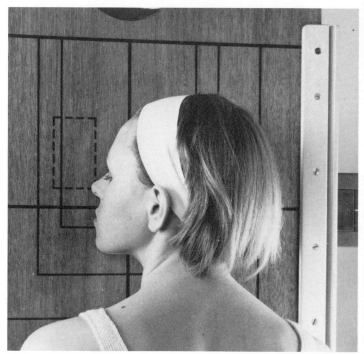

1871

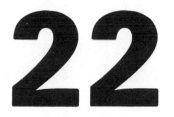

VENTRICULOGRAPHY
AND ENCEPHALOGRAPHY
STEREOTAXIS

22 SECTION 22

VENTRICULOGRAPHY AND ENCEPHALOGRAPHY

The brain and spinal cord forming the central nervous system are enclosed and protected by dense bone which incidentally acts as a radiopaque barrier for the internal soft tissues when using conventional radiography. Neither the ventricular system internally nor the subarachnoid space surrounding the brain and spinal cord, both of which contain cerebrospinal fluid, can be shown on plain films. When air is introduced as a negative contrast agent to demonstrate these spaces, the examinations are called vetriculography or air encephalography (AEG).

The ventricular system with its contained cerebrospinal fluid (CSF) lies deeply within the cerebrum, midbrain and hindbrain forming an interconnecting series of lakes and channels (1872, a, b) allowing the free flow of cerebrospinal fluid from the choroid plexuses, where it is produced, to the subarachnoid space. The two lateral ventricles lie within the cerebrum and each side opens via a foramen of Monro into the third ventricle lying between the thalami. The third ventricle is connected to the fourth ventricle by the Sylvian aqueduct running down the centre of the midbrain. The cerebellum lies behind and the pons and medulla oblongata lie in front of the fourth ventricle which communicates with the subarachnoid space surrounding the brain and spinal cord by the central foramen of Megendie and the two lateral Foramina of Luschka.

The large lateral ventricles are divided into anterior horns and body lying above and lateral to the third ventrible, the posterior horn projecting into the occipital lobe and the temporal horns below the level of the third ventricle. The third and fourth ventricles and the connecting aqueduct are midline structures, with the fourth ventricle lying anteriorly in the posterior fossa. Diagrams of the ventricular system as seen from the superior and lateral aspects are shown in (1872, a, b).

In ventriculography and air-encephalography the cerebrospinal fluid is partly replaced by air which varies in position as the head is moved. To obtain a complete examination of the ventricles the position of the head is changed to outline each part of the ventricular system with air, in turn.

For ventriculography air is introduced directly into the ventricular system after making a burr hole in the cranium but more commonly air is injected after a lumbar puncture and the examination is called air encephalography. The ventricular system can also be examined after injecting 2–3 ml metrizamide (amipaque) or iodophenyl undecylate (Myodil) into a lateral ventricle via a burr hole. The patient is positioned during fluoroscopy to run the contrast medium into the posterior part of the third ventricle and thence to the aqueduct and fourth ventricle or to the site of obstruction.

For air encephalography the patient is seated while air is injected into the lumbar theca to allow the air to rise into the ventricular system and films are taken in lateral and frontal planes to demonstrate the fourth and third ventricles and the aqueduct between. Subsequently the patient is positioned appropriately to show the various parts of the lateral ventricles.

Air encephalography is usually followed by severe headache and the examination of the ventricular system has now been almost completely replaced by computed tomography of the brain (1873), air encephalography being used occasionally for the basal cisterns. The third and fourth ventricles and aqueduct are usually examined by positive contrast ventriculography. Where computed tomography is not available, ventriculography and air encephalography are still essential investigations. Computed axial tomography (CAT) brain sections, 1 cm thick are shown in (1873, 1874).

(1873 a–f) demonstrate the normal anatomy of the ventricular system and sulci on CT.

A coronal section at two different window settings (1873 g–h) show anterior horns of the lateral ventricles in (1873g) and the bone of the face and cranium in (1873h)

In (1874 a–b) a cerebral tumour with adjacent cerebral oedema is demonstrated.

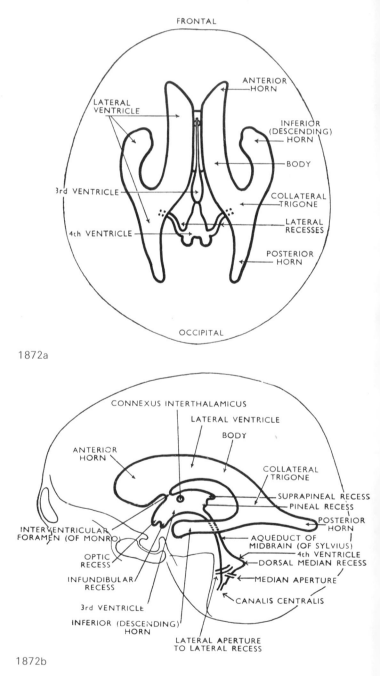

1872a

1872b

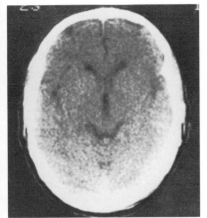

1873a

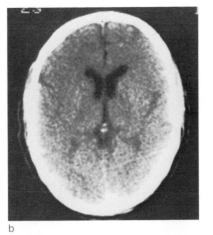

b

c

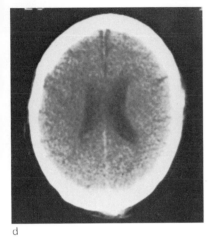

d

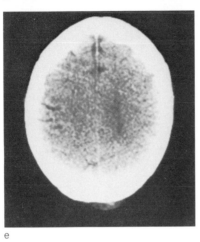

e

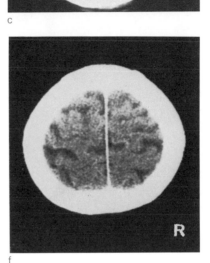

f

R

g

L

h

L

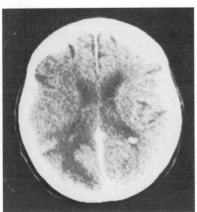

1874a

b

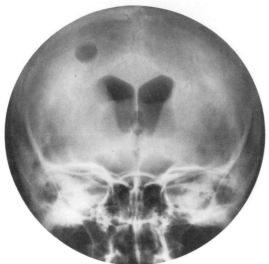

1875
SUPINE

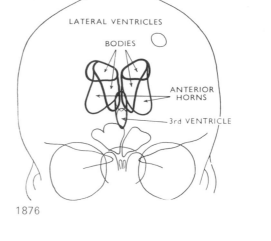

1876

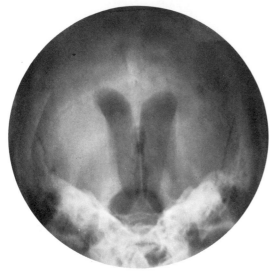

1877
SUPINE

1878

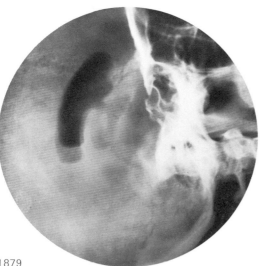

1879
SUPINE

1880

No.	Patient	Position	Tube	Ventricles shown
1875	Supine **(1903)**	Fronto-Occipital	Straight	Lateral-Anterior Horns, and Bodies. Third.
1877	Supine **(1906)**	Fronto-Occipital Half-Axial	Angled 25° to 30° (OMBL)	Lateral-Anterior Horns, and Bodies. Third.
1879	Supine **(1909)**	Lateral	Horizontal	Lateral-Anterior Horns. Interventricular Foramen. Third.
1881	Lateral Left and Right **(1923) (1924)**	Lateral	Straight	Lateral-Interventricular Foramen. Third. Aqueduct of the Midbrain. Fourth.
1883	Prone **(1913)**	Occipito-Frontal	Straight	Lateral-Inferior and Posterior Horns, and Bodies. Third.
1885	Prone **(1916)**	Occipito-Frontal Half-Axial	Angled 25° to 30° (OMBL)	Lateral-Inferior and Posterior Horns, and Bodies. Third.
1887	Prone **(1919)**	Lateral	Horizontal	Lateral-Inferior and Posterior Horns, and Bodies.
1889	Erect **(1934)**	Fronto-Occipital	Horizontal	Lateral-Upper Anterior Horns and Bodies.
1891	Erect **(1937)**	Lateral	Horizontal	Lateral-Upper Anterior Horns and Bodies.
1893	Supine Head Lowered **(1929, 1930)**	Lateral	Horizontal	Lateral-Anterior Horns. Interventricular Foramen. Third. Aqueduct of the Midbrain. Fourth.

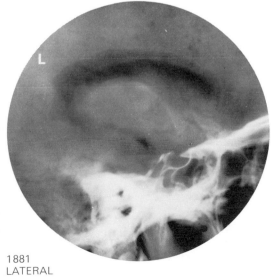

1881
LATERAL

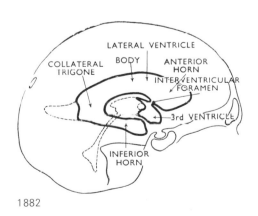

1882

22

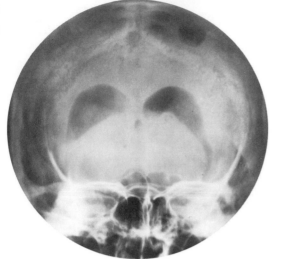

1883
PRONE

BURR HOLE

POSTERIOR HORNS

BODIES

INFERIOR HORNS

3rd VENTRICLE

1884

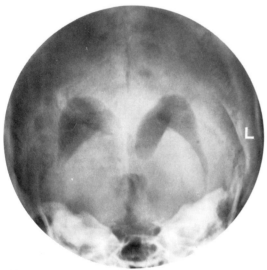

1885
PRONE

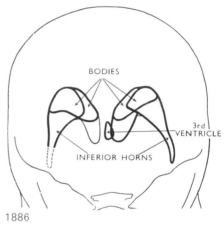

BODIES

3rd VENTRICLE

INFERIOR HORNS

1886

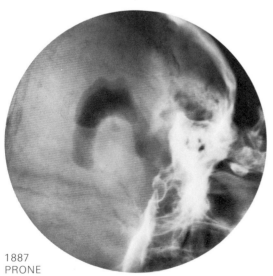

558

1887
PRONE

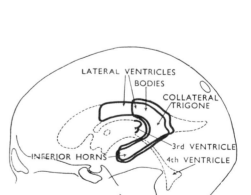

LATERAL VENTRICLES

BODIES

COLLATERAL TRIGONE

3rd VENTRICLE

4th VENTRICLE

INFERIOR HORNS

1888

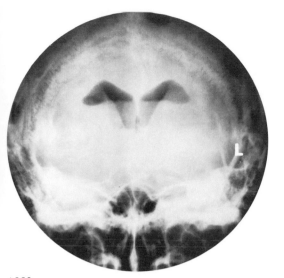

1889
VERTICAL

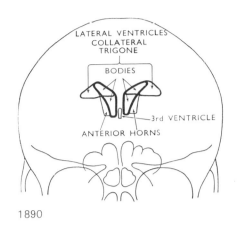

1890

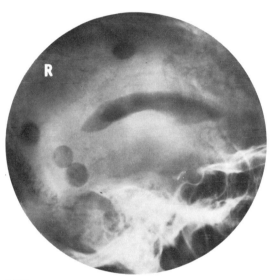

1891
VERTICAL

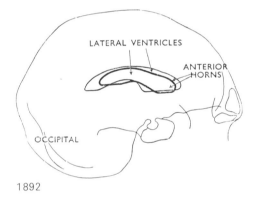

1892

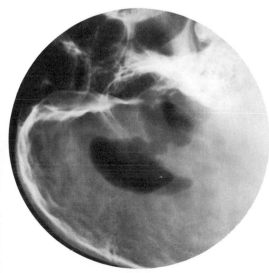

1893
SUPINE HEAD LOWERED

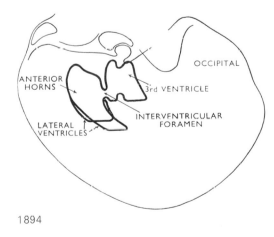

1894

22 Apparatus

The equipment used for radiography of the ventricles varies from the general couch, vertical stand and mobile tube support, to the ultramodern Mima unit specially designed for ventriculography and air encephalography with the patient strapped into the chair allowing rotation in any direction including the backward somersault. The advent of computed tomography has however led to a precipitous reduction in the number of air encelphalograms.

The skull table as illustrated in this section is suitable for examining the ventricles because the position of the tube and film can be varied without undue movement of the patient. The following features are particularly important.

A small Bucky table with a transparent top is attached to a special tube mounting to allow the central ray to be accurately adjusted to the subject and film. The unit is mounted on a substantial vertical column and there is a quite separate trolley-couch on which the patient lies.

The tube is automatically centred to the moving grid and film at all angles of the tube but the tube can be decentralised for special views. A centre finder (1900) or light marker indicates the direction of the central ray. The centre finder is hinged at its attachment and is displaced to the side before making the exposure.

The tube can be moved from the central position through 90° in three directions allowing necessary projections to be made without moving the patient's head and there is a special fitting to hold a stationary grid and cassette at right angles to the table top. When the tube and Bucky table are interlocked they can be moved together through 90° when the patient is either erect or horizontal.

The unit can also be moved vertically for the dropped head position to show the anterior parts of the lateral and third ventricles (1929, 1930, 1931) and the grid can be rotated to adjust the grid slats to the direction of the X-ray beam for unusual tube angulations.

For complicated positioning of the head in relation to the film there are reflecting mirrors under the transparent table top which can be seen when the hinged grid is either removed or allowed to hang vertically beside the table (1899).

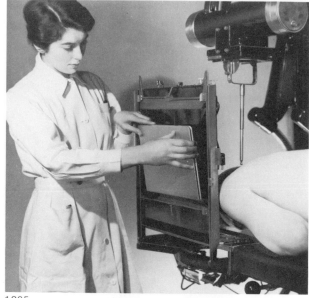

1895

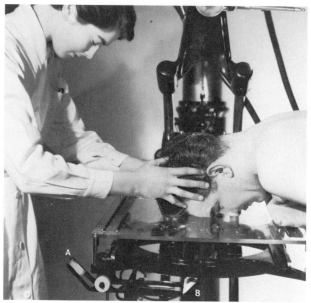

1896

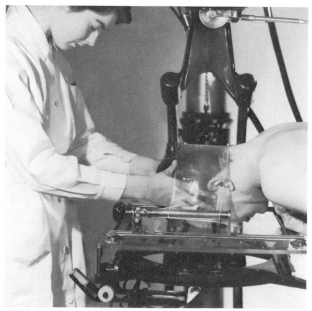

1897

The head is immobilised by a linen band attached to spring rollers and can be tightened from both sides simultaneously (1899). In the earlier illustrations a transparent plastic band is shown but later the band has been omitted so as not to obscure the position of the head.

There is a slot near the tube aperture for holding a flat primary diaphragm (1898) and a set of eight diaphragms are provided for circular and rectangular fields for the various skull projections.

The series of photographs (1895–1900) illustrate some of the features of the skull table.

(1895) shows how a cassette can be placed in position beneath the grid, after being withdrawn and hinged upwards.

(1896) The grid assembly has been removed to show details of the positioning system. Two small electric bulbs illuminate the head through the transparent table top and there are two mirrors (A & B) by which the radiographer can see the patient's position relative to the cross lines on the table top allowing the head to be easily and accurately adjusted.

(1897) Two metal runners are now in position and are used to hold the immobilizing head band. The head is adjusted with the head band over the head.

(1898) The radiographer steadies the head with one hand while tightening the band on one side.

(1899) The immobilizing band is commonly tightened from both spring rollers simultaneously while checking the position of the head in the mirror. The moving grid assembly is hinged downward after inserting the cassette as shown in (1895).

(1900) The grid is in position under the transparent table top and the immobilizing band finally tightened over the head.

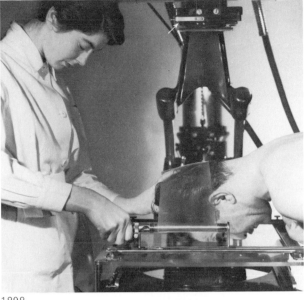

1898

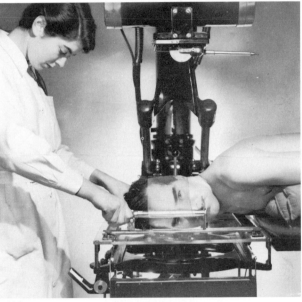

1899

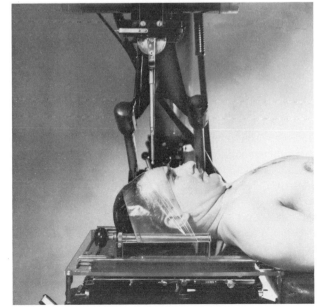

1900

Positioning

For ventriculography films are first done with the patient supine and viewed before turning the patient prone as the air leaves the ventricular system via the fourth ventricle in the prone position. In each position of the head several views are required to adequately demonstrate the ventricular system. The usual sequence is:

PATIENT SUPINE: 1. Fronto-occipital—tube straight (vertical ray)

2. Fronto-occipital—30° tube tilt to feet

3. Lateral—tube horizontal

PATIENT PRONE: 4. Occipito-frontal—tube straight (vertical ray)

5. Occipito-frontal—30° tube tilt to head

6. Lateral—tube straight (horizontal ray)

HEAD LATERAL: 7. Left and
(table top
horizontal)   8. Right—tube straight (vertical ray)

PATIENT SUPINE: 9. Lateral—tube straight (horizontal
Head lowered   ray)

PATIENT ERECT 10. Occipito-frontal—tube straight (horizontal ray)

11. Lateral—tube straight (horizontal ray)

A gentle rocking movement will help the air to fill the appropriate ventricle but jerkiness must be avoided as it intensifies the headache, provoking nausea and vomiting. A brief interval after moving the patient to a new position allows the air to move in the ventricles.

The ventricles vary considerably in size often being larger in the elderly, so that the air required for a particular examination varies with the subject. Less than 10 ml of air is unsatisfactory and the average is 20–30 ml.

A photograph, radiograph and a diagram are used to illustrate each projection and on pages 556–559 there are radiographs and accompanying diagram of a common series of projections for ventriculography. Autotomography is used to show the third and fourth ventricles (page 575).

Planes, lines and landmarks

To use the skull table properly, positioning the patient to the cross lines on the transparent table top must be meticulous and the planes, lines and landmarks recommended by the Commission of Neuroradiology in Milan in 1961* must be followed. Two illustrations from the report (1901, 1902) show the lines for the frontal and lateral aspects and regions.

In this section the orbito-meatal line is used for positioning and centring and the degrees of tube angulation must be adjusted accordingly if the anthropomorphic base line is used.

*Projections and Nomenclature in Neuroradiology (Report of World Federation), Milan, 1961.

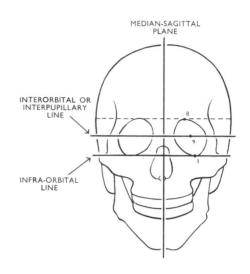

1901

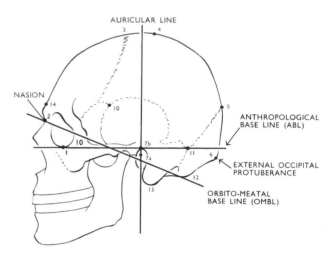

1902

1. Infra-orbital point
2. Nasion
3. Bregma
4. Vertex
5. Lambda
6. Inion
7. (a) Centre of external auditory meatus and axis of external auditory canal
   (b) Superior border of external auditory meatus
8. Superior border of orbit
9. Centre of orbit
10. Pterion
11. Asterion
12. Lowest point of the occiput
13. Mastoid tip
14. Glabella

(1) Supine—fronto-occipital

With the patient supine the median plane and base line must be at right angles and the centring point, 3·5 cm (1½ ins) above the nasion, must coincide with the centre of the table top.

■ Centre 3·5 cm (1½ ins) above the nasion (1903, 1904, 1905)

A primary diaphragm with a suitable aperture is selected in advance and the moving grid is set for the appropriate exposure. The immobilizing band is tightened and the pointer moved to one side before making the exposure.

Note—The air rises to fill the anterior horns and bodies of the lateral ventricles and anterior part of the third ventricle with the head in this position (1903, 1904, 1905).

Supine fronto-occipital

kVp	mAs	FFD	Film ILFORD	Screen ILFORD	Grid
75	25	90 cm (36")	RAPID R	FT	Grid

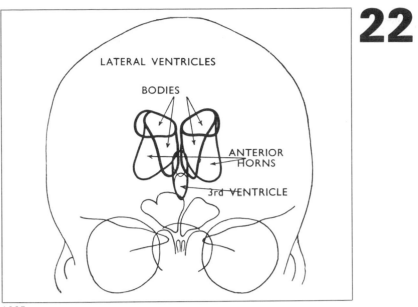

1905

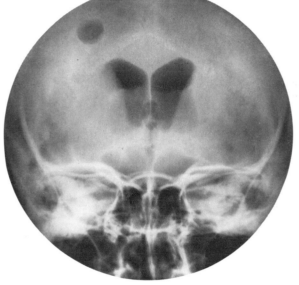

1904

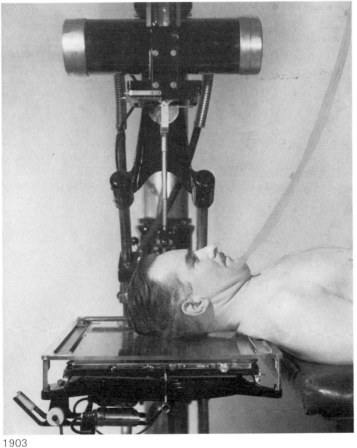

1903

(2) Supine—fronto-occipital with tube angled 30° (half axial)

With the patient supine as for the previous previous projection angle the tube 30° towards the feet. Because the tube is automatically centred to the centre of the skull table top, the patient must be moved to bring the centring point 5 cm (2 ins) above the nasion. The film is displaced 5 cm (2 ins) toward the feet to offset the effects of the tube angulation.

■ Centre 5 cm (2 ins) above the nasion with the tube angled 30° toward the feet and move the centring pointer to one side before making the exposure (1906, 1907, 1908)

Varying the tube angulation produces a different view of the air filled anterior horns and bodies of the lateral ventricle and of the anterior part of the third ventricle.

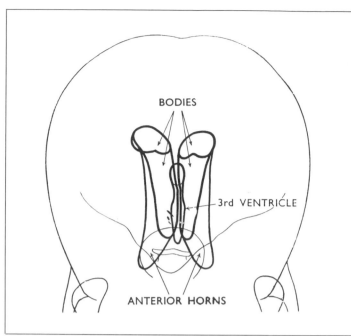

1908

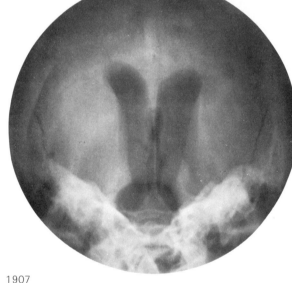

1907

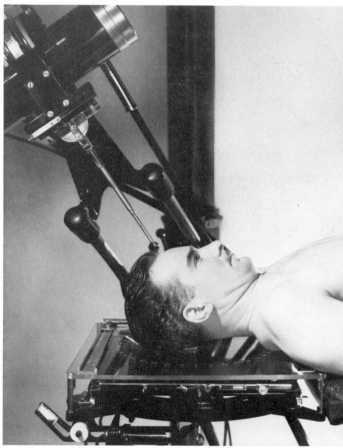

1906

Supine—fronto-occipital 30° tube tilt

kVp	mAs	FFD	Film ILFORD	Screen ILFORD	Grid
80	25	90 cm (36″)	RAPID R	FT	Grid

(3) Supine—lateral

The head is rocked gently backwards and forwards to move the air into the third ventricle and with the head in the same position as for the two previous projections the tube is moved through 90° to the horizontal position (1909). The vertical cassette support, is slid into position on the rails which normally holds the immobilizing band, but now holds the cassette and stationary grid vertically against the lateral side of the head. The head and tube are adjusted to bring the centring point 6 cm (2½ ins) above and 2·5 cm (1 ins) in front of the external auditory meatus.

■ Centre 6 cm (2½ ins) above and 2·5 cm (1 ins) in front of the external auditory meatus and move the centring pointer to one side before the exposure is made (1909, 1910, 1911, 1912)

The exposure factors are on page 568. The anterior part of the body and anterior horns of the lateral ventricles and most of the third ventricle are shown in this projection (1910) in the position in which the film was exposed, as shown by the air-fluid levels. However (1911) and the accompanying diagram (1912) have been turned for viewing in the conventional position.

The lateral projection produces the key view in case of doubt as to the degree of filling of the ventricular system and completes the supine series. The films must be seen by the radiologist before moving the patient into the prone position for the occipito-frontal views.

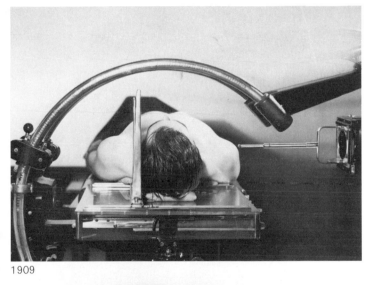

1909

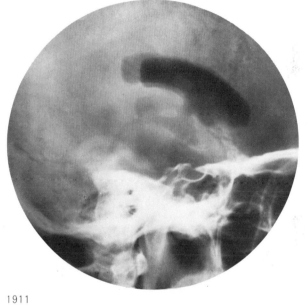

1911

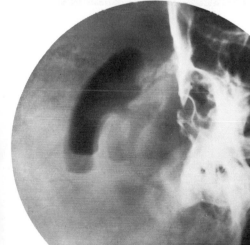

1910

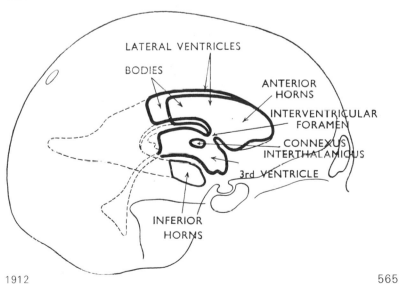

LATERAL VENTRICLES

BODIES

ANTERIOR HORNS

INTERVENTRICULAR FORAMEN

CONNEXUS INTERTHALAMICUS

3rd VENTRICLE

INFERIOR HORNS

1912

(4) Prone—occipito-frontal

The grid assembly is withdrawn from the table top and is hinged downward, after removing the cassette. The mirror viewing system can then be used. The patient is slowly turned into the prone position with the base line and the median sagittal plane adjusted to right angles to the table top and the nasion 3·5 cm (1½ ins) below the cross lines as seen in the viewing mirror. The immobilising head band is tightened, the hinged centre pointer is moved out of the way and the grid assembly replaced into the table top.

■ Centre 3·5 cm (1½ ins) above the nasion, the tube is automatically centred to the crossed lines on the table top (1913, 1914, 1915)

Note—The air rises to fill the posterior parts of the bodies and the posterior horns of the lateral ventricles (1914, 1915).

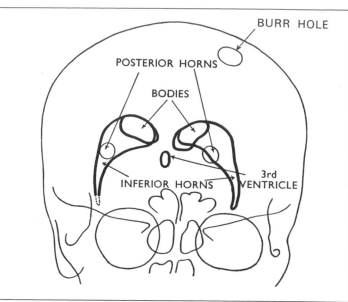

1915

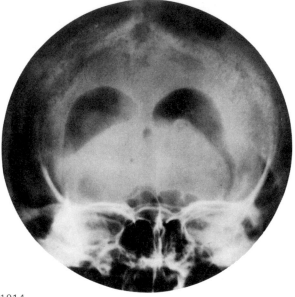

1914

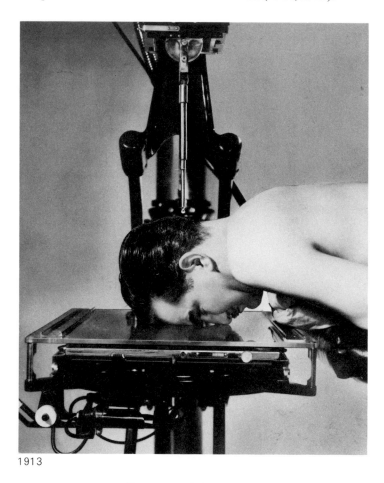

1913

Prone—occipito-frontal

kVp	mAs	FFD	Film ILFORD	Screens ILFORD	Grid
75	25	90 cm (36″)	RAPID R	FT	Grid

(5) Prone—occipito-frontal with 30°

With the head in the same position as in the previous projection (1913) the tube is angled 30° towards the head. The head is adjusted to bring the centring point 6 cm (2¾ ins) above the nasion onto the cross lines on the table top. The cassette is moved 6 cm (2½ ins) upwards to offset the tube angulation.

■ Centre to 6 cm (2½ ins) above the nasion in the midline and to the cross lines on the table top as seen in the viewing mirror, with the tube angled 30° towards the head (1916).

After immobilising the head, set the grid, hinge back centring point and replace the grid assembly into the table top before making the exposure.

Note—The tube angulation shows the posterior parts of the bodies and the posterior horns in a different view (1917, 1918).

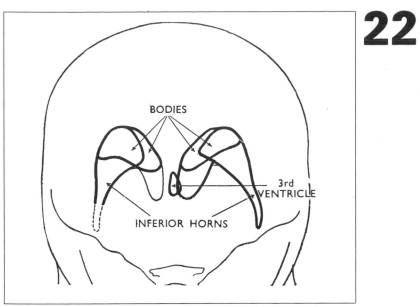

1918

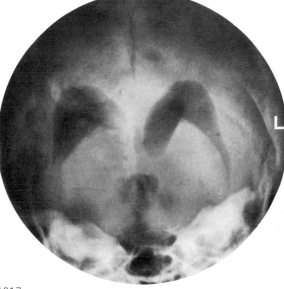

1917

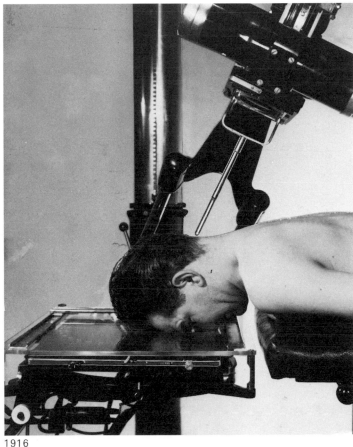

1916

Prone—occipito-frontal with 30° tube tilt

kVp	mAs	FFD	Film ILFORD	Screens ILFORD	Grid
80	25	90 cm (36″)	RAPID	FT	Grid

(6) Prone—lateral

With the patient in the same position as in the previous two projections (1913, 1916) the tube is rotated through 90° into the horizontal position. Slide the cassette and grid into the vertical cassette support and then against the lateral side of the head. The head and tube are adjusted to bring the centring point 6 cm (2½ ins) above 3·5 cm (1½ ins) behind the external auditory meatus.

■ Centre with a horizontal beam to a point 6 cm (2½ ins) above and 3·5 cm (1½ ins) behind the external auditory meatus (1919, 1920, 1921, 1922)

Note—This projection usually shows the posterior part of the body and posterior horns although in (1921) the posterior horns are truncated. However, the inferior or temporal horn and a small posterior part of the third ventricle are seen. In (1920) the film is shown in the position in which it was exposed but (1921) and the accompanying diagram (1922) are in the conventional position for viewing.

This projection completes the usual prone series and must be shown to the radiologist before moving the patient.

The prone-lateral film (1921) should be compared with the supine-lateral (1911) on page 565.

Prone—lateral

kVp	mAs	FFD	Film ILFORD	Screens ILFORD	Grid
80	25	90 cm (36″)	RAPID R	FT	Grid

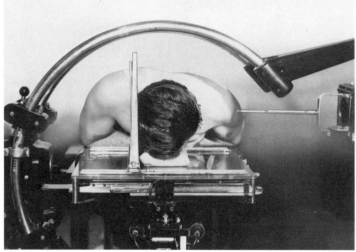

1919

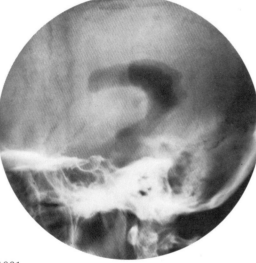

1921

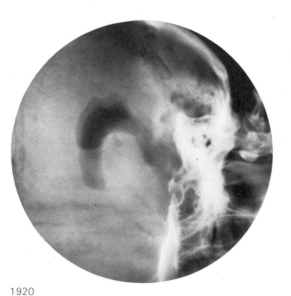

1920

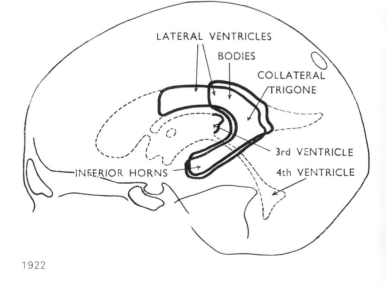

LATERAL VENTRICLES

BODIES

COLLATERAL TRIGONE

3rd VENTRICLE

4th VENTRICLE

INFERIOR HORNS

1922

(7) Lateral—right and left

From the previous position the head is turned to the true lateral position, right and left in turn with the interorbital line at right angles and the median sagittal plane parallel to the table top (1923, 1924). There should be a short interval between positioning and exposure to allow the air to enter the uppermost ventricle. The head is adjusted under the immobilis-ing band to bring the centring point to the cross lines on the table top using the viewing mirror.

■ Centre 5 cm (2 ins) above and 2·5 cm (1 ins) in front of the external auditory meatus (1923, 1924, 1925)

Note—With the head in the lateral position (1924) the air fills the lateral ventricle away from the film and may also show the third and possibly the fourth ventricles (1925, 1926, 1927, 1928).

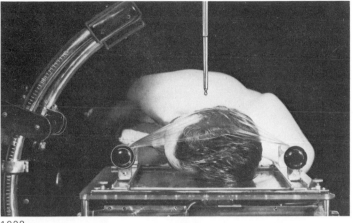

1923

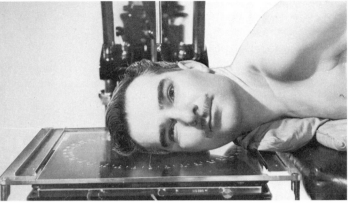

1924

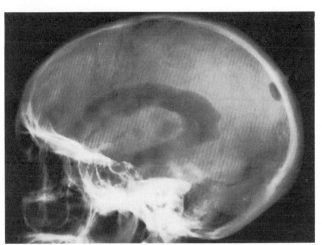

1925

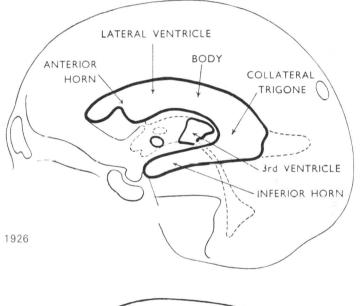

1926

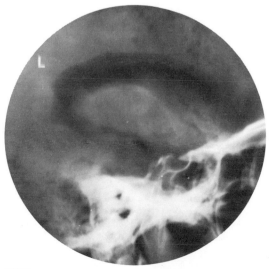

1927

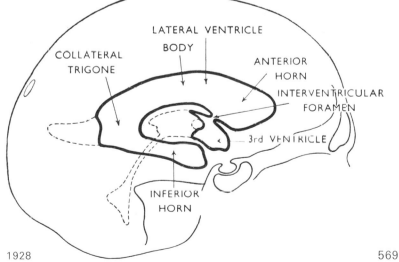

1928

(8) Supine—lateral—head lowered

With the patient supine, the skull table below the level of the couch and the neck in extension, the vertex of the head rests on a wool pad on the table top with the base line 5°–10° to the horizontal.

The head should be moved slowly and gently without excessive extension at the neck as the air tends to pass into the fourth ventricle and out of the ventricular system in this position and will then end the examination.

The cassette and stationary grid in the vertical support are placed against the lateral aspect of the head and the tube is swung through 90° into the horizontal position.

■ Centre 5 cm (2 ins) above and 2·5 cm (1 in) in front of the external auditory meatus (1929, 1930, 1931, 1932)

The exposure factors are the same as on p. 568.

Note—The air passes into the third ventricle and may enter the fourth ventricle in this position which however shows the anterior horns of the lateral ventricles, the interventricular

foramina of Monro, the anterior half of the third ventricle and with further extension of the head may show the aqueduct of Sylvius and the fourth ventricle.

Radiograph (1933) is shown in the position the film was exposed and (1931) and the accompanying diagram (1932) in the conventional viewing position.

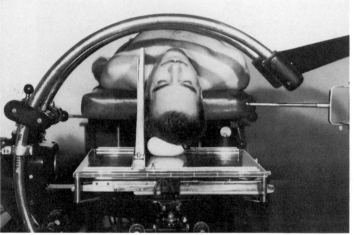

1929

1930

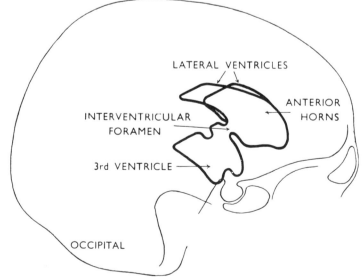

1932

1931   SUPINE HEAD LOWERED

(9) Erect—fronto-occipital

The patient is seated using the supporting back rest of the couch and the interlocked grid. The table and tube are turned through 90° to bring the centre pointer horizontal. The patient faces the tube with the chin well down and the base line and median sagittal plane at right angles to the table top. The centre pointer must be directed 3·5 cm (1½ ins) above the nasion (1934).

■ Centre 3·5 cm (1½ ins) above the nasion using a horizontal central ray.

Erect—fronto-lateral

kVp	mAs	FFD	Film ILFORD	Screens ILFORD	Grid
75	25	90 cm (36")	RAPID R	FT	Grid

Note—In the erect position the air rises to the top of the ventricles showing the anterior horns and bodies of the lateral ventricles and the lateral trigones (1935, 1936).

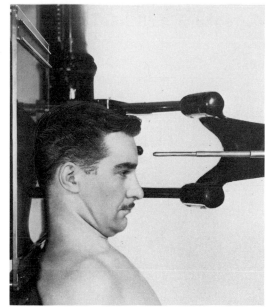

1934

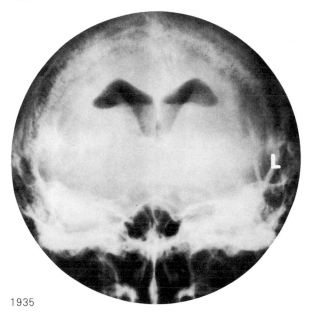

1935

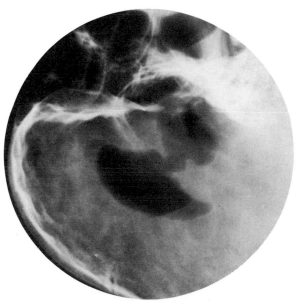

1933

LATERAL VENTRICLES
COLLATERAL TRIGONE
BODIES
3rd VENTRICLE
ANTERIOR HORNS

1936

571

(10) Erect—lateral

Without changing the position of the patient from the previous projection, the tube is swung through 90° on its semicircular arms with the centre pointer horizontal. The cassette and stationary grid in their special fitting must be against the side of the head and adjusted to bring the centre pointer 5 cm (2 ins) above and 2·5 cm (1 ins) in front of the external auditory meatus.

■ Centre 5 cm (2 ins) above and 2·5 cm (1 in) in front of the external auditory meatus (1937, 1938, 1939)

Note—The uppermost parts of the bodies and anterior horns of the lateral ventricles are shown in this projection.

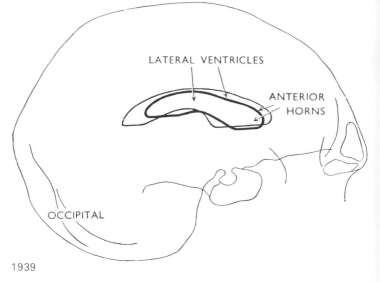

1939

			Erect lateral		
kVp	mAs	FFD	Film ILFORD	Screens ILFORD	
70	15	90 cm (36″)	RAPID R	FT	Grid

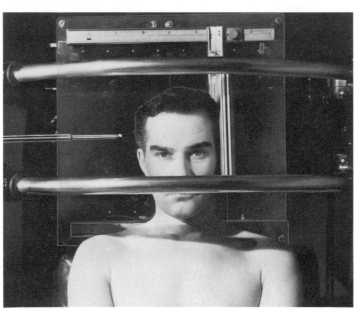

1937

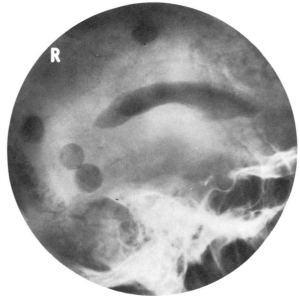

1938

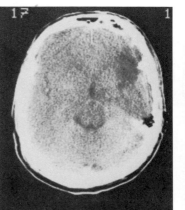

1940

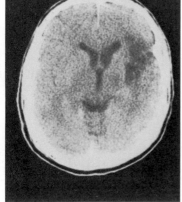

1941

Encephalography

In air encephalography the patient is in a sitting position for the lumbar puncture, facing the vertical table top. The occipito-frontal and lateral views taken in this position (1942, 1943) are preferred and can replace the two projections with the patient antero-posterior (1934) and lateral (1937). For the posterior fossa, however, with air in the fourth ventricle taken during the injection, the chin is lowered bringing the base line to 80° to the horizontal.

Two films (1948, 1949) from a series of radiographs of a child taken during general anaesthesia show views of an air encephalogram and are similar to those shown previously taken during ventriculography (1948, 1949), on p. 551.

However, children, particularly are now examined with CT (1944–1947) which shows the ventricular system quite clearly but in axial section.

In (1940, 1941) a right fronto-parietal infarct is shown as an area of low attenuation adjacent to a slightly dilated lateral ventricle.

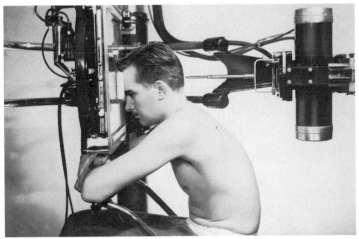

1942

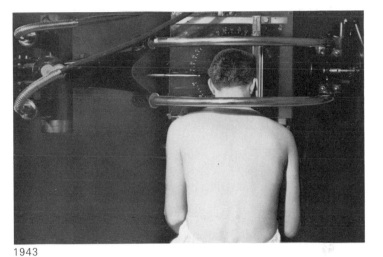

1943

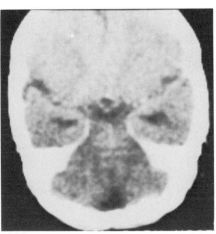

1944

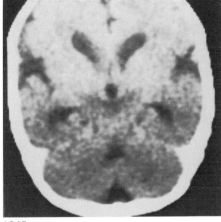

1945

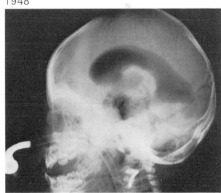

1948

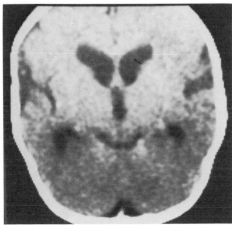

1946

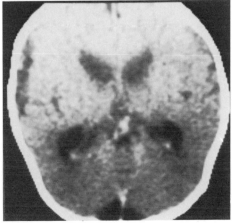

1947

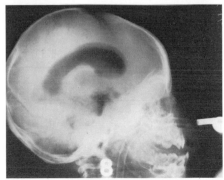

1949

Ventriculography—positive contrast

The third ventricle, aqueduct and fourth ventricle or an obstruction to the cerebro spinal fluid (C.S.F.) pathway in this region are best shown after the injection of opaque contrast medium into a lateral ventricle. Previously 2 ml of ethyl iodophenydecylate (Myodil) which is an oily contrast medium was used but has recently been replaced by metrizamide (Amipaque), a water soluble, anionic organic iodine compound. The contrast medium is injected through a burr hole into a lateral ventricle and then manipulated under fluoroscopy with image intensification to pass from the lateral ventricle, through the interventricular foramen into the third ventricle and thence down the aqueduct into the fourth ventricle or until the site of obstruction is reached. Frontal, half axial and lateral spot films are taken as a record of the examination (1950).

Radiographs

In (1950a) there is contrast medium in the left temporal horn and the third and fourth ventricles on the frontal view and by correct positioning flows into the third and fourth ventricles as shown on the lateral views.

In (1950b) the aqueduct and fourth ventricle are displaced to the right and forwards by a posterior fossa tumour.

In (1950c) there is contrast medium in the posterior part of the third ventricle, in the aqueduct and fourth ventricle which are displaced.

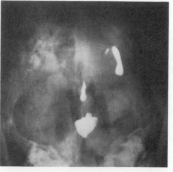
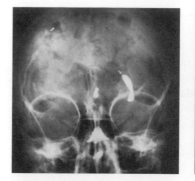
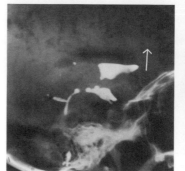
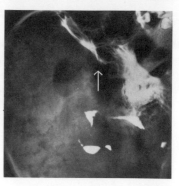

1950a

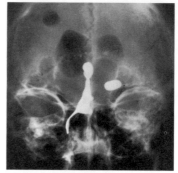
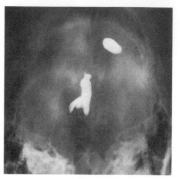

1950b

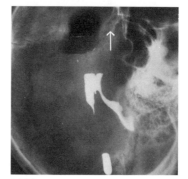
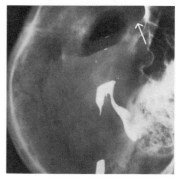

1950c

Autotomography

Autotomography is produced by blurring out overlying structure with gentle side to side movements of the head, using a long exposure time. The midline structures remain in focus and are thus clearly shown free of superimposed bone shadows particularly of the mastoid air cells. Automography is especially useful for demonstrating the third and fourth ventricles and the connecting aqueduct, during lumbar air encephalography. Although the patient's head can be rotated with a mechanical attachment, a sling harness is more commonly used in unconscious or uncooperative patients but active rotation of the head by a cooperative patient is by far the best method.

The patient is seated facing the skull table with the head well flexed to bring the base line (OMBL) 80° to the horizontal, keeping the median sagittal plane at right angles to the table top. A preliminary practice of the rotary movement of the head is essential. The head is moved 5° to either side of the midline keeping the base line (OMBL) 80° to the horizontal (1951).

With the patient correctly positioned and the tip of the lumbar puncture needle in the spinal theca 5–10 ml of air is injected and the exposure made while the head is moving slowly from side to side.

A lateral radiograph is taken with the table top, grid and cassette in position as shown in (1951) centring 1 cm behind the pinna of the ear (1953). The tube is then rotated through 90° into the occipito-frontal position and angled 30° upwards for the "reversed Towne's" or half axial occipito-frontal projection. A further 5 ml of air is injected and during a similar rotary movement of the head a further exposure is made.

Radiographs

In (1952) there is air in the lateral ventricles and the third and fourth ventricles are no longer obscured by overlying bone.

Similarly in (1953) the third and fourth ventricles are well shown.

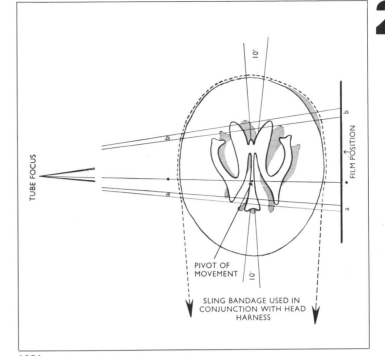

1951

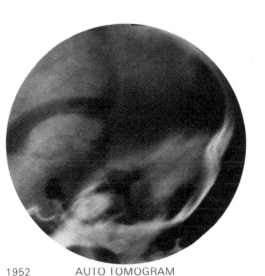

1952   AUTO TOMOGRAM

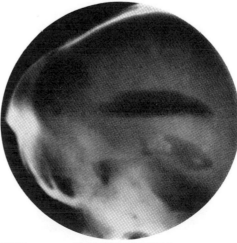

1953   AUTO TOMOGRAM

22 Stereotaxis

With stereotaxis the point of the cannula, needle or electrode can be accurately positioned in the brain by the safest route. It is used in neurosurgery and requires radiographic control. The apparatus is fixed to the skull and measurements are taken on radiographs in two or more planes at right angles to each other to determine the angle for the insertion of the needle and the depth required. There are a number of different designs of craniostat localiser.

It is the radiographer's responsibility to see that the X-ray equipment functions efficiently and correctly and exposed films are produced in the minimum time. The precise positioning required for this procedure is prearranged for the type of stereotaxis in use or any modification needed for a particular case.

Two methods of craniostat localisation are described and the part radiography plays in the procedure. In the first method, used to treat Parkinson's disease, localised injection is made into the globus pallidus of the basal nucleus. Head markers are used for accurate centring in the antero-posterior and lateral projections.

The localiser is firmly attached into a single burr hole in the anterior parietal region and carries a small external protractor which can be rotated through 90° which shows on the antero-posterior and lateral radiographs. The exact angle required for the needle can thus be shown and the depth calculated from the enlargement factor for the standard distances used. The needle has centimeter notches to read off the depth to which the needle is inserted.

A small quantity of air is injected into the ventricles for their visualisation and radiographs are taken at a focus-film distance of 76 cm (30 ins) with the median sagittal plane at 18 cm (7 ins) from the film in the lateral position, centring to the marked head positions (1954a, b). A similar antero-posterior film is taken and the required direction of the needle is carefully checked on both views and inserted to the required depth. Further films are then taken (1955a, b) and if the tip is correctly placed the injection is made. There is often an immediate and dramatic relief of symptoms in selected cases of Parkinson's disease.

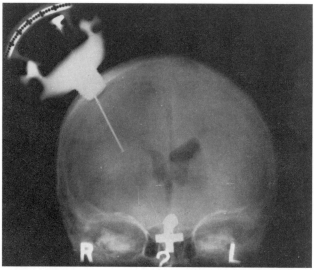

1954a

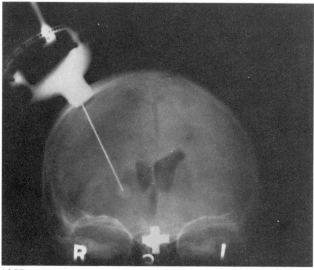

1955a

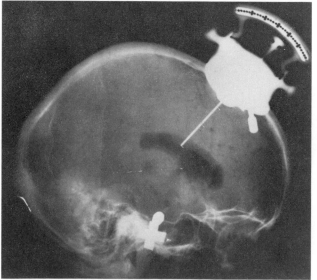

1954 b

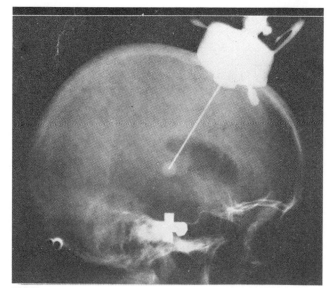

1955b

In the second method two adjacent burr holes in the cranial vault are occupied by metal cap and ball structures (1956a) through which a needle or probe can be inserted in the correct direction and to the correct depth.

The craniostat made up of a rectangular framework of light metal tubes and castings is securely fixed to the cranium by four screws (1956b) and is placed symetrically around the head. A semicircular localiser is attached to the frame around the head and can be adjusted over the burr holes (1956c).

A small amount of contrast medium such as Amipaque is injected into a lateral ventricle with the chin well tucked in bringing the base line 30° below the horizontal. The flow of contrast medium into the 3rd ventricle shows the position of the foramen of Monro.

A double grid of wires forming 1 mm squares (1956d) on the tube side of the skull overlies a selected part of the cranium. Meticulous care is required in adjusting the head, craniostat and X-ray tube even to the extent of using a spirit level. A focus-film distance of 4 metres (12 feet) minimises geometric distortion and the central ray is focussed to the centre of the wire grids by a telescopic device. If centring is correct the images of the two wire grids are superimposed as shown on radiographs in antero-posterior and lateral projections taken on a dried skull specimen (1956d).

A point on the 1 mm square grid is selected, the trunnions of the semicircular localiser are positioned to coincide with the selected point and the wire grid is then removed. The localiser is similarly positioned in the antero-posterior plane. The point selected will now be at the centre of the radius of the semicircular localiser and can be approached from any point on the hemisphere. The most suitable angles in the sagittal and coronal planes are measured on the radiographs.

Three radiographs (1957, a, b, c) show the grids with a probe through a burr hole and its tip correctly positioned. To confirm the position two lateral radiographs are taken (1957b) with direct centring and (1957c) with lateral tube displacement.

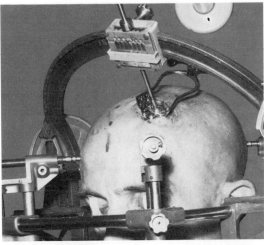

1956a

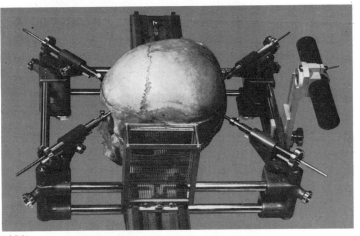

1956b

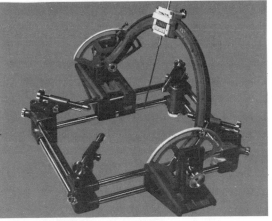

1956c

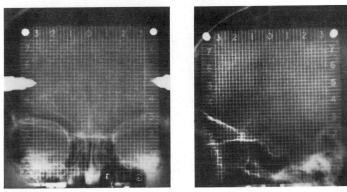

1956d

577

22

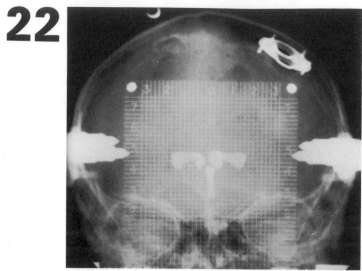

1957a

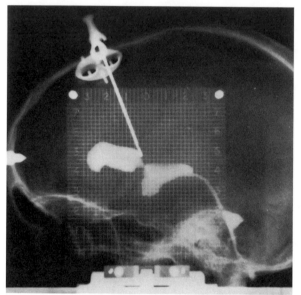

1957b

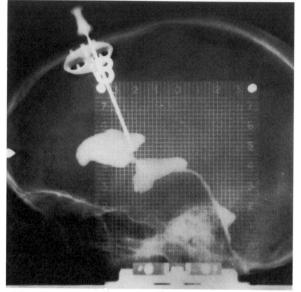

1957c

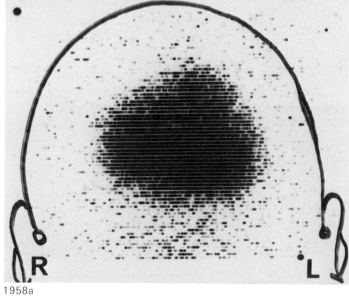

R   L

1958a

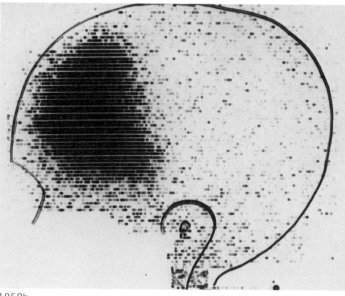

1958b

Isotope scanning

Minute amounts of radiopharmaccuticals such as technetium pertechnetate (99 m Tc) are concentrated in various lesions such as haemorrhage, tumours or abscesses and by giving off gamma rays can be detected by instruments with scintillation counters.

There are a number of different scanners, the most commonly used in brain scanning is a gamma camera. The patient is given 200 mgm of potassium perchlorate orally, 20–30 minutes before to block uptake of the isotope by the choroid plexuses. Twenty mCi (millicuries) of technetium pertechnetate is given intravenously and one to two hours later five views of the skull are taken, a frontal, occipital, two lateral a right and left (1959) and a vertex view.

The gamma ray photons are detected by an array of phototubes in the circular head of the gamma camera which are between 25 and 45 cm in diameter. The phototubes are connected by an electronic network to locate the scintillation crystals and display the accumulation of these impulses by generating light dots on a cathode ray tube producing an image. The image is recorded on film or photographic plates such as polaroid or bromide paper.

The impulses generated from phototubes can also be stored in a mini computer, the data can be processed to increase the sensitivity of the instrument.

Emission computed tomography

With two facing scintillation cameras rotating around the patient's head using the computed tomography principle, tomographic sections of gamma-ray images can be produced. The sensitivity is greatly increased with this system, approaching that of transmission computed tomography in brain lesions and is especially valuable for diagnosing subdural haematomas.

Conventional gamma camera imaging of brain pathology has however been largely superceded by computed tomography (CT) because of its greater specificity and anatomical resolution.

Isotope images

(1958a, b) were taken on a rectilinear scanner and (1959) on a gamma camera.

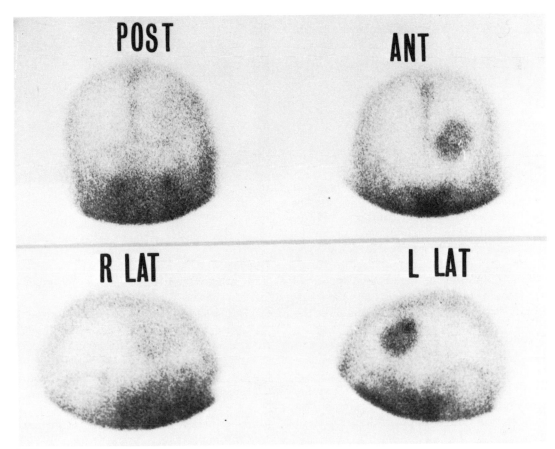

1959

22 Ultrasonography

Ultrasonography has now almost no part to play in diagnosis of intracranial pathology in adults but is extremely valuable in the neonatal period particularly in demonstrating intracranial haemorrhage. Previously this modality was only used to assess midline shift in space occupying lesions.

The mechanical vibrations used for ultrasonography have frequencies well above the range of human hearing but there is otherwise no essential difference between the mechanical vibrations producing sound and those required for scanning with ultrasound. Ultrasonographic transducers use the Piezo-electric effect which allows the production of mechanical vibrations through electrical activity and conversely can also transform mechanical vibrations back into electrical activity. The transducers therefore both produce and receive the ultrasonic vibrations using frequencies of 3–5 MHz (mega-herz).

The ultrasonic waves are reflected back from the interface or boundaries between tissues with different densities which occurs in the newborn skull at the margins of the ventricular system and at the falx cerebri or midline. Distortion of the ventricular system, fluid collections such as subdural haemorrhage and blood in the ventricles can thus be recognised.

The B-mode or brightness mode is used for neonatal brain imaging and each scan produced is essentially a tomographic section giving a two dimensional view of the brain. Air acts as a barrier to ultrasonic waves and therefore to establish intimate acoustic contact between the transducer and the baby's head olive oil is used as a coupling agent.

The great advantage of ultrasonography in neonatal brain imaging is that it is a non-invasive procedure, can be done with portable apparatus and does not use X-radiation.

Computed tomography

Computed tomography was invented by Godfrey Hounsfield and the first device installed at the Atkinson Morley Hospital in London was used for brain scanning by Dr. Ambrose in 1970.

An X-ray tube, interlinked with a system of detectors, scans the head to take some 200,000 readings from at least 180°. The photons emerging from the X-ray tube are measured as well as the number of photons falling on the detectors. Computers using mathematical techniques of reconstruction, then calculate tissue attention values in a 1 cm thick axial section of the brain.

Once the tissue attenuation values in an axial section through the skull have been computed, a corresponding anatomical picture can be produced, using the same computers, for display on a cathode ray tube. The images are recorded on radiographic or photographic plates but the original tissue attenuation values are stored as numerical data on tapes or floppy discs to be viewed as required.

Images that closely resemble anatomical sections of the brain are produced by computed tomography because of the good spatial and contrast resolution possible with the system (1960).

Tumours, cerebral infarcts, abscesses and surrounding cerebral oedema are accurately displayed, the actual lesions usually showing considerable contrast enhancement after an intravenous injection of a urographic type water soluble contrast medium.

Six to eight sections at 1 cm intervals are needed to show the brain from base to vertex. The original brain scanner and some body scanners take two adjacent sections simultaneously, using two X-ray tubes and sets of detectors.

Brain scans are in the vast majority of cases done with 26 cm (10 ins) wedges which effectively limits the radiation field and reconstruction programme to this size. For body scans 33 cm (13 ins) and 40 cm (16 ins) wedges are also available (1961).

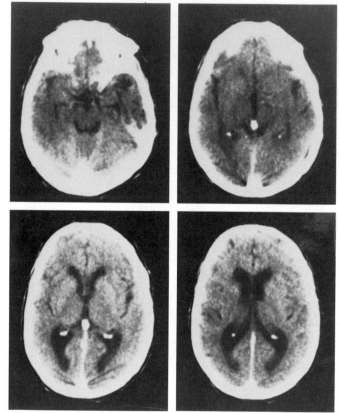

1960

(1960)

Four sections from a normal examination with the base line at 20° and shows
(a) The superior orbital plates, temporal lobes, chiasmatic cistern, quadrigeminal plate cistern and cerebellum.
(b) The 3rd ventricle, sylvian fissures, pineal, choroid plexuses and posterior horns of the lateral ventricles.
(c) The 3rd ventricle, anterior and posterior horns of the lateral ventricles, pineal and choroid plexuses and Sylvian fissures.
(d) Anterior and posterior horns of the lateral ventricles and choroid plexuses.

Positioning

Most brain scans are done with the patient supine (1962) and at 1 cm intervals using a 10–13 mm thick section.

1. Posterior fossa. To show the cerebellum (1963) and other structures in the posterior fossa the chin is well tucked in to bring the orbito-meatal line or base line 25°–30° to the vertical, keeping the median sagittal plane at right angles to the table top.

The fourth ventricle appears as a dark semilunar low density area and the ambient cisterns encircling the brain stem with the corpora quadrigemina are shown lying anterior to the cerebellum (1964).

2. Supratentorial structures. With the patient supine the base line (OMBL) should be only 10°–15° to the vertical.

The lowest sections show the chiasmatic cistern and after contrast enhancement, the arteries of the circle of Willis (1965). Above this level the third ventricle and anterior horns of the lateral ventricles become visible and then further sections show the body of the ventricles, posterior horns and finally the sulci of the surface of the brain.

3. The orbits. With the patient supine the base line (OMBL) should be parallel to the vertical. Three to four sections at 1 cm intervals cover the orbital cavities.

The eyeball, lens, optic nerve, eye muscles and the surrounding bone, are clearly visible (1966).

4. The pituitary fossa. The base line (OMBL) should be at − 15° to the vertical to bring the floor of the middle fossa parallel to the plane of section.

The section should be reduced to 0·5 cm thickness and contrast enhancement should be used for examining pituitary tumours (1967). Six to eight sections are required for the pituitary fossa but further sections will be needed if there is suprasella extension of a tumour. Coronal sections are very valuable in this region (1968).

5. The petrous temporal and base of skull. With the patient supine and the base line (OMBL) at − 15° to the vertical as for the pituitary fossa axial sections are taken parallel to the floor of the middle fossa but must include the external auditory meatus, mastoids and jugular foramen.

6. Paranasal sinuses. With the patient supine the base line (OMBL) is at − 10° to the vertical (or the anthropomorphic (Reid's) base line at right angles to the table top) 1 cm adjacent sections are taken from just above the level of the inferior orbital margin to below the level of the maxillary antra or below the level of the tumour being investigated (1969). Sections which include the teeth are likely to produce unacceptable streak artefacts if metallic fillings are present. The angle of the base line must then be varied to move the fillings in the teeth out of the section being scanned to obtain worthwhile diagnostic information.

7. Examination for radiotherapy planning. All computed tomography examinations performed for radiotherapy planning must be done with the patient in a similar position to that assumed on the radiotherapy couch and in the individualised radiotherapy shell.

8. Coronal sections. The whole body scanner has an aperture sufficiently large to perform sections in the coronal plane.

(i) **Prone Coronal sections.** With the patient prone and the neck markedly extended the base line must be as near to parallel with the table top as possible for the patient.

(ii) **Supine Coronal sections.** For thick set patients with short necks the supine position with neck extension may be more practical. Again the orbito-meatal line should be as nearly parallel to the table top as is comfortable for the patient.

Coronal sections frequently pass through fillings in teeth to produce marked streak artefacts. When possible the head should be adjusted to exclude metallic tooth fillings from the section.

With coronal sections tumours can be more accurately localised particularly for surgery (1970).

9. Off lateral sagittal sections. With lateral flexion at the neck and using an angled support, off lateral sections of the cranium become possible with the whole body scanner.

10. Coronal and sagittal reconstruction. The data of computed tomography is stored in digital form and suitable reconstruction programmes can be used to form pictures in coronal and sagittal planes. However, the original sections taken in the axial plane must be contiguous with no gaps between or preferably overlapping. At present the detail in routine reconstruction pictures is not nearly as good as in direct coronal or off lateral sagittal sections but is certainly adequate for preoperative localisation.

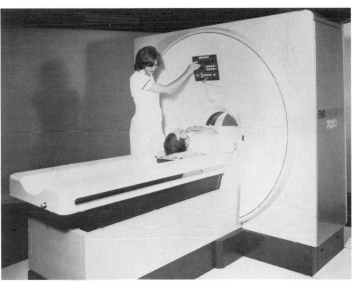

1961

(1961)
The whole body scanner has an aperture large enough to perform coronal head scans. For most body sections the patient is supine and enters scanner feet first.

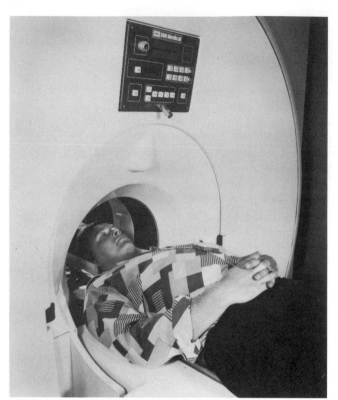

1962

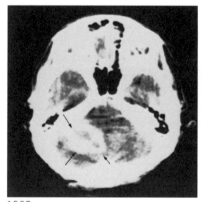

1963

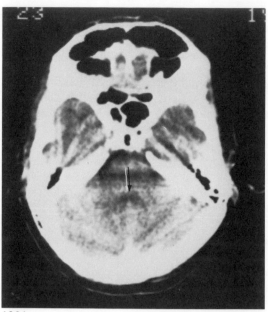

1964a

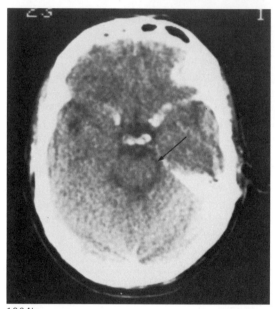

1964b

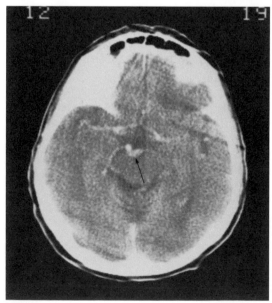

1965

(1962)

A head band or bolsters and a special head rest help to keep the head immobilised for the relatively long exposure times of 3 seconds to two minutes, compared with conventional radiography.

(1963)

The baseline is at 30° for sections of the posterior fossa, which in this patient shows a cerebellar metastasis after contrast enhancement. (arrows).

(1964)

(a) Sections through the posterior fossa and cerebellum show the 4th ventricle as a crescentic low density or black area (arrow).

(b) A section 1 cm above, is through the anterior and posterior clinoids and brainstem demarcated by the surrounding ambient cisterns. (arrow).

582

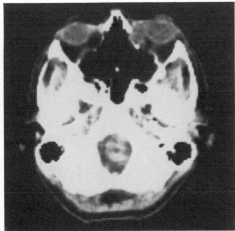
1966a

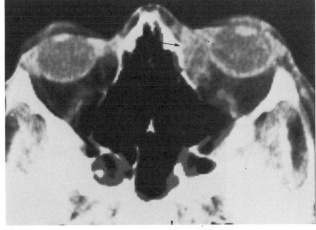
1966b

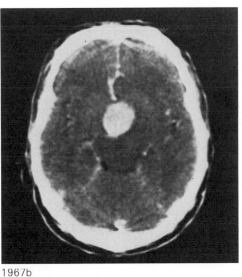
1967a

1967b

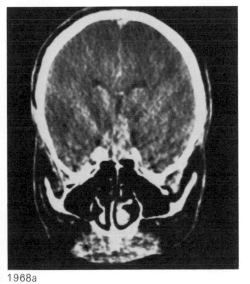
1968a

1968b

(1965)
The Circle of Willis is frequently shown on CT after intravenous contrast enhancement. There is a small aneurysm on the basilar artery. (arrow).

(1966)
A right proptosis caused by an abscess in the lacrimal sac, appears as a low density area adjacent to the orbit (arrow), well seen in the enlarged view taken from the independent viewing console. The eyeball with its lens and sclera are clearly seen and displaced by the lacrimal abscess.

(1967)
Pituitary tumour after contrast enhancement in a case of acromegaly.

(1968)
Coronal sections are important in pituitary tumours to show its upward extension and relationship to the 3rd ventricle.

22

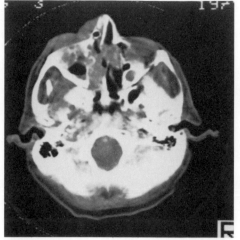

1969

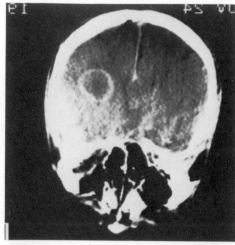

1970a

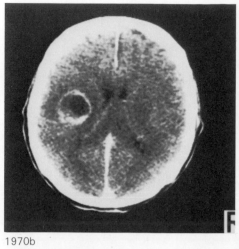

1970b

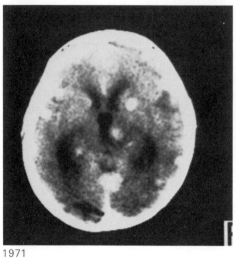

1971

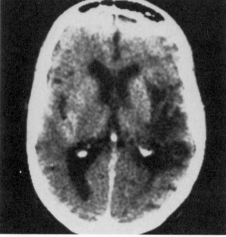

1972

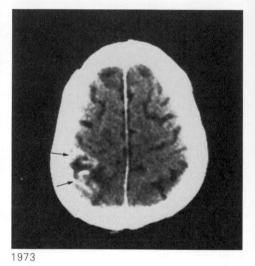

1973

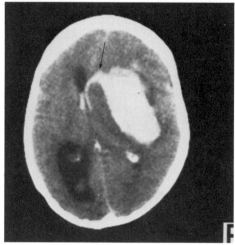

1974

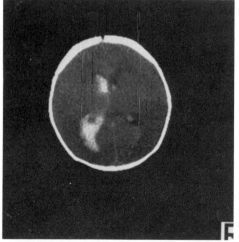

1975a

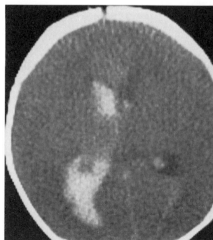

1975b

584

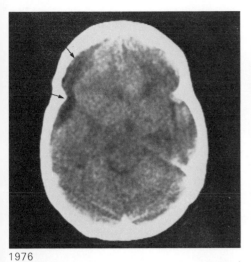

1976

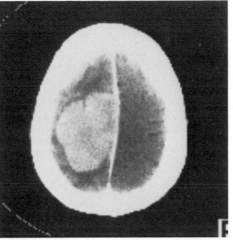

1977

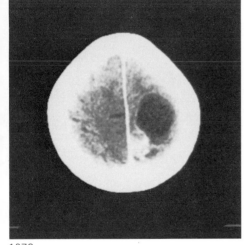

1978

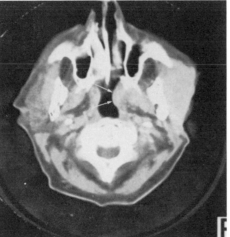

1979

(1969)
Carcinoma of the ethmoidal sinuses with bone destruction and extending across the midline onto the right side and into the left maxillary antrum.

(1970a, b)
Ring enhancement of a cerebral glioma. The coronal section is extremely valuable for preoperative localisation.

(1971)
Multiple cerebral metastases shown after contrast enhancement.

(1972)
A large cerebral infarct, appearing as an area of low tissue attenuation (black area) in the distribution of the middle cerebral artery.

(1973)
Luxury perfusion (arrows), in an area of cerebral infarction associated with prominent sulci in ischaemic cerebral disease.

(1974)
Cerebral haemorrhage causing marked midline displacement, with a leak of the blood into the right lateral ventricle which is entering the third ventricle through the foramen of Monro (arrow). Recent haemorrhage has high attenuation values (white area).

(1975a, b)
Neonatal haemorrhage into the left lateral ventricle appearing as an area of high attenuation. (b) Shows enlarged view taken from independent viewing console.

(1976)
Subdural haematoma appearing as an area of low attenuation in the left fronto-parietal region. (arrows). With time water is absorbed into the blood clot which liquefies and changes to an area of low attenuation.

(1977)
Para-falcine meningioma, without contrast enhancement, has high tissue attenuation values.

(1978)
Cystic glioma seen on the uppermost section. Small lesions can be completely missed unless the uppermost sections are included in the examination.

(1979)
Parotid tumour with extension deep to the mandible producing a bulge into the lateral wall of the naso-pharynx, (arrow).

22 Scanning methods

The scanning methods are considered in more detail in separate sections with Isotope Scanning (Nuclear Medicine) in Section 37, page 807; Ultrasonography, Section 38, page 831 and Computed Tomography, Section 39, page 856. Nuclear Magnetic Resonance Scanning is only now being developed, and limited examples are available and described in Section 40 page 885.

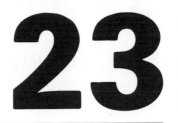

MYELOGRAPHY

MYELOGRAPHY

The spinal cord is the prolongation of the central nervous system from the medulla oblongata and extends from the uppermost cervical region to its termination in the filum terminale at the level of the second lumbar vertebra. The membranous coverings of the spinal cord and the spaces between are continuous with those around the brain. The subarachnoid space lies between the pia mater, the thin innermost layer closely attached to the brain and spinal cord, and the next layer the arachnoid mater. The space between the arachnoid mater and the outer layer or dura mater is the subdural space and is considerably smaller than the subarachnoid space (1980). The cerebro-spinal fluid is contained in the subarachnoid space into which contrast medium is injected for myelography.

The dura mater, a thick external covering of the spinal cord, is separated from the bone of the spine by the subdural space and contains a plexus of veins in loose fatty connective tissue.

Myelography is the radiographic investigation of the spinal canal for the diagnosis of space occupying and obstructive lesions and requires the injection of a contrast agent into the subarachnoid space usually following a lumbar puncture. Either a negative contrast agent such as air or oxygen is used or more usually a positive non-reactive organic iodine compound. Recently a water soluble anionic iodine compound 'Amipaque' (metrizamide) has been introduced for myelography and ventriculography replacing myodil (iophendylate). Metrizamide has many advantages being freely miscible with cerebro spinal fluid, it flows along the subarachnoid spaces around the nerve roots and is absorbed from the subarachnoid space within forty eight hours. There is thus no need to aspirate the contrast medium following myelography as is the case with iophendylate. Metrizamide also has a low viscosity and thus a narrow bore needle (22-gauge) can be used. Toxic reactions such as headache and nausea may follow but seldom last for longer than 24 hours. Rarely convulsions and arachnoiditis leading to paralysis may occur. The compound is isotonic with cerebrospinal fluid in the concentration usually used for lumbar myelography (170 mgI/ml) made up to a volume of 10 ml. For thoracic and cervical myelography a slightly more concentrated solution is usually used, namely up to 250 mgI/ml in a volume of 10 ml.

The subarachnoid space

Positive myelographic contrast agents have a higher specific gravity than cerebrospinal fluid and can therefore be positioned in the theca by tilting or rotating the patient (1981, 1982, 1983). The two diagrams in longitudinal section (1981a and b) and the diagrams in axial section (1982a) show how the position of the contrast medium in the theca can change when the patient is turned supine from the prone horizontal position. Similarly if oxygen is used it will rise to the top and change position with rotation of the patient as represented by the light areas in the

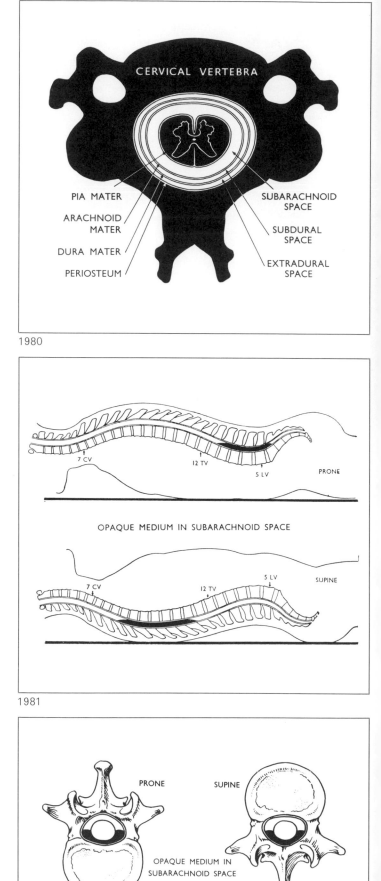

CERVICAL VERTEBRA

PIA MATER
ARACHNOID MATER
DURA MATER
PERIOSTEUM

SUBARACHNOID SPACE
SUBDURAL SPACE
EXTRADURAL SPACE

1980

OPAQUE MEDIUM IN SUBARACHNOID SPACE

7 CV   12 TV   5 LV   PRONE

7 CV   12 TV   5 LV   SUPINE

1981

PRONE   SUPINE

OPAQUE MEDIUM IN SUBARACHNOID SPACE

1982a

axial diagrams (1982a, b and c). When oxygen is used for myelography (1996), 30–50 ml replaces a similar quantity of cerebrospinal fluid removed and the injection is performed with the patient horizontal. Subsequently, under fluoroscopy with image intensification, the patient is positioned to manipulate the gas into the required position but not into the ventricular system in the brain which will occur with too much feet down tilt.

Thus with both negative and positive myelography careful tilting and rotation of the patient under fluoroscopy is required for the examination and the appropriate films are taken, including localised views at the site of the pathology. In the lumbar region, frontal, oblique and lateral views are done routinely.

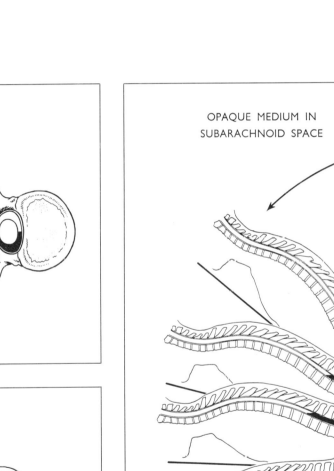

1982b

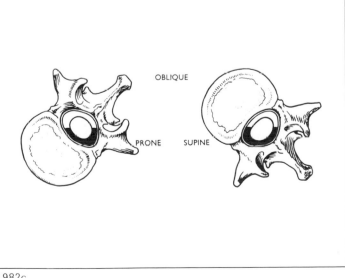

1982c

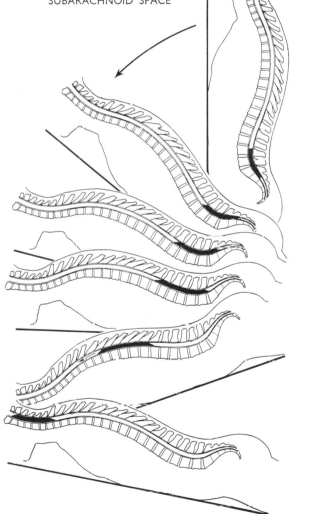

OPAQUE MEDIUM IN SUBARACHNOID SPACE

1983

Positioning

The curvature of the spine is extremely important in moving the contrast medium up the subarachnoid space and in maintaining it in the required region. With the patient prone the lordosis produces a natural reservoir for the contrast medium in the lumbar region (1983a) and considerable head down tilt is required to move the contrast over the dorsal curve. However, with the patient supine the dorsal curve then acts as the natural reservoir for the contrast. The contrast flows much more easily with much less table tilt when the patient is lateral.

To prevent the contrast medium running into the intracranial subarachnoid space, the neck must be extended with the patient prone, the chin resting on the couch top and the median sagittal plane of the head at right angles to the couch, in line with the rest of the body. When the contrast medium is in the cervical region the couch can again be placed horizontally and gentle tilting allows examination of each segment in turn.

The position of the contrast medium in the spinal theca is shown diagrammatically (1983) as the body is tilted in the prone position from erect to head down and then brought back to a slight feet down tilt.

Some of the positions required for myelography are shown in the series of photographs (1984a–d). In (1984a) the patient is in the horizontal, prone oblique position, in (1984b) lateral with slight feet down table tilt, in (1984c) supine with the feet lowered and in (1984d) supine with the head lowered. In (1985) the patient is prone with head turned sideways and (1986) shows the tube and cassette in position for a horizontal ray film which may be needed in any position, prone or supine and with the head or feet down.

The new water soluble contrast medium usually leaks past all but the most complete block in the subarachnoid space. If there is a complete block contrast medium must be injected above the level of the block to show its upper limit.

Films are taken at various levels to show the progress of the contrast medium and any local pathology. An intramedullary lesion may produce a complete block in the cervical region as in (1987) but after a cisternal puncture there is also contrast medium above the tumour as shown on the lateral view (1990). In (1987–1989) contrast medium is moving up the spinal cord with progressive head down tilt.

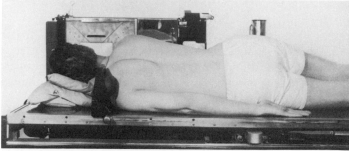

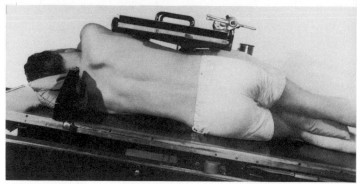

1984a

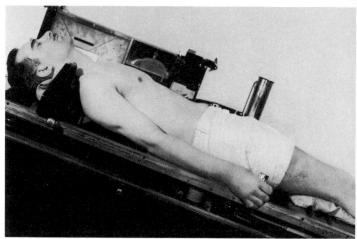

1984b

1984c

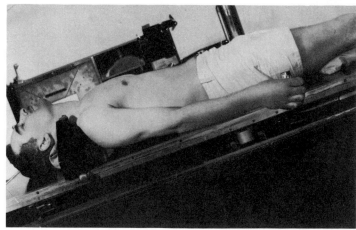

1984d

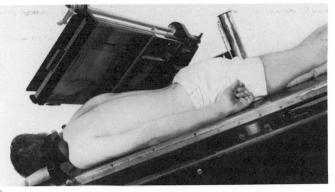

1985

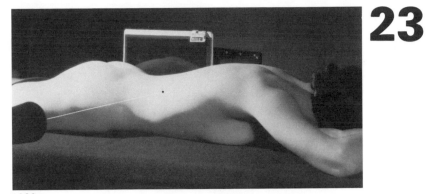

1986

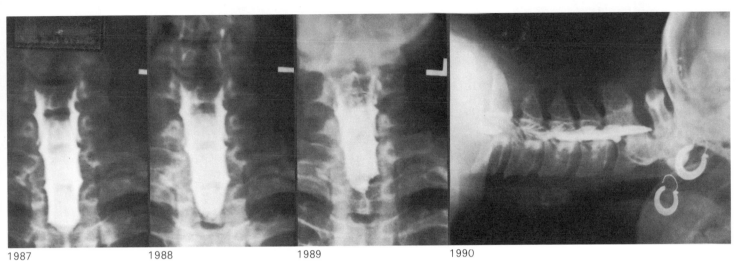

1987   1988   1989   1990

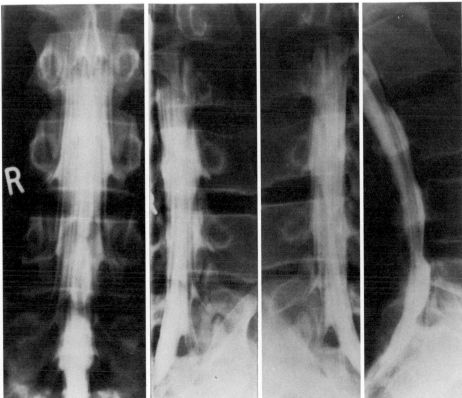

1991   1992   1993   1994

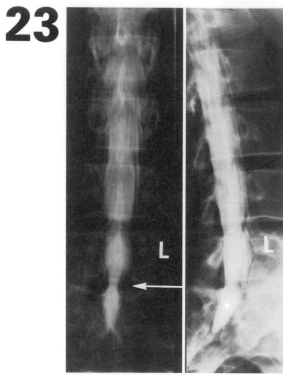

1995

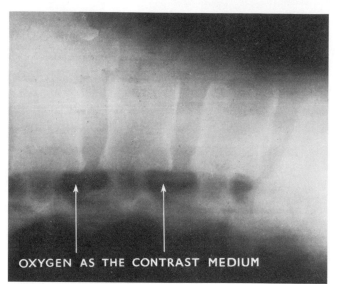

OXYGEN AS THE CONTRAST MEDIUM

1996

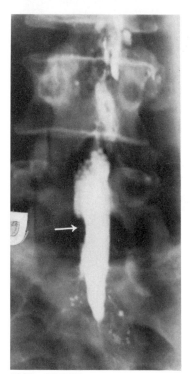

1997   PRONE

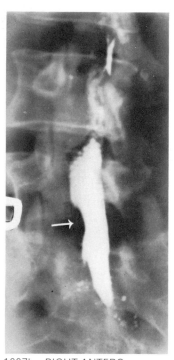

1997b   RIGHT ANTERO-
POSTERIOR OBLIQUE

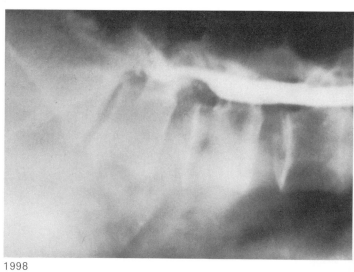

1998

Metrizamide (Amipaque) myelography is also called radiculography because the contrast medium runs into the subarachnoid spaces of the nerve root sheaths, showing the nerve roots in profile (1991–1995). Being water soluble it is largely absorbed within 48 hours and aspiration of contrast medium following myelography is no longer needed as previously when iophendylate (Myodil) was used which also sometimes went into the nerve sheaths but would then remain there for years.

A dorsal decubitus view (1996) shows a gas myelogram which appears as a dark band in the spinal theca.

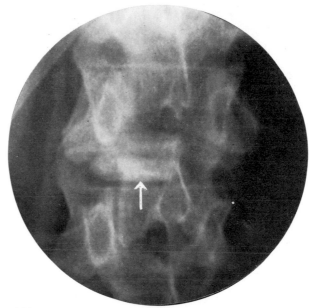

1999a

Intervertebral discs

Disc protrusion into the spinal canal or impinging on a nerve root is a common cause of backache especially when associated with sciatica or pain radiating down the back of the leg. On myelography the disc protrusion shows as an extrinsic filling defect on anterior (1998) or antero-lateral margins of the contrast medium at the level of an intervertebral disc (1997a and b). Enlargement of the nerve root or pressure on the nerve root sheath may be shown with metrizamide radicullography. Oblique views (1997a and b) and the prone horizontal ray lateral are thus most important in posterior or postero-lateral intervertebral disc protrusions.

Occasionally disc calcification occurs in the lumbar region and is then visible on radiographs of the spine (1999).

Discography

The intervertebral discs can also be examined by the direct injection of contrast medium into the intervertebral disc space.

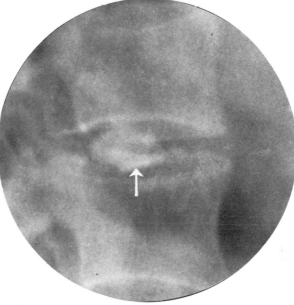

1999b

24

ANGIOGRAPHY

ANGIOGRAPHY

Harvey's description of the circulation of the blood in 1628 came a year after the discovery of lymphatics by Asellius. However, it was not till 300 years later that aortography was initiated by dos Santos and his colleagues in Portugal and in 1952 lymphography was introduced by Kinmonth of St. Thomas' Hospital, London. Opaque cathers and safe contrast agents were subsequently developed and angiography is now a commonly used radiographic procedure.

Angiography includes both the radiographic demonstration of the arterial (aortography and arteriography) and the venous systems (phlebography or venography) by contrast injections either by direct needle puncture or after insertion of a catheter.

Contrast agents

Water soluble organic iodine compounds are used for arteriography and venography and are essentially similar to urographic contrast agents. Whereas for lymphography ultrafluid lipiodol is usually used.

The water soluble compounds that have emerged as having low toxicity are tri-iodinated monobenzoic acid derivatives with the iodine atoms in the 2·4·6 position on the benzene ring as either methylglucamine or sodium salts.

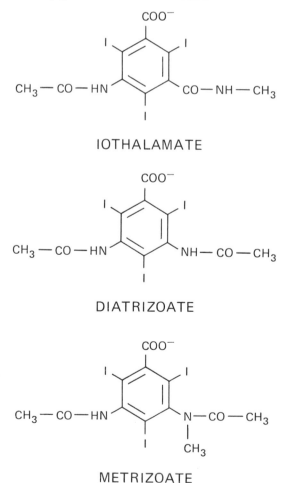

IOTHALAMATE

DIATRIZOATE

METRIZOATE

The methylglucamine or meglumine salts are much less irritant to blood vessels than the sodium salts which occasionally cause intense pain even with slow intravenous injections. Recently compounds of even lower osmolality have been introduced which cause even less reaction than the monobasic tri-odinated meglumine salts. These new compounds have two linked benzene rings to produce a larger molecule known as a dimer, with six iodine atoms attached

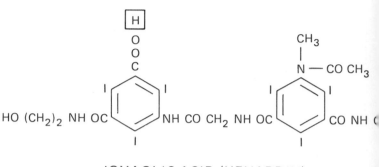

IOXAGLIC ACID (HEXABRIX)

Angiographic contrast media are available in varying concentrations from 60 % to 80 % w/v solutions and containing between 28 grammes of iodine per 100 ml and 42 grammes under various trade name, Hypaque, Renografin, Renovist (diatrizoate), Conray (iothalamate), Triosil (metrizoate) and Hexabrix (ioxaglate).

The compounds with lower osmolality such as the meglamine salts or dimer molecules have higher viscosities than sodium salts but the viscosity can be greatly reduced by warming the contrast medium to 37°C before injection.

While toxic reactions are uncommon and fatalities rare, occurring in 1 in 40,000 cases, nevertheless, basic precautions are still essential. A previous hypersensitivity reaction to contrast medium is a contraindication to angiography and great caution should be exercised in asthmatic and allergic subjects. A resuscitation kit must be available in the angiography room, all personnel trained in resuscitation procedures and the patient must not be left unattended for any part of the examination.

Injection of Contrast Medium

The volume of contrast medium injected varies from 10 ml for "selective" angiography when the tip of a catheter is in an artery supplying the organ being examined to 60 ml for a "free" flush aortogram. A hand injection for selective arteriography of 10–15 ml of contrast medium is quite suitable but a pump injection is needed for aortography. Many different kinds of injector pumps are now available from the simple Talley to the complex Cordis which is integrated with the film changer and electrocardiograph. It is thus possible to inject variable amounts of contrast medium, at different pressures with varying film programmes depending on the type of examination being performed.

Needles, Catheters and Guide Wires

A wide variety of needles, catheters and guide wires are available, supplied by manufacturers in sterile packs. The catheters and guide wires are disposable and used only once and a supply is kept in the radiology department preferably in a separate catheter store room. In most modern hospitals pre-sterilised packs containing gowns, dressing towels and swabs are prepared by the Central Sterilising Supply Unit (CSSU) and thus available not only for routine use but also for emergency arteriography.

Viewing

Angiography is performed using image intensification and television monitoring with over head lights dimmed during fluoroscopy but otherwise the room is lit normally. In some centres biplane viewing is also possible and all viewing recorded on video for instant playback with picture "freeze" or "stop".

There should also be fast automatic processing available and an adequate number of viewing boxes for selected films within the angiographic room as well as close to the processor for the whole examination.

Film Changers

The examination may be recorded on full-sized cut film or roll film, on 100 or 70 mm film or on 35 mm by cineradiography.

In the early days of angiography hand changers were used with pull out cassettes after each exposure (2000). Up to two exposures per second could be obtained often only to a maximum of eight. Now however there are many varieties of automatic film changers many of which are also biplane.

A simple manually operated changer for peripheral arteriography can operate with either 35×35 cm (14×14 ins) or 35×38 cm (12×15 ins) cassettes and can also be used in association with a long cassette and a second tube to show the arteries of the thighs and legs (2001). The cassettes must be backed with lead to prevent fogging of the films in the lower cassettes.

Simple automatic changers move loaded cassettes beneath the table top (2002) into the required position for an exposure and then away, being replaced by the next cassette. In cut film changers such as the Schönander (2003) unexposed film is stacked within the changer and moved one film at a time into position between intensifying screens over a roller. There is a grid overlying the uppermost screen. The changers are mobile, can be fitted to take horizontal, vertical or biplane exposures and for 25×30 cm (10×12 ins) or 35×35 cm (14×14 ins) film at rates of up to 6 per second.

As the cut film passes between the intensifying screens they are compressed to obtain good contact with the film and then released. The films pass on into a light-tight container (2003) which is used to transport the film to the dark room where they are removed for automatic processing. Exposures are preset with varying programmes to suit particular examinations.

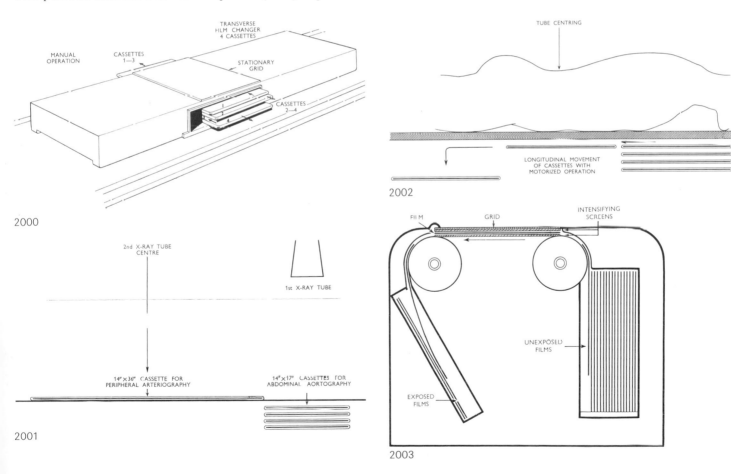

2000

2001

2002

2003

Roll film changers (2004) such as the Elema operate similarly and can also be positioned at right angles for biplane examinations in either antero-posterior and lateral or oblique projections. The roll film is 30·5 cm (12 ins wide) and up to 15 metres (50 ft) long. As the film passes between the intensifying screens compression is applied for each exposure and is capable of up to 12 exposures per second, preset for any required programme for up to 40 exposures.

After completing an examination the spools are removed, in complete darkness, into a light-tight container to be taken to the dark room. The rolls of film are threaded onto large spindles for automatic processing. With rapid processing (90 sec) it is possible to view the examination for quality control and whether the examination has been completed. Special viewing facilities are required which has spindles to hold the roll film, wide viewing and light coning.

Subtraction

If there is an exactly matching control exposure obtained before the injection of contrast medium the unwanted overlying bone shadow can be removed from angiograms by a photographic technique. The initial control exposure is reversed to show the bones as grey-to-black images and exactly superimposed on the angiogram which cancels out the image of the bone (2054c, 2055b, 2056b, 2057).

Miniature angiography

Angiography can also be recorded on 100 mm and 70 mm film with up to 6 exposures per second by using image amplification. With the Rapidex cassette up to 40 exposures can be taken. As with the cut film and roll film changers, pre-set programmes for variously spaced exposures are available. For cerebral angiography the apparatus is modified for the cranium to fill a 25 × 25 cm (10 × 10 ins) screen providing a maximum image for the 70 mm film and viewed directly or after enlargement.

Cineradiography

Biplane 35 mm cineradiography via image intensification is particularly used for coronary angiography and paediatric angiocardiography. Exposure speeds of up to 50 frames per second are available but usually 25 frames per second is sufficient. Special viewers such as the Tagiano are now available for playback at various speeds in both forward and reversed directions and for "stop" or "freeze" viewing of individual frames.

The radiation dosage is greatly reduced and the quality of the image improved by pulsed exposures synchronised with the camera; radiation exposures occur only when the film is stationary within the cine camera.

Video recording

The television image can be monitored by videotape recording for instant replay, remote viewing, slow motion or still images and is especially valuable for showing the position of the catheter tip or to study the results of a test injection.

Precautions

In the last decade safe contrast agents were introduced but basic precautions are still most important. Patients undergoing angiography must not be dehydrated particularly when they have diminished renal or liver function. Previous contrast medium hypersensitivity is a contra-indication and particular care must be taken with patients who have asthma or allergies. The angiographic room must have a resuscitation kit in a prominent position and radiographers must be trained in resuscitation procedures with an alarm system available to call for further aid in an emergency. Under no circumstances must the patient be left unattended during or after the procedure and following the examination must be monitored for vital signs.

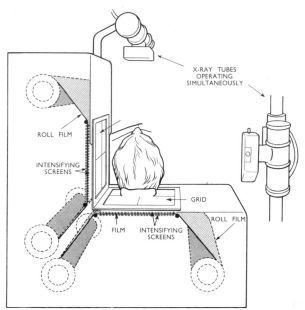

2004

Cerebral Angiography

The angiographic anatomy of the major cerebral arteries (2005, 2006, 2008) and veins (2007) are shown in lateral (2005, 2007 and 2008) and in frontal view (2006) in annotated diagrams to be compared later with illustrated radiographs.

Opaque medium

Methyl glucamine tri-iodinated compounds such as Conray '280' or the newer dimer compound Hexabrix '320' are suitable for cerebral angiography.

The examination is performed either under general anaesthesia often when direct needle puncture of the carotid artery is used or with local anaesthetic particularly for the transfemoral selective carotid artery injections. The cerebral vessels are shown with 6–8 ml of contrast medium and the contrast injection is repeated for each additional sequence.

The first exposure is taken at the end of the injection and further exposures over a six second period to cover the capillary and venous phases, requiring a minimum of 3 films. Contrast medium injected into the internal carotid artery demonstrates the anterior and middle cerebral arteries (2010) and into the vertebral artery, the posterior cerebral artery and cerebellar arteries (2022).

Between contrast injections the needle or catheter is kept patent by saline infusions.

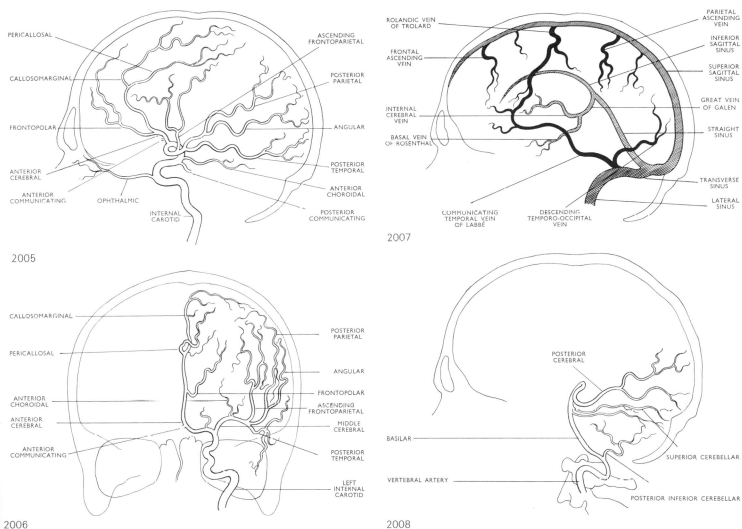

Technique with the skull table

For many years cerebral arteriography was performed on a skull unit using a magazine containing 3 or 5 cassettes (2009) each being exposed in turn and extracted manually. This method requires considerable team work with a good rapport between radiologist and radiographer. The magazine is spring loaded and each cassette has lead backing to prevent exposure of the next cassette, the first film being exposed at the end of the injection of 6–8 ml of contrast medium and thereafter at approximately 1½ to 2 second intervals. Following the lateral series a further contrast injection is needed for the antero-posterior series.

Automatic film changer

Two 30×25 cm (12×10 ins) film changers at right angles to each other are needed for simultaneous biplane angiography or a single changer can be used which can be positioned horizontally as well as being turned through a right angle for the lateral projection. Films are exposed at two per second for 5 seconds to show the arterial, capillary and venous phase of the angiogram.

The patient is supine with the head extended either by having foam pads under the shoulders or by lowering the head support. The head band is placed loosely over the forehead and tightened later for immobilisation.

The radiologist injecting the contrast medium must be shielded by adequate lead protection and just prior to the injection the patient's head is adjusted and immobilised by tightening the head band.

Timing of exposures

For subtraction radiography a film must be taken immediately before the contrast medium is injected. The arterial phase is shown at the end of the injection of 6–8 ml of contrast (2010) the capillary phase $2\frac{1}{2}$ seconds later (2011) and the venous phase 5 seconds after the end of the injection (2012). The comparable arterial and venous phase antero-posterior films (2013, 2014) require similar timing of exposures.

Exposure factors

The exposure times must be short to eliminate movement blurring and the kilovoltage should be at least 10 kV higher than for similar routine skull projections. The films should be sufficiently penetrated to show the contrast filled carotid artery as it passes through the dense petrous temporal bone.

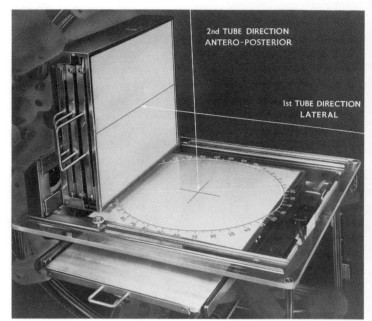

2009

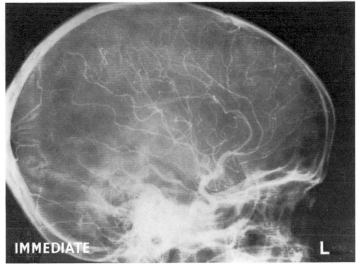

IMMEDIATE L

2010

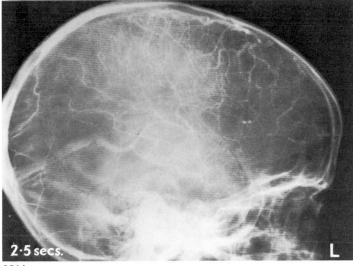

2·5 secs. L

2011

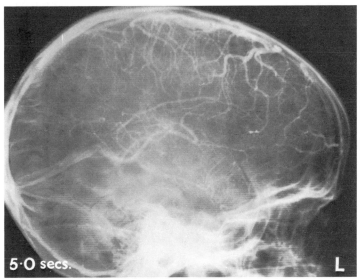

5·O secs. L

2012

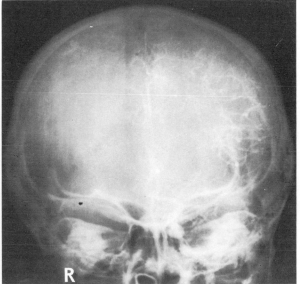

R

2013

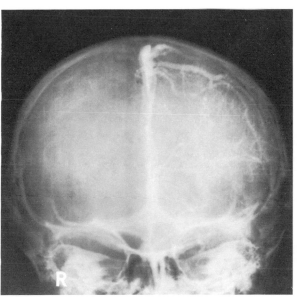

R

2014

Positioning

A single examination for the cerebral vessels of one side usually consists of a lateral and antero-posterior view which may have a 25° caudal tilt. Both antero-posterior and antero-posterior with a caudal tilt may be needed together with an oblique view for demonstrating cerebral aneurysms. Each position will require a further injection of 6–8 ml of contrast medium.

Lateral view

The patient is supine with the neck extended either by placing foam pads under the shoulders or by lowering the head support of the skull table. With a foam pad under the occiput the whole head will be shown in the lateral position. The median sagittal plane must be at right angles to the table top and parallel to the film. A horizontal ray at right angles to the film is centred 1 cm above and in front of the external auditory meatus and the X-ray beam collimated to just include the skull (2015–2017).

Antero-posterior

If the lateral series is satisfactory after being viewed, the tube is rotated through 90° and angled 25° caudally. The Patient's head is supported while both the head and shoulder pads are removed. A 15° foam sponge wedge under the head keeps the chin well tucked in to bring the base line vertical.

The X-ray beam is well collimated to just cover the skull and centred 5 cm (2 ins) above the glabella in the midline. A further 6–8 ml of contrast medium injected and a series of films taken (2018).

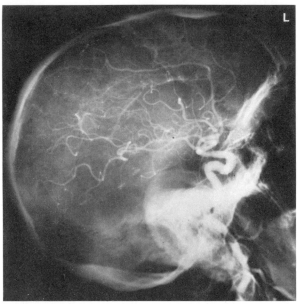

2015

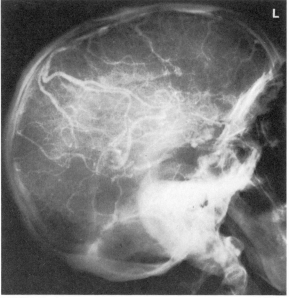

2016

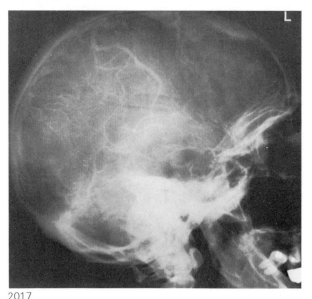

2017

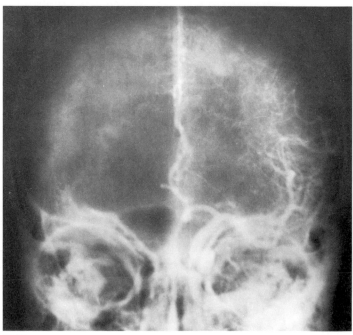

2018

Oblique projections

The head is rotated 30–45° away from the side being injected and the tube centred 5 cm (2 ins) above the mid-point of the uppermost superior orbital margin with a 25° caudal tilt. In some cases the tube is perpendicular and centred directly over the superior orbital margin.

In this projection the carotid syphon is "opened out", the curves of which are otherwise superimposed (2019, 2020).

Vertebral arteriography

Vertebral angiography is performed either by direct needle puncture of the vertebral artery or by catheterisation from below by way of the femoral artery and aorta. Vertebral angiography shows the posterior cerebral artery and cerebellar circulation (2022). The lateral projection is similar to the lateral carotid series but for the fronto-occipital view the caudal tube tilt must be increased to 30°.

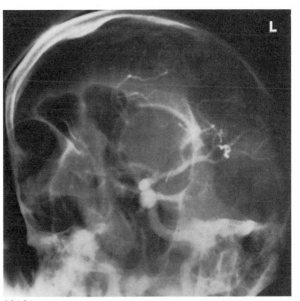

2019

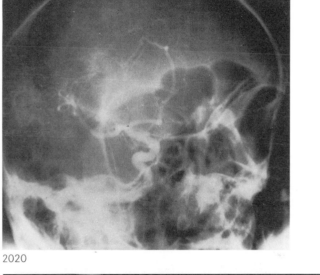

2020

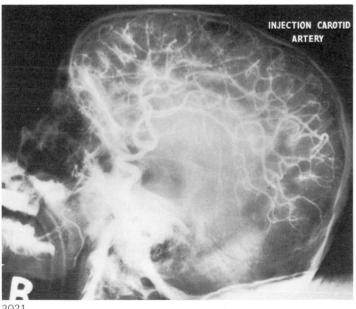

2021

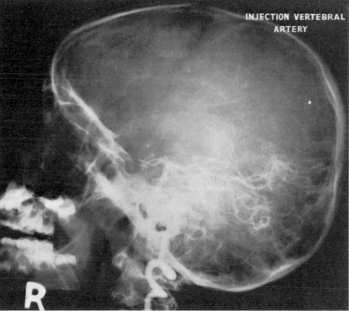

2022

24 Cardiac angiography

Contrast examinations of the heart and great vessels are usually combined with pressure studies of individual heart chambers and blood gas analysis of oxygen and carbon dioxide, to detect shunts and calculate cardiac output.

Opaque medium

To visualise the cardiac chambers and great vessels in the adult large volumes of high concentration contrast agents are injected rapidly under pressure (50–70 lbs/sq. ins) with a pump. But to show the coronary arteries each orifice is selectively catheterised and small quantities of a non-reactive contrast agent such as the dimer Hexabrix or the anionic compound Amipaque are injected by hand. During cardio-angiography or coronary angiography the patient is closely monitored, especially for ECG abnormalities. Resuscitation equipment and trained personnel must be immediately available.

The contrast medium used includes diatrizoate (Hypaque 75–80%), iothalamate (angio-conray '420'), metrizoate (Triosil 75%) which are warmed to 38°C before injection. The usual precautions for contrast agents must be taken particularly in excluding patients who have had previous hypersensitivity reactions.

Two or even three injections will be required if the two planes are exposed separately or an oblique projection is needed in addition.

Cardiac angiography

In cardiac angiography a catheter is passed into the appropriate vessel or cardiac chamber, the contrast medium injected and a rapid filming sequence demonstrates its passage through the heart and great vessels.

The catheter is positioned using fluoroscopy with image amplification and television control. Filming is by single or biplane roll film or cut film changer or by cine angiography. The roll film changers can expose at up to 10 films per second, the cut film changers up to 6 films per second and with cine angiography up to 50 frames per second.

Cardiac angiography is used in congenital heart disease, valvular heart disease especially due to rheumatic fever and in ischaemic heart disease to show ventricular dysfunction, cardiac aneurysms and valvular incompetence. Coronary arteriography demonstrates any narrowing of coronary vessels due to atheromatous plaques and selective pulmonary angiography shows the presence of pulmonary infarcts or emboli.

A diagram of the anatomy of the heart and great vessels (2023) shows the circulation of the blood through the cardiac chambers.

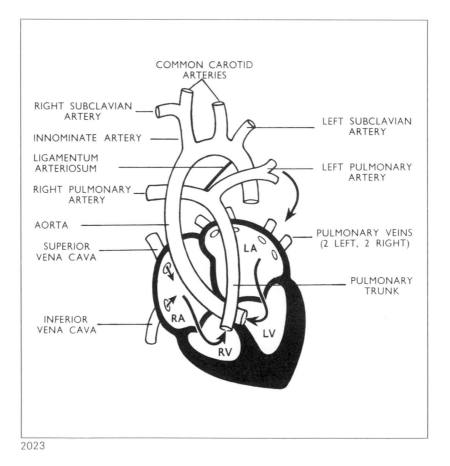

2023

Selective angiography

The catheter is introduced either into a peripheral vein or artery and passed toward the heart.

The ante-cubital vein at the elbow or the femoral vein at the groin are usually selected for right heart catheterisation (2024) to show the vena cava, right atrium, right ventricle or pulmonary artery. In children the catheter often passes through a patent foramen ovale between the atria (2025) and then the left atrium and ventricle can also be examined.

In adults the aorta and left ventricle are approached by retrograde arterial catheterisation usually from the femoral artery.

The vena cavae and right heart can also be shown by a rapid injection of contrast medium into a peripheral vein such as the median cubital vein in the arm (2026) or the femoral vein from the thigh.

General Principles

Preliminary radiographs on the film changer are essential to establish correct exposures. With roll film units this must be done on the previous day because of the inconvenience of removing the exposed film in the dark. The kilovoltage is 10 kV higher to adequately display the contrast filled heart and great vessels.

A meticulous technique is needed in cardiac angiography with unstinting attention to detail for a satisfactory diagnostic result. The procedure is planned beforehand to suit the particular problem and the factors to be considered include radiographic projections, injection site, type and quantity of contrast medium, injection pressure, type of catheter, exposure factors and filming programme. An increased exposure is required for the necessary penetration when dense contrast medium is being used.

Although the filming often only lasts 10–12 seconds it is the culmination of a well planned procedure for which every detail must be arranged in advance; with cassettes or film magazines loaded and in position, exposure factors checked and tested, tubes centred, radiation protection in order and processing equipment ready for use. The patient, often under general anaesthesia, is then positioned to the tubes and films. For the lateral projection foam sponge blocks raise the patient to the correct height relative to the film area.

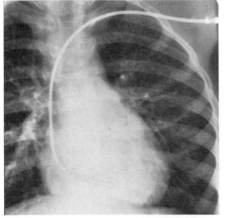
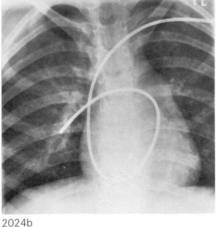

2024a   2024b

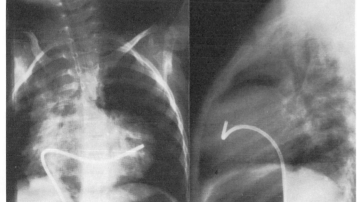
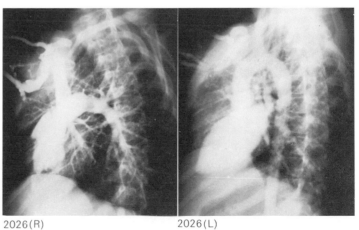

2025a   2025b   2026(R)   2026(L)

X-ray equipment

Simultaneous biplane film changers produce corresponding views at right angles to each other either in lateral and antero-posterior (2028, 2029) or oblique projections (2033a, b) with one injection of contrast medium. Exactly corresponding views are a great advantage in diagnosis, a single contrast injection is much safer for the patient and the procedure is completed more quickly.

The two X-ray tubes, firing simultaneously at right angles to each other can be operated from a single six valve high tension unit using the same kilovoltage and time but dividing the milliamperage approximately between the two tubes. The lateral tube usually requires double the mA of the antero-posterior tube for example 400 mA for the lateral and 200 mA for the antero-posterior tube. It is however an advantage to have two transformers to select quite independent factors for each projection.

Cross hatched grids in front of the film areas eliminate secondary radiation (2027) which is further diminished by selective filtration with thin sheets of tin or lead at the back of each grid. The X-ray beam must be well collimated in each projection to the area being examined to further reduce unwanted scattered radiation.

Cardiac radiographic units have programme selectors which are set in advance to operate the filming automatically, such as three exposures per second for 3 seconds (for the right heart), then two exposures per second for 2 seconds (for the pulmonary circulation) and finally four exposures per second for 4 seconds (for the left heart).

The contrast injection or pump is also automated and interlinked with the filming exposures. Triggering the film sequence thus also triggers the pump to deliver the appropriate quantity of contrast medium at the required pressure.

Positioning and timing

The choice of projections, usually antero-posterior and lateral or right and left antero-posterior obliques depends on the abnormality being investigated and exposures may vary from two to ten per second.

In coarctation of the aorta (2030–2032) projections include the whole length of the thoracic aorta to below the diaphragm particularly for the lateral view and can be covered by two films per second for 8 seconds. An example of coarctation of the aorta in a child is shown in the antero-posterior and oblique views (2030–2032). The arrow indicates the narrowed segment which is usually present at the attachment of the ligamentum arteriosum.

In pulmonary stenosis the antero-posterior and lateral projections are preferred and again filming is at two per second for 8 seconds.

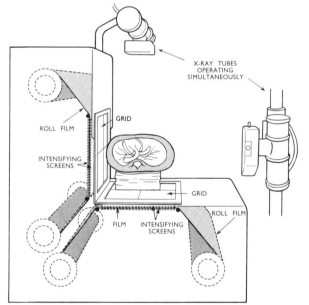

2027

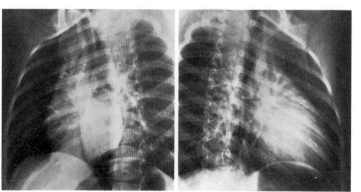

2033a   2033b

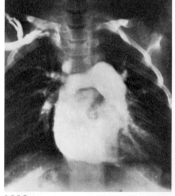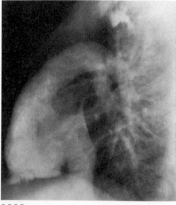

2028   2029

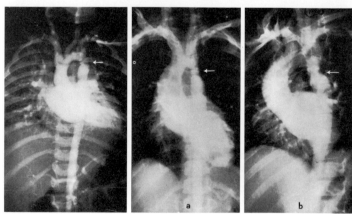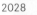

2030   2031   2032

Selective cardiac angiography

The injection of contrast medium as close as possible to the abnormality being investigated has considerable practical and theoretical advantages. The length and time of the examination is reduced with considerably less radiation to the patient using less contrast medium.

For the right heart or pulmonary artery, the catheter is introduced into a large vein such as the antecubital vein at the elbow or the femoral vein in the groin and passed upwards towards the heart, being monitored by fluoroscopy with image intensification. The catheter is positioned for the particular examination required, and may pass through the defect being investigated such as a patent ductus arteriosus (2034, 2035) but requires to be seen in two views for confirmation.

The tip of the catheter is followed fluoroscopically often passing through the superior vena cava, right atrium, right ventricle (2036), across the pulmonary valve and into the pulmonary artery (2037). Pressure recordings and blood samples are taken for gas analysis as required from each position.

The contrast medium is delivered by an automatic pressure injector which also triggers the programmed film sequence with exposures being made at a rate of up to 10 films per second on roll film or 50 per second on cine-angiography.

There is a great variation in the amount of contrast medium required especially with age and with the condition being investigated. In infants of 3–4 weeks with a weight of 4–6 lbs (1·5–3.7 kilo) 8–10 ml of metrizoate 75 % is quite common, at 5–7 years and a weight of about 40 lbs (18 kilo), 30 ml and in adults 50–60 ml.

Typical exposures for an infant (1), child (2) and adult (3), are as follows

	kVp		MAS	FFD	Film ILFORD	Screens ILFORD	Grid
	AP	Lat					
(1)	65	85	2	100 cm (40″)	RAPID R	FT	Grid
(2)	75	95	2	100 cm (40″)	RAPID R	FT	Grid
(3)	105	125	5	100 cm (40″)	RAPID R	FT	Grid

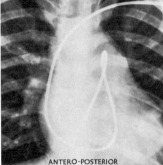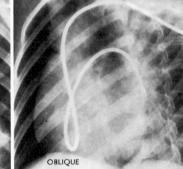

ANTERO-POSTERIOR OBLIQUE

2034 2035

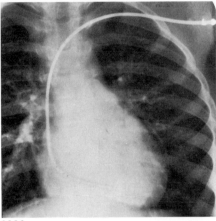

2036

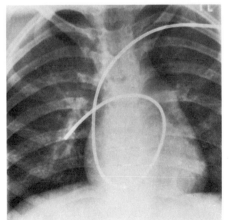

2037

In infants the catheter is commonly passed upwards from the femoral vein and inferior vena cava to the right heart (2038) but may pass into the left heart either through a patent foramen ovale or interventricular septal defect. The position of the tip of the catheter is confirmed fluoroscopically by viewing in two planes at right angles to each other.

After injection of contrast medium films were taken at 8 films per second and selected films at one second (2039) shows contrast medium in the right ventricle passing through a ventricular septal defect into the aorta with only minimal contrast medium passing into the pulmonary artery (2040, 2041) at $1\frac{1}{2}$ and $1\frac{3}{4}$ seconds.

Coronary angiography

Selective coronary angiography is often a routine procedure in cardiac centres but occasional examinations in any department are contraindicated. A practiced and well prepared team is essential. Percutaneous catheterisation is usually used with the left and right coronary arteries requiring different shaped, preformed catheters.

Rapid sequence cine with either the patient or the tube rotating is needed to show the coronary artery in its entire length to exclude asymmetrical stenoses or those hidden by toruosity of the artery.

Repeat angiography may be required following by-pass surgery and the technique is modified according to the procedure used.

Left ventricular angiography is often also performed prior to operation to exclude significant left ventricular dyskinesia or an actual left ventricular aneurysm.

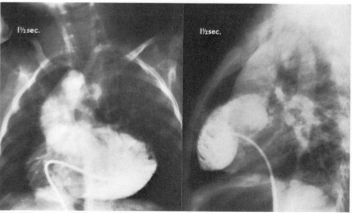

2038

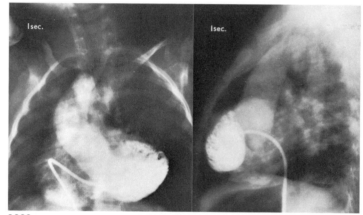

2039

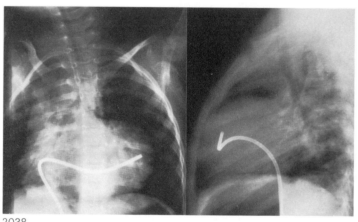

2040

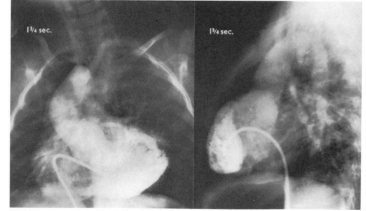

2041

Superior vena cavography or Veno-cardiography

The superior vena cava can be shown by contrast injection into either one or both median antecubital veins. For veno-cardiography (2042–2049) a wide bore cannula is inserted into a median antecubital vein and strapped into position. A large rapidly injected bolus of contrast medium is needed but the dilution nevertheless results in a poor demonstration of the cardiac chambers and pulmonary arteries.

The contrast medium reaches the pulmonary artery in $2\frac{1}{2}$–3 seconds and the aorta in 4–6 seconds. Filming is therefore continued for 8–10 seconds.

The contrast medium can be shown to pass down the superior vena cava into the right atrium (2042), right ventricle (2043, 0·5 sec) into the pulmonary arteries (2044–2047, 1·3–3·5 secs) back into the left atrium (2048, 7 secs) and thence into the aorta (2049, 8·5 secs). However, the opacification of the left ventricle and aorta is usually too poor for diagnostic purposes (2048, 2049).

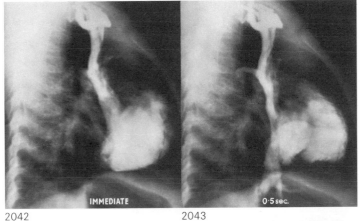

2042   2043

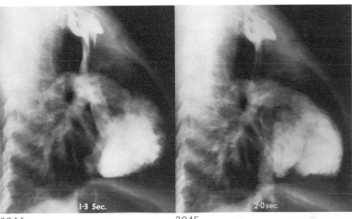

2044   2045

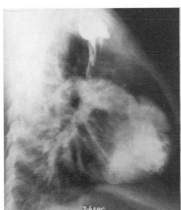

2046   2047

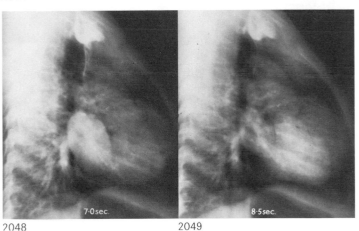

2048   2049

Veno-cardiography

Films may be taken in the frontal (2050, 2051) and oblique projections (2052, 2053) and annotated diagrams at the side of each radiograph shows the relevant anatomy. In the frontal view at 3 seconds the superior vena cava, right atrium and pulmonary arteries contain contrast medium (2050) and at 6 seconds the left atrium, left ventricle and aorta (2051).

In the left anterior oblique position (2052, 2053) the left subclavian artery, superior vena cava, right atrium, right ventricle and left pulmonary artery are shown at 3 seconds and at 7½ seconds, the left atrium, left ventricle and aorta contain contrast medium but the shadow of the right ventricle persists suggesting the presence of an interventricular septal defect causing a left to right shunt (2053). However veno-cardiography produces poor opacification of the left atrium. left, ventricle and aorta and therefore selective angiography is preferred.

For all cardio-angiography strict aseptic precautions are essential together with monitoring of vital signs especially the ECG and blood pressure.

Cine angiography

Cine angiography is particularly useful in paediatric cases and in coronary angiography. The recording is through image amplification, with pulsed exposures to minimise radiation, onto 35 mm film with a cine camera, and with simultaneous video recording, immediate playback is possible.

Modern 35 mm film can be processed by departmental automatic processors and are viewed on special equipment such as the Tagiano or Steenberg which allows playback at various speeds in both forward and backward directions and the viewing of single frames as stills or sequentially.

Subtraction
Subtraction technique

Dense bone shadows frequently overlie opacified arteries in angiography, obscuring detail and degrading the diagnostic information. By a photographic process it is possible to remove the unwanted bone shadows, showing the blood vessels more clearly—a process called subtraction.

Photographic subtraction consists essentially of 4 stages, taking a control radiograph for the bone, forming a reversed image, exactly superimposing the reversed image on the arteriogram to subtract the bone and then making a final copy of the subtracted angiogram.

Stage 1

The **plain film** (2054a) of the bone image is taken immediately before the contrast is injected and the patient must be immobilised so that no movement occurs otherwise subsequent superimposition of the bone shadows will be poor or completely ineffective.

The technical factors must be the same in the preliminary exposure as in the arteriogram and must give good penetration of bone.

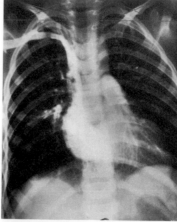
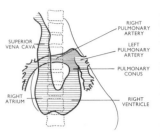

2050

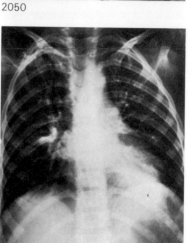
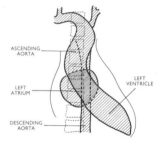

2051

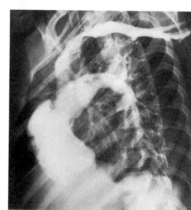
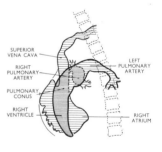

2052

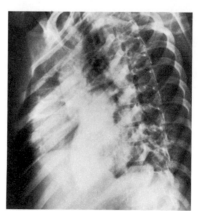
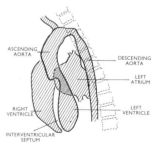

2053

Stage 2

A reversal contact print of the initial or control film is made to give a **positive transparency** with an overall dark grey appearance. The film should have a contrast scale which can record the complete tone range of the original radiograph such as Ilford fine-grain ordinary photographic film. The image must be fully exposed and developed.

Stage 3

The film showing the contrast filled blood vessels (2054b) and the positive transparency are **exactly superimposed** (2054c) to cancel out the bone shadows and show the contrast filled blood vessels unobscured by the overlying bone.

Stage 4

The exactly superimposed films are kept in position and a contact print onto a fine grain standard film is made. Unless the two films are kept perfectly superimposed, the detail in the subtraction arteriogram will be lost.

The positive transparency can also be produced by a X-ray exposure screen method.

Screen method

Formation of positive transparency

The front fluorescent screen in a cassette is blacked out and the initial or plain film is in contact with an unexposed film in the cassette.

Exposure factors

The cassette is then exposed at 50 kilovolts, 3 mAs at 120 cm and has standard processing to produce the positive transparency or mask. This is then used to superimpose on the selected film of the arteriogram.

The two superimposed films with the bone subtracted can then be printed for a permanent record of the arteriogram.

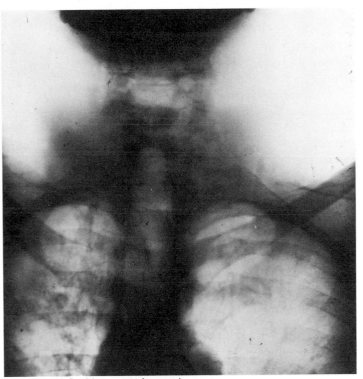

2054a　　(1) Positive copy of control

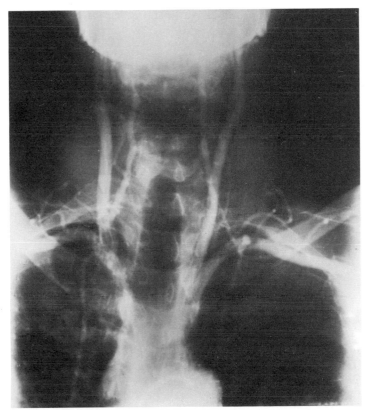

2054b　　(2) Angiogram

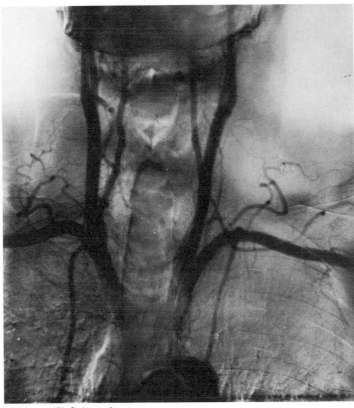

2054c　　(3) Subtraction

In cerebral angiography subtraction radiography is particularly valuable to show angiographic detail at the skull base and in the orbit, as illustrated in (2055a, b) in a boy aged 13 who developed a post-traumatic carotico-cavernous fistula. The cavernous sinus and orbital veins become clearly visible on the subtraction film when not obscured by bone. Similarly in a woman of 53 years the orbital meningioma is shown on the subtraction film (2055d) when poorly seen on the arteriogram (2055c). The final film is usually shown as a positive print to accentuate the contrast filled blood vessels.

Further examples of the value of subtraction radiography in a four vessel angiogram (2056a, b) and in an aortogram for renal arteries (2057, 2058) indicate the value of this photographic method to bring out the full information inherent in arteriography.

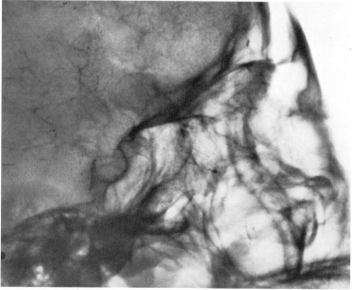

2055a (1) Angiogram

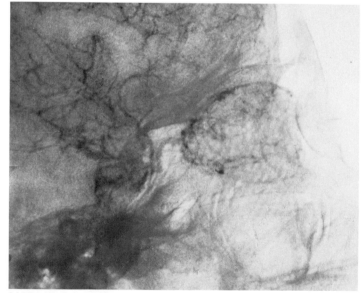

2055b (2) Subtraction

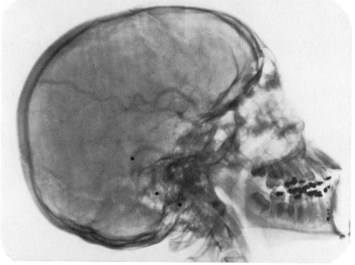

2055c (1) Angiogram

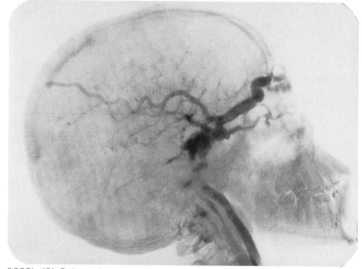

2055d (2) Subtraction

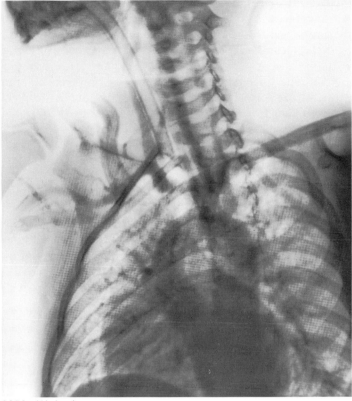

2056a (1) Angiogram

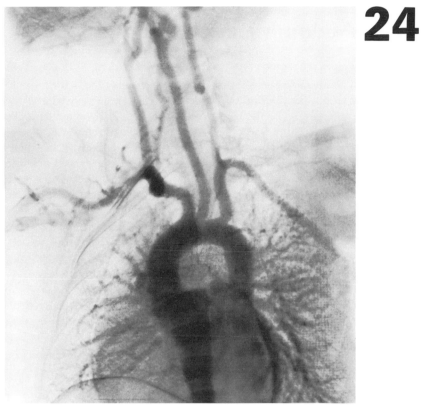

2056b (2) Subtraction

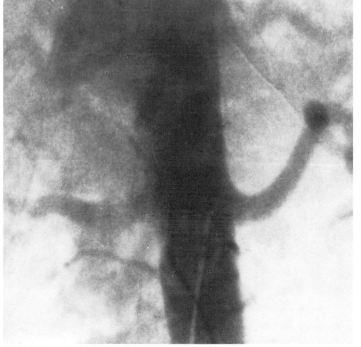

2057 Subtraction

2058 Aortogram

24 Abdominal aortography

The thoracic aorta passes below the crura of the diaphragm to become the abdominal aorta at the level of $D_{11/12}$ behind the oesophagus and then lies close to the vertebral bodies just to the left of the midline. The aorta continues downwards in this position to about $L_{4/5}$ when it divides into common iliac arteries (2059). The aorta commonly calcifies in the elderly and the walls become visible especially on the lateral view but otherwise will only be demonstrated on radiographs when containing contrast medium. However ultrasonography and computed tomography, especially the former is now preferred as the initial examination for the aorta because no catheterisation is needed.

With abdominal aortography, atheromatous stenoses and aneurysms can be localised pre-operatively with accurate delineation of major branches such as the renal arteries and the collateral circulation. However, for the angiographic demonstration of masses within organs, selective catheterisation of the feeding artery is advised.

Aortography shows not only the aortic calibre which may be markedly reduced (2059) but also the major branches namely the renal arteries, coeliac axis and mesenteric arteries as well as the lumbar arteries and finally the bifarcation to form the common iliac arteries. The common iliac arteries divide into external and internal iliacs and the external iliac into the superficial and deep femoral arteries (2059, 2060).

Contrast agents
Aortography usually produces a marked burning sensation in the buttocks and down the legs which is much less marked with methyl glucamine (meglumine) salts (Conray '280') and virtually absent with the dimer ioxaglate (Hexabrix) or metrizamide (Amipaque). Amipaque is however far too expensive for aortography but the dimer compounds are likely to be available for arteriography in the near future. 30–40 ml of contrast medium is used preferably injected with a pressure pump.

Methods
Contrast medium is injected into the aorta by either direct needle puncture using the translumbar approach (2059, 2067–2069) or percutaneous catheterisation usually from below via the femoral artery (2065, 2066). For the translumbar direct needle puncture, the patient is in the prone position and the examination is usually performed under general anaesthesia. The percutaneous femoral approach is done with the patient supine using a local anaesthetic.

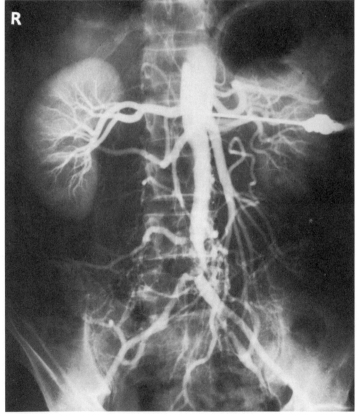

2059

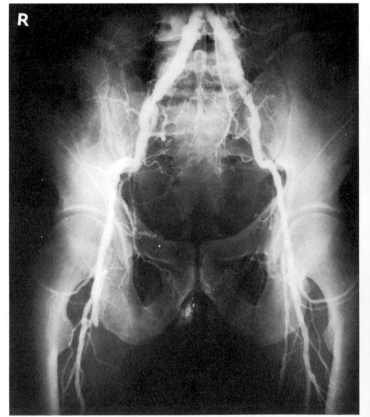

2060

Cassette and film changers

Multiple exposures are used to show the aorta and its branches; a minimum of 4–5 with a manual cassette changer and 8–10 with an automatic film changer.

The Schönander film changer (2061) can take up to thirty 35 × 35 cm (14 × 14 ins) films which are stored in a steel box inside the changer and fed over a roller into position between two intensifying screens lying behind a grid. Just before each exposure the intensifying screens are compressed onto the film and released after the exposure. The exposed film is moved on by a roller to be stored in a light tight box within the changer which is removed at the end of the procedure.

The automatic changer is programmed for each examination and varies with different patients depending on the clinical problem and therefore the examination must be planned in advance.

Cassette changers may be automated or may be manually operated, and are frequently designed for both abdominal and lower limb arteriography (2063). In the example shown three 35 × 43 cm (14 × 17 ins) and three 35 × 92 cm (14 × 36 ins) cassettes are held in brass trays which are sufficiently radiopaque to protect films below and further brass

plates are positioned on either side of the radiographic window, the lower plate being movable (2063). Both the cassette trays and lower brass plate have attached cords to move them into and out of the exposed field. In the upper diagram the changer is prepared for an abdominal aortogram and in the lower diagram for a lower limb arteriogram. The lower limb exposures require a wide tube aperture and a long focal-film distance. A graduated aluminium wedge filter (2064) at the tube aperture compensates for the differences in tissue density from hip to the ankle while for the abdominal films there is a small square aperture in the double diaphragm (2064). Two 35 × 43 cm (14 × 17 ins) cassettes placed end-to-end may be used in place of the long 35 × 92 cm (14 × 36 ins) cassette.

Similar cassette changers have been automated bringing the cassettes and protective plates into position during the examination. This system was originally developed at St. Bartholomew's Hospital in London.

A simple cassette changer for abdominal aortography moves a 35 × 35 cm (14 × 14 ins) cassette longitudinally into position for each exposure and then out of the field to be replaced by the next cassette (2062).

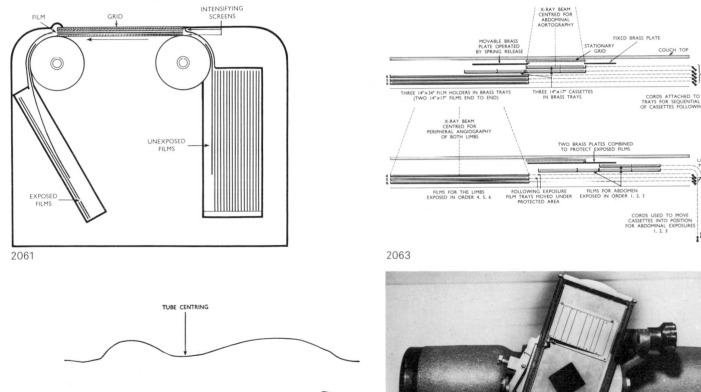

2061

2063

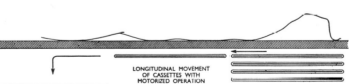

2062

2064

Retrograde femoral catheterisation

In catheter aortography the patient is supine and local anaesthesia is used, making this the preferred examination. A preliminary film of the required region is taken with the patient positioned over the film changer and should be 8–10 kVp higher than the usual abdominal film to show the aorta filled with contrast medium over the spine.

After the area has been anaesthetised the femoral artery is punctured under strict aseptic conditions and a flexible guide wire is passed into the artery through the needle. The needle is removed leaving the guide wire in position and then an opaque catheter is threaded over the guide wire up the iliac artery into the aorta to the required position. The guide wire is removed and the position of the catheter checked fluoroscopically.

When the catheter has been satisfactorily positioned 20–30 ml of contrast medium is injected usually with a pressure injector and a series of films are exposed in rapid succession to show the aorta, its major branches and the smaller peripheral arteries especially to the kidneys (2065). In a late film at 7–10 seconds the renal parenchyma is 'stained' with contrast medium producing the nephrogram phase of the examination (2066).

The early film (2065) at 0·5 sec shows the aorta, splenic, hepatic, superior mesenteric and renal arteries, at 2·0 secs the small arteries are visible and on the late film at 7 secs the nephrogram or tissue staining phase (2066).

Translumbar aortography

The aorta and iliac arteries can also be demonstrated by direct needle puncture from the back, the translumbar route. The patient is therefore in the prone position for this examination. A general anaesthetic is required and the contrast medium is injected by hand (2067–2069).

A preliminary film is taken with the patient prone over a suitable film changer and a long needle is inserted from the left side to enter the aorta at the level of the first or second lumbar vertebra. A small test injection is given for a further control film to show the position of the needle tip and if satisfactory following viewing 20–30 ml of contrast medium is injected by hand. A series of films are exposed in rapid sequence using a film or cassette changer.

A typical series for translumbar aortography (2067–2068) shows the long needle inserted from the left side, the very early film (2067) with minimal contrast above the level of the needle tip, contrast in the splenic, hepatic, superior mesenteric and renal arteries (2068a, 2069) the aortic bifurcation and smaller arteries (2068a) and the late film after the contrast has been cleared from the aorta and iliac arteries shows the early nephrogram phase (2068b).

Close co-operation and team work is needed particularly for the manually operated changer as after each exposure the top cassette must be removed ready for the next exposure. For a typical aortogram 5–10 films are taken at one or two per

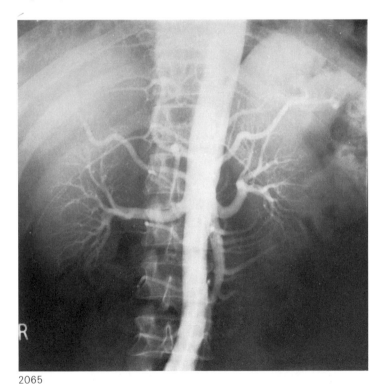

2065

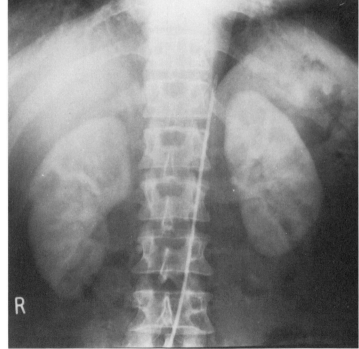

2066

second. The first film is exposed after 15 ml of contrast medium has been injected and usually a total of 25–30 ml of contrast medium is used.

Typical exposure factors for abdominal arteriography are as follows

kVp	mAs	FFD	Film ILFORD	Screen ILFORD	Grid
90	20	100 cm (40″)	RAPID R	FT	Moving

Lateral aortography

Lateral aortography is required to show the origins of the coeliac axis and mesenteric arteries and is usually done with the patient supine using a transfermoral percutaneous catheter technique. A horizontal beam with a lateral film changer will be needed in this position. If not available, the patient must be turned onto his side following insertion of the abdominal aortic catheter. (2070)

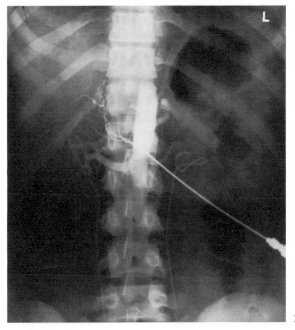

2067

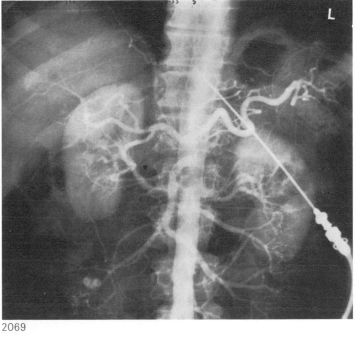

2069

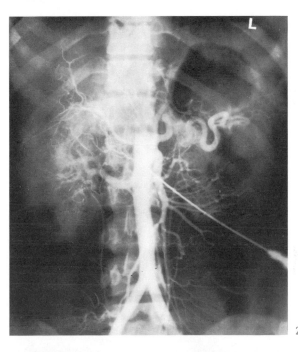

2068a

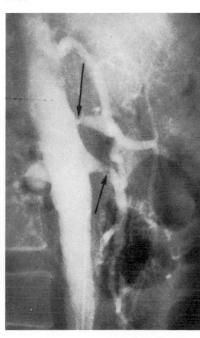

2070

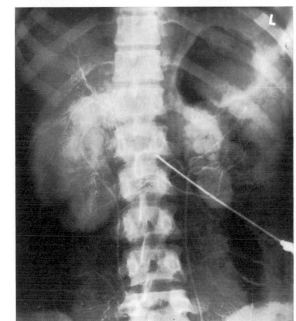

2068b

Renal arteriography

Although the renal arteries and their branches can be shown by translumbar aortography (2059–2069) a transfermoral catheter technique is now almost invariably used. Catheter arteriography has the major advantage of allowing both a free flush intraluminal injection of contrast medium (2065) and selective injection into a single renal artery (2071, 2074, 2075). For renal arteriography the needle or catheter tip is somewhat higher than for aortography, being at the $D_{11/12}$ level and the coeliac axis with its hepatic and splenic artery branches are usually also shown (2065, 2069).

The film sequence for renal arteriography is essentially similar to aortography but an early film to show the origin of the renal arteries unobscured by the superior mesenteric artery and a late film at 10–15 secs for the nephrogram phase are particularly important.

Selective renal arteriography

With midstream injections or "free-flush" aortograms the renal arteries are often partially obscured by overlying mesenteric arteries degrading the diagnostic information. With selective renal arteriography only the renal vessels and branches are shown (2071, 2074, 2075).

A pre-shaped catheter is introduced into the aorta as for catheter aortography. However when the guide wire is removed from within the catheter it reverts to its hook or C-shaped curve (2073, 2075) and under fluoroscopic control is manipulated into a renal artery. With a small test injection of contrast medium its position is checked on the television monitor (2074).

The X-ray beam is well collimated to just cover the renal area and catheter (2071) and a series of films are exposed to show the major renal vessels, intrarenal arterioles, capillary and venous phase (2071–2073) and a late film for the nephrogram.

Not infrequently a kidney has two renal arteries (2077) and then each must be catheterised and examined in turn.

Much smaller quantities of contrast medium are used in selective arteriography, 8–10 ml being sufficient for a renal artery and usually injected by hand.

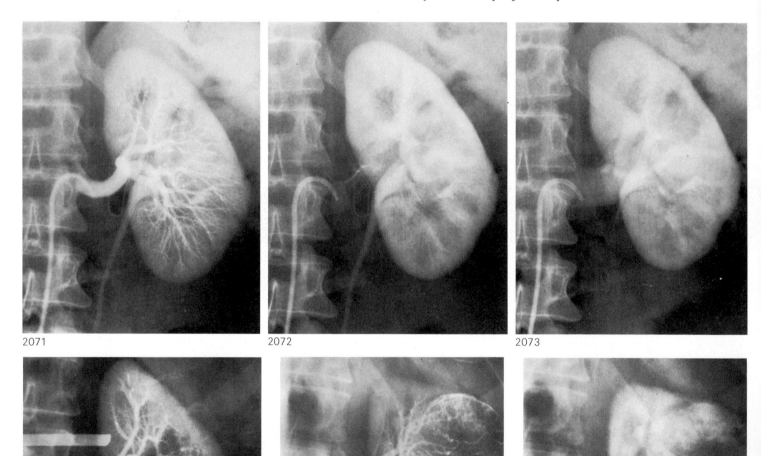

2071

2072

2073

2074

2075

2076

Angio-tomography

Where overlying structures obscure detail it is possible to obtain better definition by tomography (2078, 2079) but has been superseded by subtraction radiography and selective angiography.

Spleno-portography

The splenic and portal veins can be shown by the injection of contrast medium directly into the splenic pulp (spleno-portography), after selective arteriography of the splenic or superior mesenteric arteries to show the venous phase (arterio-portography) or after transhepatic injection into the portal venous system (transhepatic portography).

Precautions

Before splenic or hepatic punctures are undertaken any bleeding tendency must be excluded by the appropriate tests.

Spleno-portography

With the patient supine the spleen is punctured and the splenic pressure measured. 30–40 ml of contrast medium is injected and a series of film of the upper abdomen are exposed. One film per second for 10 seconds and then one film every other second for a further 5 seconds is a typical sequence. The splenic and portal veins are shown and any collateral vessels especially the para-oesophageal group which produce oesophageal varices in portal hypertension (2080).

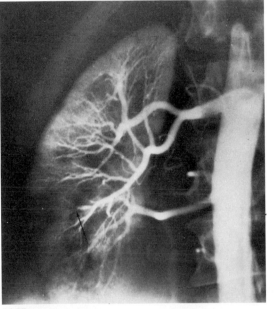

2077

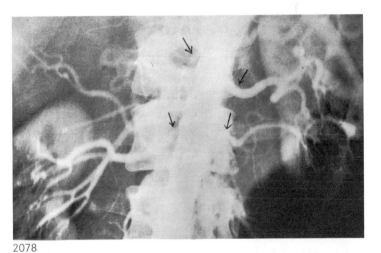

2078

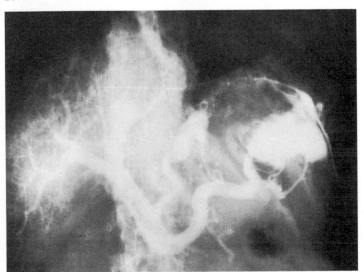

2080

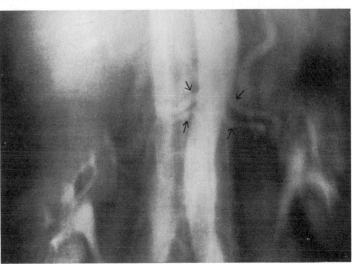

2079

Arterio-venography of the portal system

Selective catheterisation of the coeliac axis or superior mesenteric arteries (2081) is performed, usually by the transfermoral percutaneous method as for selective renal arteriography. After positioning the catheter well into the splenic or mesenteric artery 50–60 ml of contrast medium is injected with a pressure injector. A film series on an automatic film changer taken at one per second for 10 seconds followed by one every other second for 10 seconds will show both the arterial and venous phase (2081,2082). A preliminary film immediately prior to the contrast injection should always be done for subsequent subtraction radiography.

Transhepatic portography

The portal venous system can also be examined by direct needle puncture of the liver to locate a large intrahepatic vein. A flexible guide wire is then passed into the portal vein, the needle removed and a catheter threaded over the guide wire in the same way as percutaneous femoral arteriography.

Retrograde injections of contrast medium show the portal venous system and any collateral veins.

This method has also been used to selectively catheterise the collateral left gastric oesophageal venous plexus for obliteration therapy in bleeding oesophageal varices.

Selective visceral arteriography

Selective coeliac axis arteriography (2083)
(hepatic and splenic arteriography)

The coleiac axis arises from the anterior aspect of the aorta at the level of D12/L1 and divides in the hepatic, left gastric and splenic arteries. Selective coeliac axis arteriography shows both the liver and spleen but for even greater detail the tip of the catheter is passed further into either the hepatic or splenic arteries. Hepatic, splenic and left gastric selective arteriography is used to show vascular lesions, the site of haemorrhage in upper gastrointestinal bleeding, tumour pathology (2084) and the size and patency of the spleno-portal venous system (2085).

Selective superior and inferior mesenteric arteriography

The superior mesenteric artery arises about 2 cm below the coeliac axis at about the level of the first lumbar vertebral body and the inferior mesenteric at the L4/5 level. Both arteries come off the anterior aspect of the aorta.

Selective mesenteric arteriography (2086) is similar to coeliac axis arteriography but shows the arterial and venous supply to the small and large bowel.

Selective pancreatic arteriography

The pancreatic arteries can be demonstrated by catheterising the gastroduodenal artery, a branch of the hepatic artery or the dorsal pancreatic artery which often arises from the coeliac axis (2087).

Small pancreatic tumours especially endocrine adenomas such as insulinomas are well shown by selective pancreatic arteriography. Antero-posterior and left-anterior oblique views are needed and a preliminary non-contrast film for radiographic subtraction must always be taken.

Radiographs

2081 Selective arteriography of a common splenic-superior mesenteric artery with a replaced right hepatic.

2082 is the venous phase with a clearly visible splenic and portal vein. Thus, the combined examination (2081, 2082) is known as arterio-portography.

2083 is a normal coeliac axis arteriogram for showing hepatic, splenic and left gastric arteries.

2084 malignant circulation of a right hepatoma is demonstrated from a selective coeliac axis arteriogram.

2085 is the venous phase of a selective coeliac axis arteriovenogram showing a patent splenic and portal vein which drains into the inferior vena cava following a porto-caval shunt operation for portal hypertension.

2086 Selective arteriogram of the superior mesenteric artery in the supine right anterior oblique position.

2087 Selective coeliac axis arteriogram (subtraction radiography) showing a pancreatic carcinoma. (By kind permission of Dr H. Herlinger.)

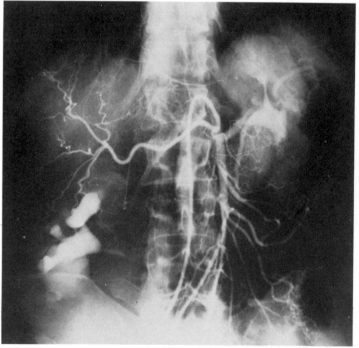

2081

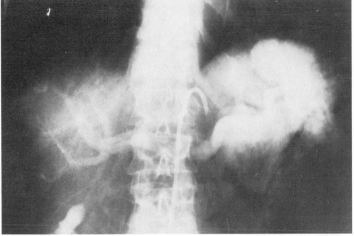

2082

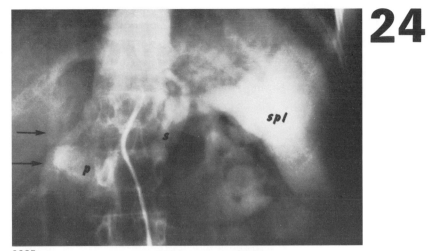

2085

Key to 2085
spl spleen
s splenic vein
p portal vein

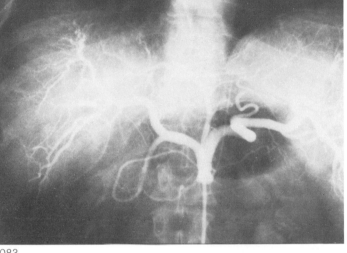

2083

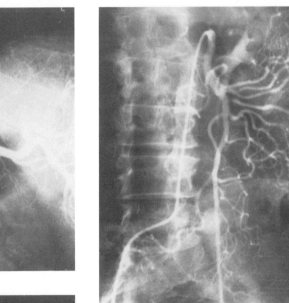

2086

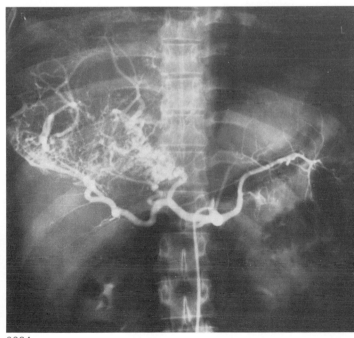

2084

2087

Lower limb arteriography

For atheromatous disease producing arterial narrowing and occlusion, bilateral lower limb arteriography is invariably indicated and most commonly performed by retrograde catheterisation of the femoral artery with the tip of the catheter in the lower aorta. The examination must include the pelvis showing the lower aorta, and the thighs down to the ankles.

However, for focal pathology such as bone tumours only one side needs to be examined and often a downstream selective catheterisation is performed.

For a bilateral lower limb arteriogram 20–30 ml of contrast medium is used and for a unilateral examination 15–20 ml. A non-reactive, normo- or low osmolar tri-odinated compound such as meglumine iothalamate or diatrizoate 60% or a dimer such as meglumine ioxaglate 60% should be used.

Scanography method

A slit diaphragm $\frac{1}{16}$ in wide providing 1 cm ($\frac{1}{2}$ in) cover on the film at 100 cm (40 ins) FFD with its long axis at right angles to the long axis of the limb, limits the tube aperture and X-ray beam. To compensate for the varying tissue thickness from thigh to foot the speed of the continuously exposing tube is increased below the knee. The total exposure is approximately 8 secs, 5 secs for the tube movement from hip to knee and 3 secs from knee to foot (2088). The examination is usually done with a local anaesthetic.

With the patient supine and the lower limb over a single 102×30 cm (40×12 ins) cassette or two 51×30 cm (20×12 ins) cassettes placed end to end, the exposure starts after 10 ml of contrast has been injected. For lateral or oblique views a further injection is needed.

Alternatively with a moving top table the tube can remain stationary, central over the hip region and the table top moved at a similar speed towards the tube.

The scanography method can be used for one limb or both lower limbs simultaneously, for the latter a wide slit beam and cassette is needed. If a long film is not available, 3 or 4 single films can be placed end to end in the cassette (2089, 2090).

The depth of the slit should at least be the size of the width to avoid the effects of penumbra.

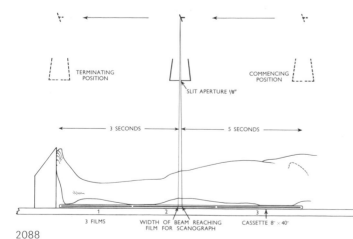

2088

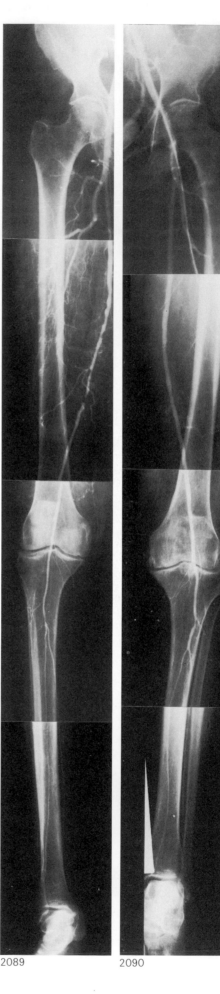

2089   2090

Manual changer

A simple manual changer can be coupled to the tube and both the tube and changer can move together to take separate exposures of each part of the lower limb in turn namely, pelvis and upper thigh, middle thigh, and leg to ankle.

Serial changer and moving table top

Peripheral arteriography is now usually carried out with an automatic film changer and automated movement of the table top. However when an automated table top is not available the table top can be moved manually across the serial changer.

An alternative method is shown in (2063) which uses movable cassettes.

Where separate cassettes are used for each region comparable radiographic density can be obtained by changing the exposure factors, by using screens of different speeds or by a balance of screen and non-screen film.

The examination must show the whole length of the artery. The contrast medium will be markedly slowed if the artery is obstructed (2091–2093) and the timing of the exposures must be varied accordingly.

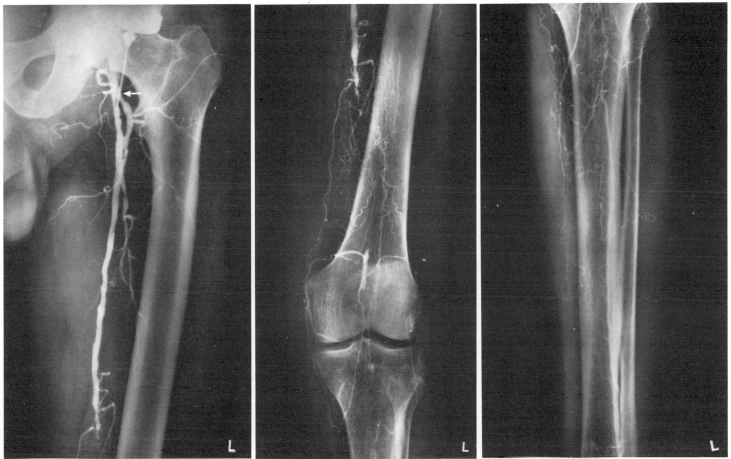

2091   2092   2093

Xero-radiography with veno-arteriography

The lower limb arteries below the pubic ramus can be shown from a contrast injection into an antecubital vein with the use of a special changer for xero-radiography which takes one exposure per second for eight seconds. 55–65 ml of 70% contrast medium is injected in 7–10 secs after warming to 38°C. For the popliteal region and leg the films are taken in the lateral position and the interval between films is 3 seconds thus covering a 24 second period.

Exposure factors are 80 kV, FFD at 120 cm (50 ins) with varying mAs, for thigh 100–120 and calf 80–10 mAs using Xerox system 125, with contrast selector at D and density selector at C.

Post-mortem radiography

Injection of contrast medium into arteries after death fills many more small vessels (2094) than is usually shown by in life angiography.

Brachial arteriography

Contrast medium is injected either by direct needle puncture into the brachial or subclavian or by a catheter introduced into the subclavian artery (2095) via the transfermoral-aortic route. 10–15 ml of a non-reactive contrast medium such as meglumine dimer (Hexabrix) or anionic contrast (Amipaque) is used and the examination can then be done under local anaesthetic.

A film changer with exposures taken one per second for 5–10 seconds will show both the arterial and venous phase and is used for angiomatous malformations (2096a—arterial phase; 2096b venous phase) and embolic occlusion.

Macroradiography

Direct enlargement radiography using a fine focus tube of 0·1 or 0·3 mm can give ×2 enlargement and an 0·6 mm focus ×1½ enlargement with an appropriate "air-gap" to replace the grid for eliminating scattered radiation. Macroradiography is particularly useful in congenital heart disease in infants, in renal angiography and in angiography of the hand and orbit (Section 26).

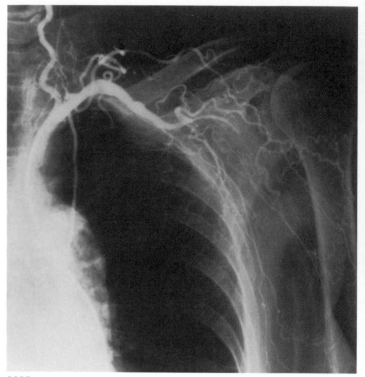

2095

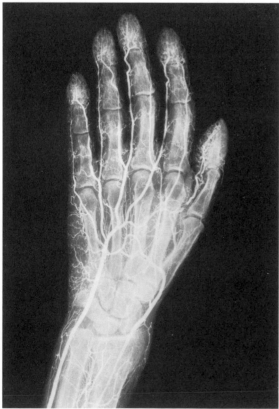

2094

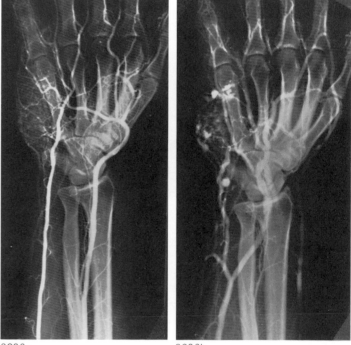

2096a   2096b

Angiography
Lower limb venography

Thrombosis in the large veins of the lower limb is a common cause of pulmonary embolism and infarction. The site and extent of venous thrombosis can be demonstrated by lower limb phlebography.

A butterfly needle is inserted into a vein on the dorsum of the foot. While the superficial veins around the ankle are compressed with a Velcro band or narrow sphygmomanometer cuff, 50 ml of contrast medium such as Conray '280' or Hexabrix 60% is injected with the patient supine and tilted feet down to about 45°. Films are taken of the leg in the frontal and lateral projections using fluroscopic control with image amplification and television monitoring. The table is brought to the horizontal position to move the contrast medium up the limb into the pelvis, while further films are taken of the popliteal femoral and iliac veins. Immediately afterwards the cuff is released and all the contrast medium flushed out of the veins with half strength saline or 5% glucose solution and no more is injected till the veins are no longer visible.

Venous thrombus shows as intraluminal filling defects (2097a).

Venous thrombus may also appear in the iliac veins which may show from an injection into the foot but for detailed views of the iliac veins and inferior vena cava a venous cannula is inserted into the femoral vein by percutaneous puncture using local anaesthesia (2098).

Lower limb phlebography is also used to show the site and number of incompetent perforating veins in the leg associated with varicose veins and to show incompetent venous valves in the thigh or leg (2100). Incompetent valves are demonstrated by retrograde flow of contrast medium on forced expiration with the nose and mouth closed—the Valsalva manoeuvre. The Valsalva manoeuvre normally slows the flow of contrast and accentuates the demonstration of the venous valves (2099a compared with 2099b).

Inferior vena cavography

The inferior vena cava can be displaced by retroperitoneal tumours, infiltrated by carcinoma such as a hypernephroma or occluded by thrombus (2098a). The azygos venous system then acts as a collateral venous pathway.

Contrast medium such as 50 ml of meglumine diatrizoate 60% is injected into the femoral or iliac veins by a cannula inserted under local anaesthesia and films taken at 1 per second for 6–10 seconds on a film changer (2098b).

Radiograph (2098a) shows a thrombus in the inferior vena cava with contrast medium entering the azygos venous system and (2098b) is an inferior vena cavogram with bilateral catheters in the iliac veins. There is also contrast medium in lymph nodes from a previous lymphogram and contrast medium in the spinal theca from a previous myelogram.

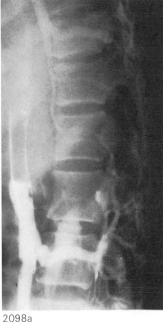
2098a

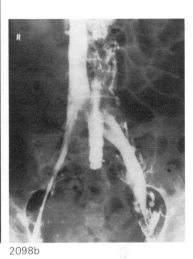
2098b

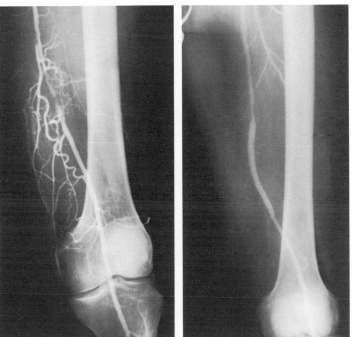
2097a

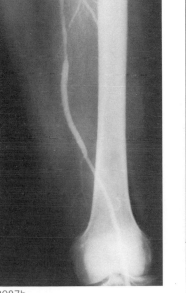
2097b

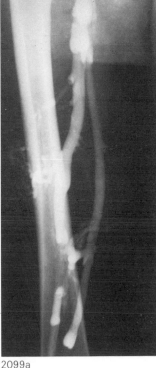
2099a

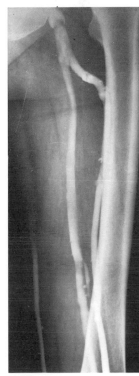
2099b

Hepatic venography

The hepatic veins drain blood from the liver into the inferior vena cava and when obstructed cause marked swelling of the liver, together with ascites (Budd-Chiari syndrome).

In "wedged" hepatic venography the catheter is manipulated into a hepatic vein from either the superior or inferior vena cava via the antecubital or femoral vein respectively, and passed into the periphery of the liver where it is wedged in a small hepatic vein. 10–15 ml of contrast medium is injected by hand to show the hepatic sinusoids and veins of the liver (2101a).

Renal venography

The renal veins become apparent in the late phase of selective renal arteriography but are usually not very densely opacified (2073). For a more detailed examination the renal vein must be catheterised and injected with contrast medium.

Selective venography (2101b) has also been used for demonstrating suprarenal tumours and thymomas but has now been largely replaced by non-invasive scanning methods such as computed tomography, ultrasonography and isotope scanning.

One of the main purposes of venous catheterisation is blood sampling for the detection of abnormal levels of endocrine substances as for example in the diagnosis of suprarenal tumours or of insulinomas in the pancreas.

Venous catheterisation like arteriography requires fluoroscopy preferably with image amplification and television monitoring.

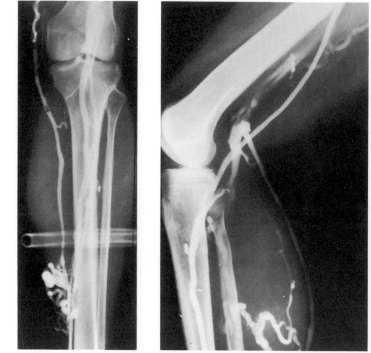

2100

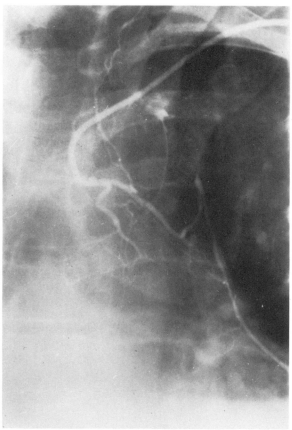

2101b

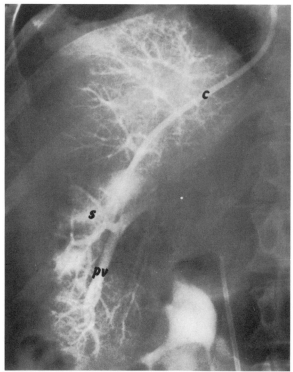

2101a

Key to 2101a
c catheter
s splenic vein
pv portal vein

Lymphography

Anatomy

All organs apart from the central nervous system have lymphatics to drain away the interstitial fluid. The lymphatic system forms an extensive network of fine capillaries which join up to form long fine vessels which have a beaded appearance due to valves at about 5 mm intervals. Lymph nodes are interpolated at varying intervals along the course of the lymphatic vessels with entering or afferent lymphatics and leaving of efferent lymphatics. The lymph nodes produce lymphocytes and also filter the clear lymphatic fluid draining into them, removing bacteria and foreign particles.

The lymphatics usually shown on lymphangiography are the subcutaneous vessels of the leg corresponding to the saphenous vein and then accompanying the iliac vessels and aorta till they drain into the cisterna chyli. The cisterna chyli drains into the thoracic duct which lies on the spine behind the aorta and eventually drains into the left subclavian vein.

Lymph is a clear colourless fluid containing lymphocytes making lymph vessels barely visible to the naked eye as fine white lines about the size of a thread of cotton but are easily seen if the lymph is stained with a dye such as patent violet blue. The subcutaneous lymph vessels are then even visible through the skin.

Lymphography is used mainly in the staging and diagnosis of lymphoma and testicular tumours for paraaortic and pelvic disease but has also been used in carcinoma cervix, melanoma and renal carcinoma. The abdominal lymph nodes are shown after contrast medium has been injected into lymphatics of the feet, but lymphography has now been largely replaced by computed tomography.

Method

Lower limb

The first two web spaces of each foot are anaesthetised and then 1 ml of 10% patent blue violet is injected into each of the anaesthetised web spaces. The patient should then move his feet and toes to and fro preferably by walking around for ten minutes, to fill the superficial lymphatics of the feet with blue dye which are seen as thin blue lines through the skin.

With the patient supine preferably on a fluoroscopy couch, local anaesthetic is injected subcutaneously around a visible lymphatic on the dorsum of the foot. The "blue" lymphatic is disected out through a small incision and cannulated with a fine needle-catheter system which is tied in position and strapped to the skin. Ultra-fluid lipiodol is injected slowly into the lymphatic with a pump, to a maximum of 7 ml of contrast medium for each leg; the injection taking 1–2 hours. Immediately the pump is connected the lymphatics in the lower leg become radiopaque with contrast medium (2102) and are visible on fluoroscopy or on filming provided the contrast medium is being injected correctly. Fluoroscopic or radiographic control is an essential part of the procedure.

The injection is stopped when the contrast medium reaches the level of $L_{1/2}$ or when 7 ml has been injected into each foot.

The lymph vessels are shown in the lower limbs and abdomen at the end of the injection (lymphangiogram) and lymph nodes free of adjacent and overlapping lymph vessels at 24 hours (lymphogram). The contrast medium remains in the lymph nodes for up to 6 months.

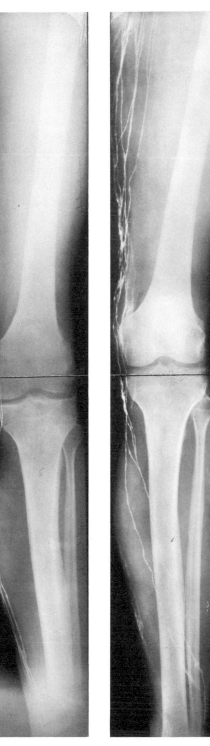

2102a

Radiographic procedures

Immediate
Supine 35 × 35 cm (14 × 14 ins) or 35 × 43 cm (14 × 17 ins) antero-posterior films of the legs, thighs (2102) and abdomen at the end of the contrast injection show the lymphatic vessels (lymphangiogram) from the ankle to the cisterna chyli and a supine right anterior oblique film of the thorax shows the thoracic duct (2102b).

Delayed films (24/48 hours)
Supine antero-posterior and both oblique films together with a lateral view of the abdomen and pelvis are taken for the lymph nodes (lymphogram) as well as penetrated postero-anterior and lateral view of the chest in case mediastinal lymph nodes have also taken up contrast medium.

Upper limb
Lymphography of the upper limb is similar to the leg with local anaesthetic and patent violet blue being injected into the first two web spaces to show blue lymphatics on the dorsum of the hand. A lymphatic is cannulated after a small skin incision but 3–5 ml of ultra-fluid lipodol is sufficient to show lymph vessels in the arm and the axillary lymph nodes (2104e, f).

Frontal and oblique films of the axilla are taken at 24 hours as well as a film of the whole chest in case lymph nodes in the mediastinum or opposite axilla have taken up contrast medium.

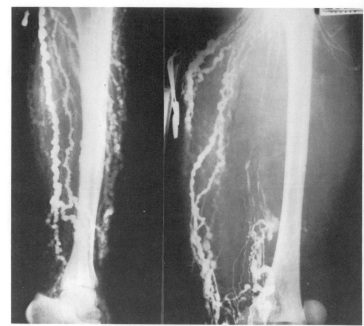

2103a   2103b

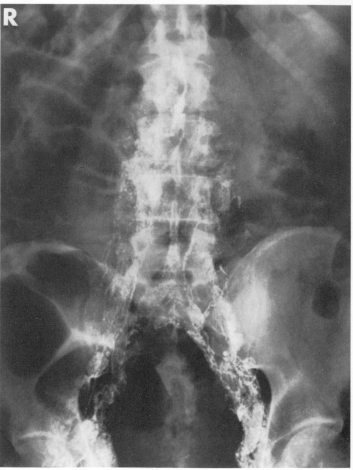

2104a

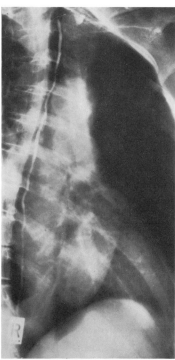

2102b   CISTERNA

Radiographs
In (2102) normal lymphatics of the lower limb from the ankle to the groin are shown in two different patients and markedly dilated lymphatics (a) in the leg and (b) in the thigh, in a case of lymphatic oedema (2103).

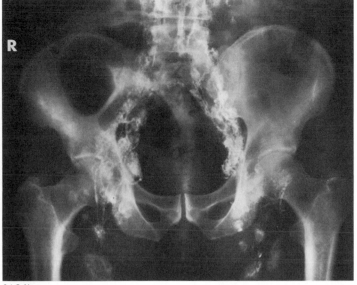

2104b

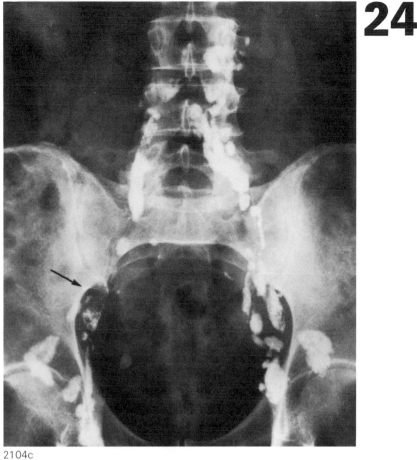

2104c

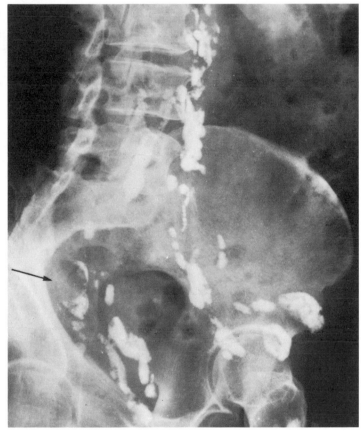

2104d

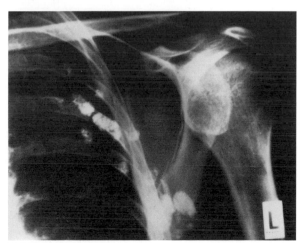

2104e

In **(2104a)** the lymphatic vessels are shown in between lymph nodes up to the level of the cisterna chyli overlying $L_{1|2}$ and in **(2104b)** lymph nodes with intervening vessels at the femoral, external iliac and common iliac regions.

(2104c, d) are frontal and oblique view of lymphograms at 24 hours after contrast has been injected into a lymphatic on the dorsum of the foot. A metastatic deposit is producing a filling defect in a lymph node (arrow).

(2104e) lymph vessels shown in forearm and arm from injection of contrast medium into a lymphatic in the hand.

(2104f) Lymphogram in the axilla showing lymph nodes. Film taken 24 hours after contrast medium injected.

2104f

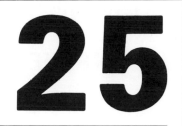

SOFT TISSUE

SOFT TISSUE

Soft tissue radiography refers by and large to muscle, skin and subcutaneous tissue, including the breasts even though all tissue in the body other than the skeleton is strictly speaking soft tissue. Radiographic contrast between the different tissues using conventional films is relatively poor and special techniques have therefore been developed, especially for mammography. Occasionally however, when cavities or fistulas are present, contrast medium can be injected (p. 646, 2151–2153).

The breasts

Mammography

Maximal contrast between the different components of soft tissue is essential for the accurate diagnosis of breast pathology particularly for the early detection of carcinoma.

Shape, size and age

In the breast there is both glandular and fatty tissue (2105), the proportions varying with age and after childbirth. In the young woman the breast is ovoid and dense (2106a) but with increasing age and after childbirth the breast increases in size with an increase in the amount of fat (2106b), becoming less dense with more inherent contrast.

The breast lies on the pectoralis major muscle but has an extension upwards and outwards towards the axilla—the axillary tail of Spence and in cross section (2105) the ducts from the milk glands can be seen to converge on the nipple as they course through the fibro-fatty tissue.

Clinical practice

Mammography is used in two different circumstances, either as a screening procedure in well women over the age of 40 years to detect presymptomatic breast carcinoma or in the investigation of lumps or otherwise suspected breast carcinoma.

As a screening procedure, repeat examinations of large numbers of patients increases the radiation hazard particularly the possible teratogenic effect. The technique must be suitably modified, taking advantage of newer methods, to reduce the radiation dose without loss of diagnostic information. The knowledge thus gained from the screening examinations can be applied in clinical practice. The ideal technique provides the minimal number of films, each of diagnostic quality with the lowest radiation dose.

THE
MAMMARY
GLAND

MUSCLE
←PECTORALS
MAJOR

LACTIFEROUS
DUCT

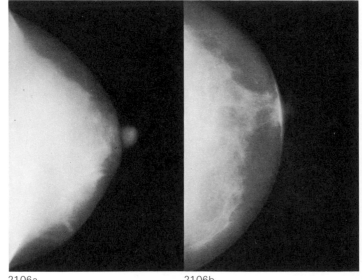

2106a   2106b

2105

General principles

A low kilovoltage is essential but in practice there is little to be gained by a kilovoltage lower than 28 kVp although it is essential to have a kilovoltage below 35 kVp.

The minimum filtration recommended by the International Committee for Radiation Protection (IRCP) is 0·5 mm aluminium but should not be above 1·1 mm because the beam hardening effect then interferes with definition essential for the visualisation of tumours.

The entrance skin dose using a non-screen film technique is approximately five times that of a vacuum packed cassette with a single back-screen being approximately 1 rad entrance dose for the cranio-caudal and 2 rads for the medio-lateral using a vacuum packed cassette with a single back screen.

It is generally accepted that the visualisation of tumours is only slightly better with Xeroradiography than with a good radiographic film technique but calcifications are much more clearly visible. Acceptable examinations are more consistently achieved with Xeroradiography, however the radiation dose is approximately 70% higher.

There appears to be no particular advantage to using a molybdenum anode tube compared with a special low kVp tungstate tube for mammography. The visualisation of tumours is about the same with the two methods but there is almost a threefold increase in the entrance dose with the molybdenum tube compared with the special tungstate tube. This is in part due to the shorter FFD used with this system.

Accurate collimation is essential to cover the whole of the breast being examined but not to include part of the opposite breast which will then increase the radiation dose. Similarly accurate labelling as to side and as to medial and lateral or cranial and caudal is essential and where a palpable nodule is being investigated a skin marker such as a lead shot should be used.

The two standard views are the cranio-caudal and medio-lateral as shown in (2107) with a lead shot skin marker on the right breast and in (2108) a cranio-caudal view of a normal breast compared with (2109) showing a carcinoma.

Occasionally carcinoma can also develop in the male breast.

Superior-inferior

With the patient seated each breast in turn rests on a cassette on the table support adjusted to a suitable height for each patient. The nipple is in profile and all puckering or creases in the skin removed. The patient leans forward against the film with her head turned away from the localising cone which is lead lined and flattened on the side in contact with the chest wall, restricting the beam to the breast and protecting the underlying lung (2110a, b). A 35 cm (14 ins) focus film distance is shown in (2110a) and a 50 cm (20 ins) in (2110b).

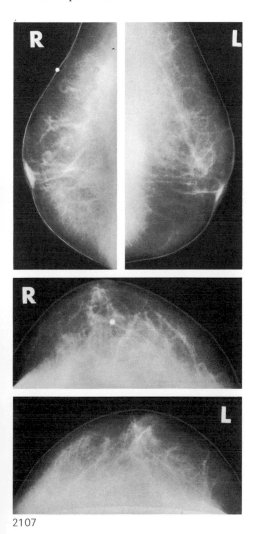

2107

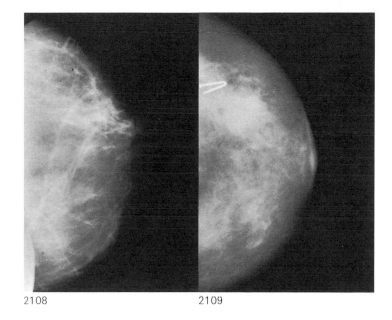

2108   2109

The cranio-caudal and medio-lateral are the classical projections for the breast with additional views to cover particular areas especially the axillary tail but recently the oblique view has been recommended as the best single view for showing breast pathology. The oblique view provides a shorter distance for the X-ray beam to travel through denser tissue giving better contrast than the cranio-caudal and medio-lateral views and furthermore includes the axillary tail of breast tissue in the area radiographed.

Specialised mammographic units having fixed centring of the tube to the platform are now available, the interlinked tube and platform rotating through 360° with the examination being carried out in the sitting position. If specialised mammographic equipment is not available, important adaptations are essential for mammography which requires a kilovoltage below 35 kVp using a minimum of 0·5 mm aluminium filtration. A variable height platform to support the breast is necessary for erect or seated patients for the cranio-caudal view together with a long localising cone flattened at one side to fit the chest wall, bringing the cone onto the breast (2110). The reclining lateral view is favoured (2112) for use with the full length couch. The skin of the breast must not be puckered or creased which will produce confusing shadows and the nipple must be in profile for each projection.

In a more elaborate projection the patient is prone with breast immersed in mineral oil to produce a uniform density. Breast compression has the advantage of providing a more uniform field and a shorter distance for the X-rays to travel through tissue producing better contrast and is especially important for the oblique view which is now often used as the projection in the "one film" technique.

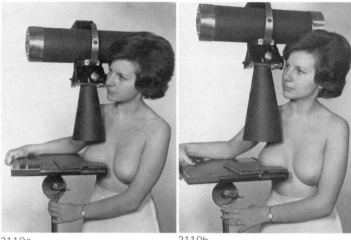

2110a   2110b

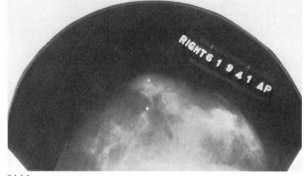

2111

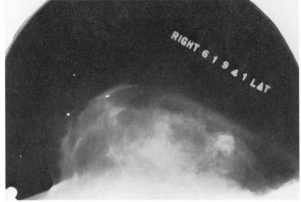

2113

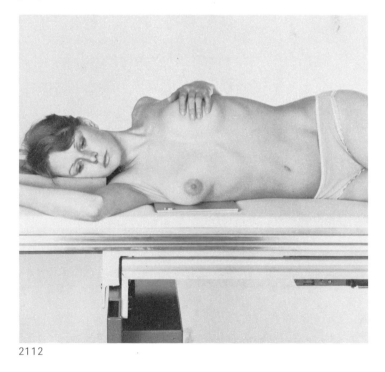

2112

Medio-lateral (supine-oblique)

With the patient lying on a foam pad on each side in turn, the arm on the side being examined is abducted, the hand is under the head and the cassette under the breast. A slight backward tilt of the patient is needed to bring the breast into the lateral position with the nipple in profile and the other breast out of the field, usually being held away from the cone by the patient's free hand (2112, 2113).

Axillary projection

With the patient sitting or horizontal she is rotated 30° to the affected side and the arm abducted to at least 90°. The scapula is thus moved out of the field and the breast away from the superimposed chest wall. The film includes both the breast and axilla.

■ Centre 5 cm (2 ins) below the axilla, both sides being examined in turn for comparison (2114, 2115).

For further detail, once a lesion has been identified a tangential projection (2116) can be helpful and the position of the lesion is marked with a small lead pellet on the skin surface (2116, 2117).

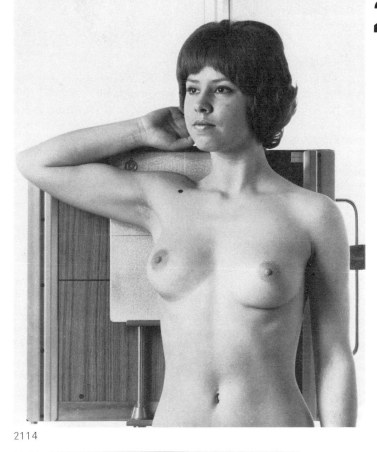

2114

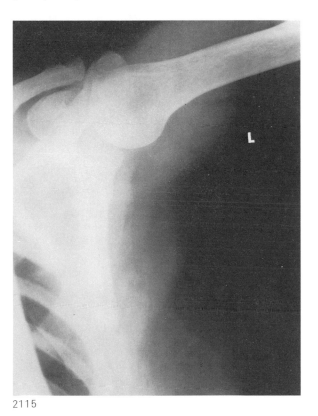

2115

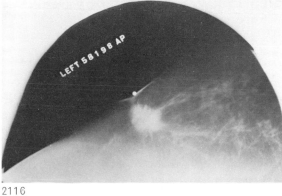

2116

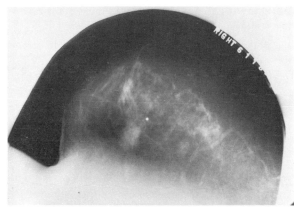

2117

Exposure technique

The minor radiological changes within tissues of low contrast which need to be shown on mammograms extends the technology to its limits. The definition must be adequate to produce films of diagnostic quality but keeping within an acceptable radiation dose especially when repeat or follow up examinations will also be needed. The system used must provide

(i) minimal unsharpness
(ii) suitable exposure factors
(iii) low grain
(iv) high subject contrast
(v) acceptable radiation dose

Type of film available

Non-screen film varies in speed by a factor of 10 from the slowest which is used for gamma radiography to the conventional-speed medical non-screen film. The fastest film has a grain size of about twice that of the slowest film.

With suitable development a high gamma can be obtained with all film with only a marginal difference in contrast. These films have a high D MAX and can record steep subject differences with increasing contrast.

Relative exposures

Slow speed films require 2000 mAs, intermediate non-screen films 500 mAs and conventional medical non-screen film 200 mAs.

Apparatus

Mammography equipment has X-ray tubes giving 25–35 kVp output but if standard equipment is to be used, the transformer must be modified accordingly. The equivalent of 0·5 mm aluminium greatly reduces the radiation dose without significantly degrading the image.

Technical factors

A small focal spot size of at most 0·6–0·8 mm is essential but the tube must be compatible with loading required for the examination using a kilovoltage of 25–35 kVp with a high contrast film suitably processed for maximum soft tissue definition. The focus film distances vary from 45 to 80 cm (18 to 32 ins) and to reduce the radiation dose a single screen vacuum packed cassette using an oblique single view technique is now routine.

Immobilisation

The patient must be as comfortable and relaxed as possible with maximum patient cooperation and breast compression for the relatively long exposure times used.

Radiation protection

Lead backing to the platform especially for the cranio-caudal view is essential for gonad protection.

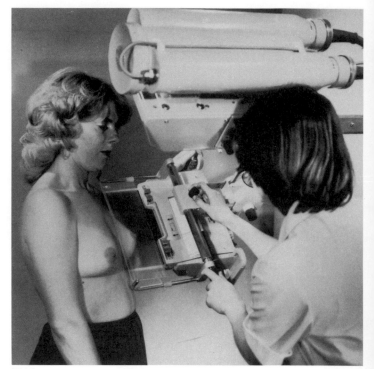
2118

Single film technique

With the latest rare earth-fine grain film combination in a vacuum packed cassette, the exposure can be reduced to 100 mAs at 30 kVp and 60 cm FFD giving an entry skin dose of 0·15–0·3 rad per exposure. Using this in conjunction with the Lundgren oblique view with compression a relatively uniform exposure field is produced and is the best combination for the "single shot" mammography technique (2118).

For the cranio-caudal and lateral projections especially without compression, there is a marked difference in tissue thickness resulting in larger contrast differences between the centre and edge of the breast. The film must then be viewed with normal illumination and also with a bright light if both the lighter inner part of the breast and the darker outer part are to be seen (2119b).

Double or tri-pack films

To overcome the differential contrast between the thin and thick parts of the breast two films of different speeds are used with a ratio of 4:1. The faster film is placed closer to the tube and with the lower kilovoltage used in mammography absorbs about 60 % of the incident radiation. If the positions of the films are reversed the exposure and radiation is considerably increased (2119b, c).

A further variation uses 3 films with a ratio of 2:1 with the fastest film closest to the tube. This system not only shows the thickest and thinnest parts of the breast but also allows considerable latitude in exposure as one of the films must be ideally exposed. However, considerably more film is being used for each examination.

Xeroradiography

Instead of film a thin layer of semiconductor becomes the detecting medium to produce a latent image. By a process similar to Xerox photocopying, the latent image is transferred onto paper. The characteristic feature of Xeroradiographic images is the marked edge enhancement which occurs at well defined contrast differences. Thus in the breast the blood vessels, ducts, skin, small calcifications and tumour edges stand out clearly. Further advantages of Xeroradiography are the small difference in radiographic density between the thick parts and the thin parts of the breast giving a more uniform exposure. Moreover it produces good images with a low kilovoltage tungsten tube. The radiation dose is however 60–100 % greater than with low dose film techniques such as with a single screen vacuum packed cassette.

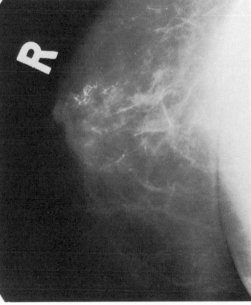

2119a

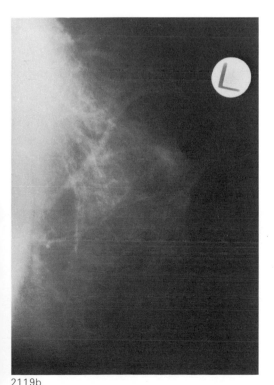

2119b

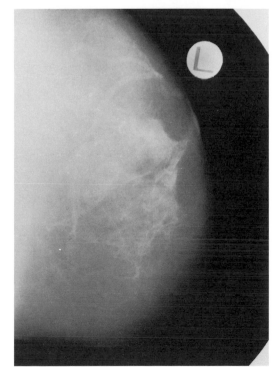

2119c

25 Soft tissue

Soft tissue radiography is used for different purposes, to show changes in soft tissues where only soft tissue contrast differences are involved, to show calcification in soft tissues as in calcific tendinitis or to show soft tissue changes adjacent to bone pathology. Clearly the three different circumstances will need quite different exposure techniques. For only soft tissue contrast a technique similar to mammography is indicated and Xeroradiography is especially suitable for calcifications. In tendons particularly at the shoulder, a double film technique in a single cassette with a ratio of 2:1 is applicable or a differential wedge filter with the thicker part over the soft tissues (2120). However when both bone detail and adjacent soft tissues are being displayed a non-screen film laid on top of the cassette, both being exposed simultaneously will show bone and soft tissue. Alternatively a high kilovoltage can be used which increases the range of tissues shown but produces a film with less contrast. A high kilovoltage technique is also valuable for showing gas shadows in tissues.

Kilovoltage

The density of soft tissue usually needs about 15 kVp less than for bone but if the region is particularly radiopaque it may be impossible to show bone and soft tissue detail on one film. A compromise solution is to increase the kilovoltage by 20–25 kVp producing less overall contrast but showing both bone and soft tissue. An alternative solution is to use more than one film in a cassette or a non-screen film on the outside of the cassette (p. 662). With this multiple film-single exposure technique bone detail as well as detail in soft tissue can be demonstrated radiographically.

Profile projections

Soft tissue lesions are shown to best effect when unobscured by overlying bone. The soft tissue exposure will then be markedly underexposed for the adjacent bone. This is well shown in (2121a) where there is post-traumatic calcification in the soft tissues shown in profile overlying the scapula. However the scapula is underexposed and no bone detail is visible. Similarly a skin papilloma is shown in (2121b) protruding from the surface but no detail in the femur is visible being underexposed for bone.

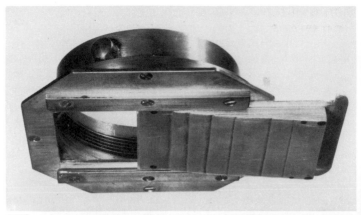

2120

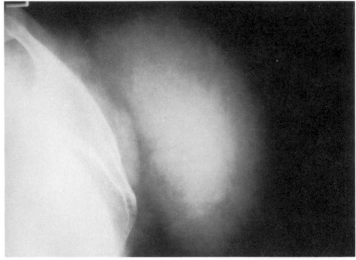

2121a

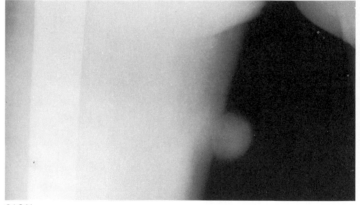

2121b

Soft tissue pathology

The adenoids are lymphoid structures in the posterior nasopharynx which are shown on lateral soft tissue films of the neck. The adenoids encroach on the posterior nasopharyngeal air space (2122a). After adenoidectomy there is no longer soft tissue encroachment on the air space (2122b).

■Centre 5 cm (2 ins) above the angle of the jaw with the head and cervical spine in the true lateral position.

In the hand arteriovenous malformations can cause marked soft tissue swelling (2123) and may be associated with small round calcifications called phleboliths.

Thyroid cysts are quite common and may calcify producing a ring shadow in the neck which displaces or indents the trachea (2124).

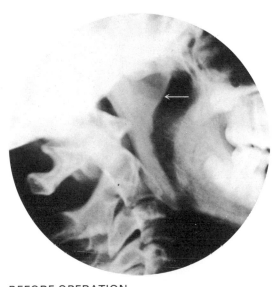

BEFORE OPERATION
2122a

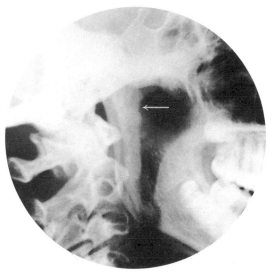

AFTER OPERATION
2122b

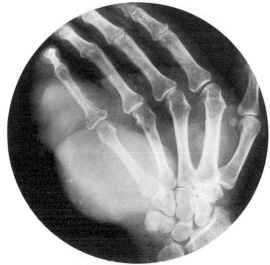

2123

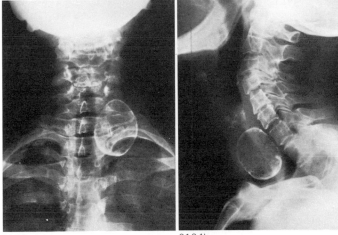

2124a   2124b

Air in the soft tissues is known as surgical emphysema and may be caused by trauma especially rib fracture (2126) or perforation of an abdominal viscus such as the rectum, the whole area must then be included on the radiograph (2125). Soft tissue trauma may also produce severe bruising or haematoma which can be seen on soft tissue radiographs (2128).

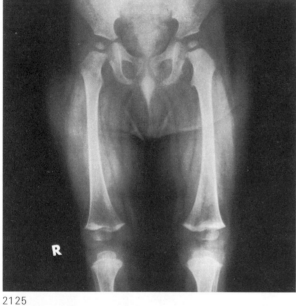

2125

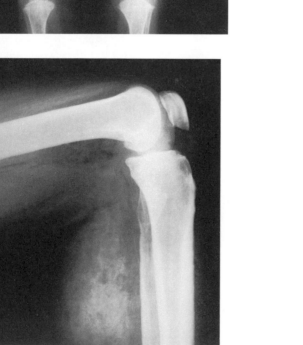

2126

2127

2128

Lipoma is a benign well defined fatty tumour which is more transradiant than adjacent tissues and therefore appears as a darker area on the radiograph as in (2129) around the shoulder joint, in (2130) on the chest wall or in (2131) in the forearm.

Note—Any soft tissue lesion on the skin such as a wart, mole or cyst must be noted by the radiographer on the request form and drawn to the attention of the radiologist as these may produce nodular shadows which could be mistaken for internal lesions.

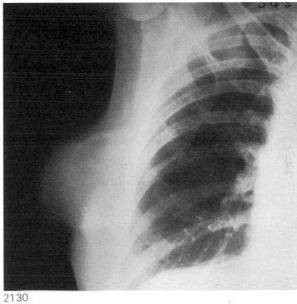

2130

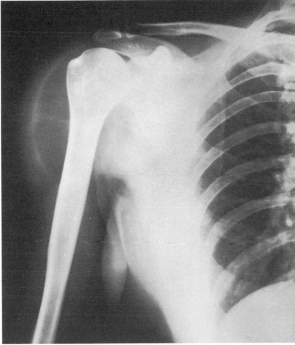

2129

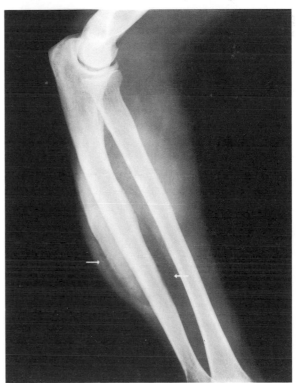

2131

Arteries

The walls of arteries commonly calcify in the elderly showing as parallel lines in the known position of arteries (2132–2135) frequently seen in the common and external arteries on a pelvic film (2132), in the femoral artery in the thigh (2133) or tibial artery in the leg (2134, 2135). Arterial calcification also occurs in chronic renal failure with hyperparathyroidism.

Phleboliths are small rounded calcifications in veins, very commonly seen in the pelvis in the paravesical venous plexus (2136) and can thus be mistaken for a ureteric calculus. Phleboliths also occur in association with angiomatous malformations (2123) and are also found in the spleen (2137).

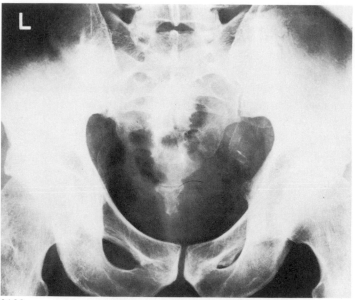

2132

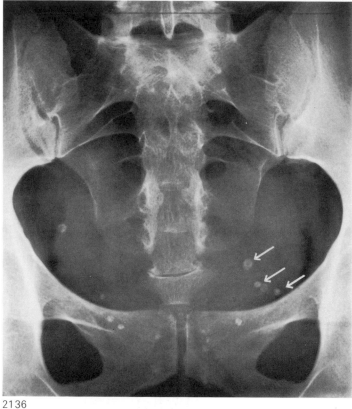

2136

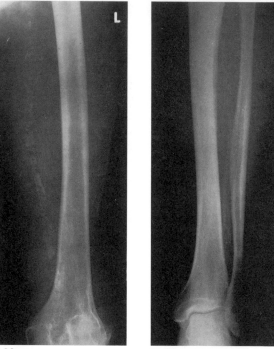

2133

2134

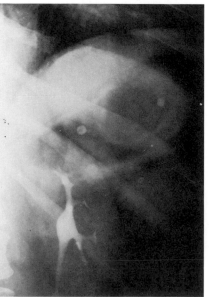

2137

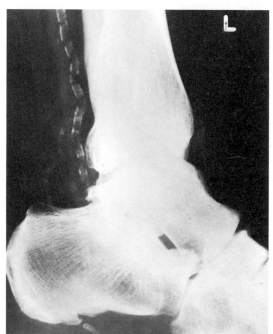

2135

Calcifications in soft tissue

In cysticercosis, the cystic form of the tapeworm Taenia solium infests the muscles, later undergoing calcification. Any muscle in the body may be involved but shows most clearly in the thigh (2139) and legs (2140) as small elongated spindle shaped calcifications, but may also be seen in the forearms (2138).

Traumatic myosities ossificans produces calcification in muscle which have been injured and can be associated with dislocation at the shoulder (2141).

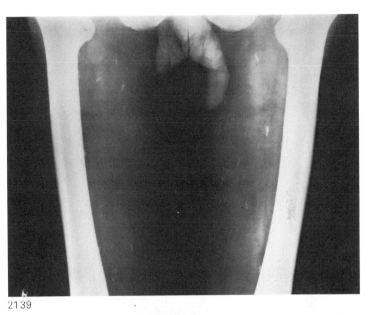

2139

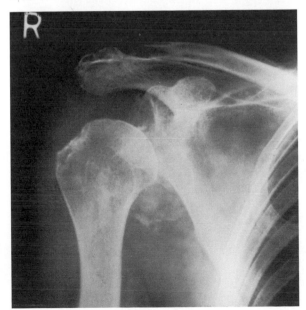

2138

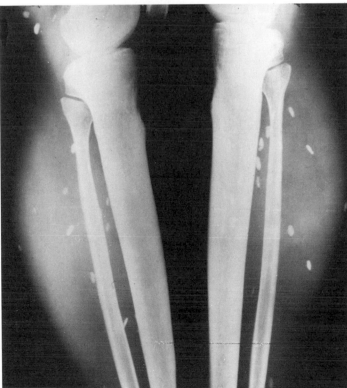

2141

2140

Traumatic myositis ossificans can occur around the shoulder (2142), in the upper arm (2144) or in the leg (2143) as the result of pressure, dislocations or fractures with injury to the adjacent muscle. There is also a progressive generalised form of myositis ossificans, unassociated with trauma causing severe limitation of movement. Bone formation may also occur in scars especially after abdominal operations.

Nodular skin lesions of neurofibromatosis may show on radiographs especially of the thorax and may be mistaken for pulmonary lesions.

Plastic prosthesis in bone (2145) as demonstrated in the upper arm may also need to be radiographed by a soft tissue technique.

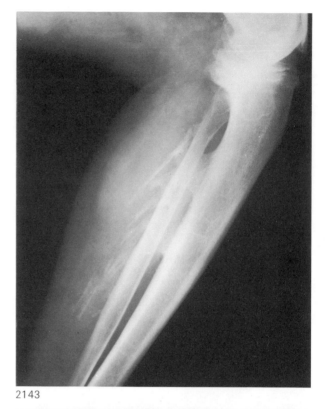

2143

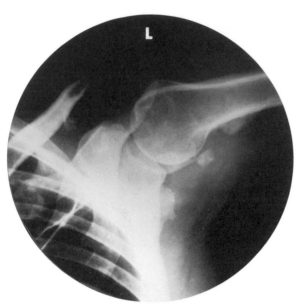

2142

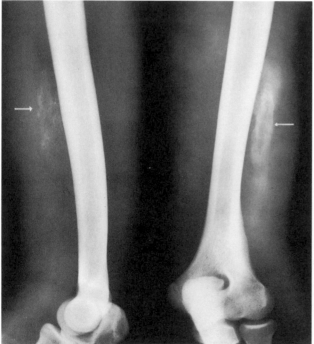

2144

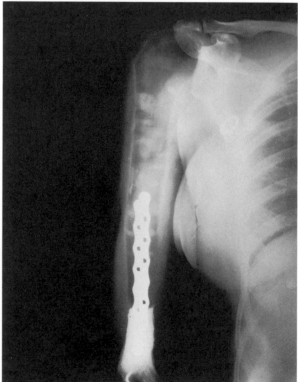

2145

Bone and adjacent soft tissues

In rheumatoid arthritis (2146) and gout (2147, 2148) there is considerable soft tissue involvement adjacent to the joint and bone disease. In rheumatoid arthritis soft tissue swelling around the joints is commonly seen on radiographs and in gout marked localised soft tissue swelling may occur and may contain irregular calcifications (2148).

In osteomyelitis or bone infection surrounding soft tissue swelling occurs and there may be a loose fragment of dead bone called a sequestrum (2149). Yaws is a chronic infection of bone occurring in the tropics often producing a marked periosteal reaction (2150).

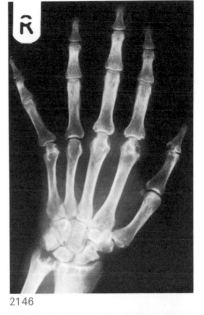

2146

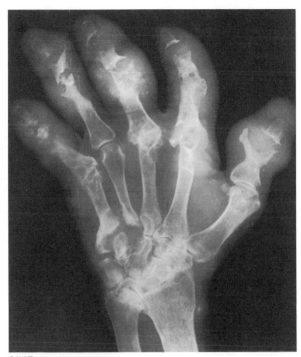

2147

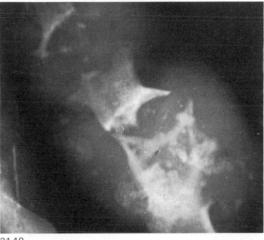

2148

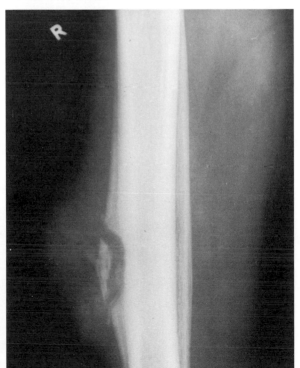

2149

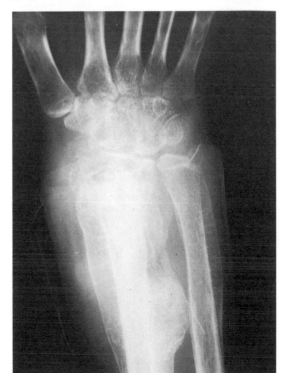

2150

Sinogram

Sinuses are soft tissue channels extending from the skin into the deeper tissues frequently down to bone and often as a result of a previous abscess. A fistula is a similar soft tissue channel but connecting the skin with an internal hollow viscus in the abdomen. These sinus or fistulous tracts can be outlined by contrast injections into the skin opening and must be radiographed in two planes at right angles to each other to show their true position.

Previously iodised oil such as lipiodol was used but now water soluble contrast agents are preferred. The contrast medium is injected through a sterile catheter inserted into the sinus or fistula which must make a watertight connection with the skin opening to prevent leakage of the contrast medium. The contrast medium is then injected under some pressure to fill the whole length of the sinus or fistula.

Radiographs are taken in frontal and lateral projections with a surface marker on the skin at the orifice of the sinus or fistula.

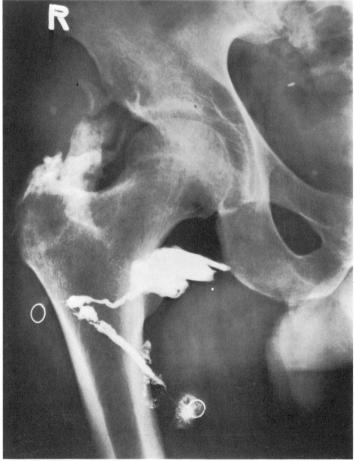

2152

Thyro-glossal fistula

A cannula or fine catheter is inserted into the track which is often at the crico-thyroid level and 5–10 ml of an anionic water soluble contrast medium is injected which usually runs upwards to the base of the tongue (arrow 2153). Lateral and frontal radiographs of the neck are taken.

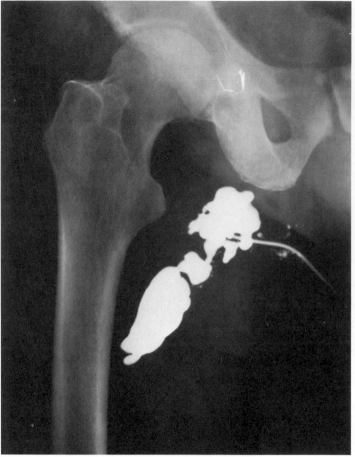

2151

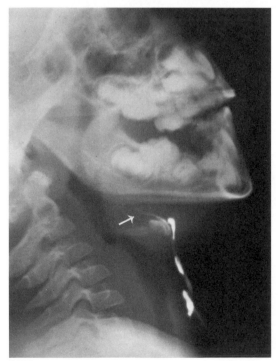

2153

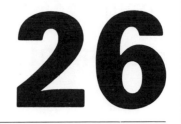

MACRORADIOGRAPHY

MACRORADIOGRAPHY

The beam of X-rays from an X-ray tube is normally divergent and even with conventional Bucky films there is some enlargement. With macroradiography there is marked enlargement of the image by decreasing the focus–object distance and increasing the object–film distance (2155, 2156). There is a simple geometric relationship between the magnification produced and the relative positions of the object and the film (2154) namely

$$M \text{ (magnification)} = \frac{D \text{ (focus–film distance)}}{d \text{ (focus–object distance)}}$$

or for any desired magnification the focus–object distance can be calculated by

$$d \text{ (focus − object distance)} = \frac{D \text{ (focus-film distance)}}{M \text{ (magnification)}}$$

Thus if the film–focus distance is 90 cm (36 ins) and a magnification of 1·5 is required

$$\text{(d) focus–object distance} = \frac{90(36'')}{1·5} = \frac{\text{(FFD)}}{M} = 60 \text{ cm } (24'')$$

If the FFD is 90 cm (36″) and the focus–object distance is 60 cm (24″) the film displacement from the object will be 90–60 cm (36″–24″) = 30 cm (12″).

When calculating the subject to film distance the mid-thickness level or level of the known lesion should be taken rather than the table top. Macroradiography has the advantage of greater definition of small structures and also enlarged objects are more easily seen. However to offset the geometric unsharpness inherent in magnification small tube foci of 0·3 mm or 0·6 mm are essential. With a 0·6 mm focus a magnification of up to × 1·5 can be obtained and with 0·3 mm up to × 2 magnification but beyond this unsharpness is unacceptable.

For thin regions of the body such as the hands and feet non-screen film will produce the best definition with good resolution up to × 2 enlargement. With increasing tissue thickness intensifying screens become necessary, high definition screens are suitable up to × 1·5 and thereafter fast tungstate screens up to × 2 enlargement. There is, of course, no enlargement of screen grain which remains constant irrespective of the degree of enlargement; the intensifying screens compensating for the lower ratings of small foci tubes.

Thus with the 0·3 mm focal spot size the tube output is severely restricted requiring long exposure times which are not suitable for the abdomen. The 0·6 mm foci have greater loading capacity and become suitable for investigations such as angiography in the kidney or brain with enlargement up to × 1·5.

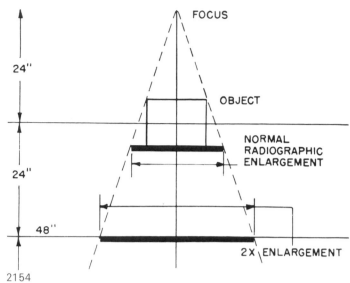

2154

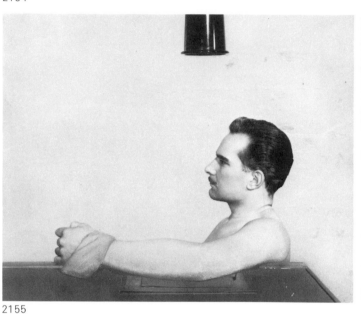

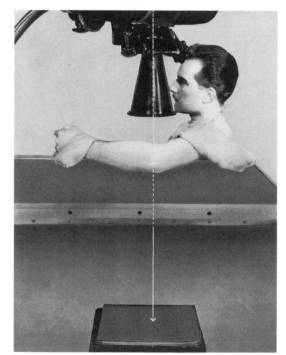

2155

2156

Meticulous radiography is essential with accurate collimation, centring and precise alignment of the tube, subject and film. Although specialised macroradiography units are available standard equipment can be suitably adapted by a trained radiographer. For subject–film alignment a transparent window is inserted into the table top and a platform supports the cassette at the usual distances beneath the table for ×1·5 or ×2 enlargement.

The added exposure needed for a grid prohibits its use in macroradiography but scattered radiation is limited by accurate collimation. The inevitable air-gap inherent in the technique nullifies the effects of the oblique rays (2157) and where non-screen films can be used, as in the hand, there is greater contrast in the enlarged radiograph. Where higher kilovoltages are possible, the exposure time can be reduced. However in the thicker parts of the body, because no grid can be used, higher kilovoltage will further reduce contrast and definition. The kilovoltage chosen will be limited by the capacity of the air-gap to deal with scattered radiation (2157).

For the extremities where the region being radiographed is normally in contact with the film the original film-focus distance say 75 cm (30 ins) does not need to be changed and only the film is then moved the required distance downward below the table. For the skull, vertebral column and renal angiography the normal focus distance of 90 cm (36 ins) will allow macroradiography with ×2 enlargement with the subject. 45 cm (18 ins) from the film and for ×1·5 enlargement 30 cm (12 ins) from the film.

If the focus-skin distances are much reduced the radiation dose to the skin will be increased. Particular care must be taken to see that the 2 mm aluminium filter is in position at the tube aperture and repeat exposures must be avoided.

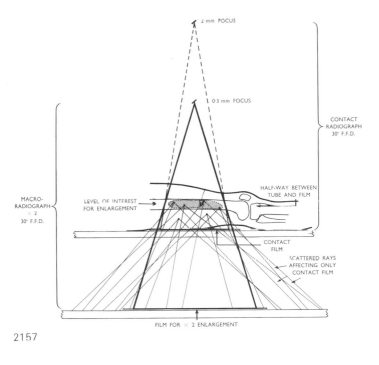

2157

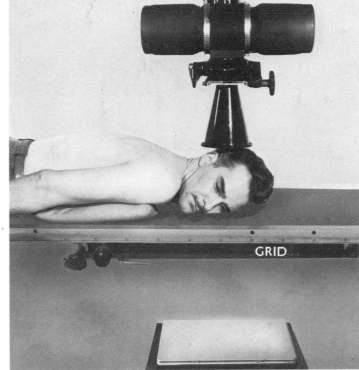

2158

Bones and joints

Conventional lateral contact and macroradiography films of the elbow joint (2159, 2160) are compared showing the increased detail obtained by ×2 enlargement. Fine bone trabeculae become clearly visible.

Various degrees of enlargement at the wrist joint are compared with the contact radiograph (2161) showing ×2 enlargement (2162), ×1½ enlargement (2163) and ×1⅔ enlargement (2164). The illustrations are the actual size of the original radiographs.

The elbow macroradiographs (2165a, b) are taken at ×1½ enlargement, in supination and pronation with full extension.

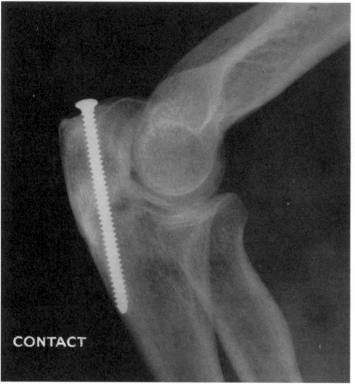

2159

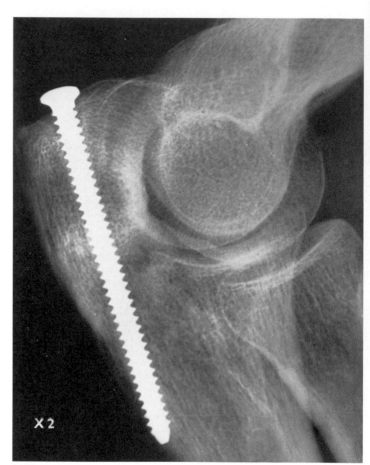

2160

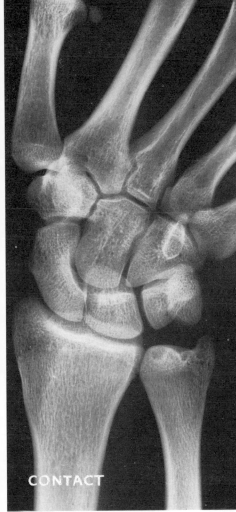

CONTACT

2161

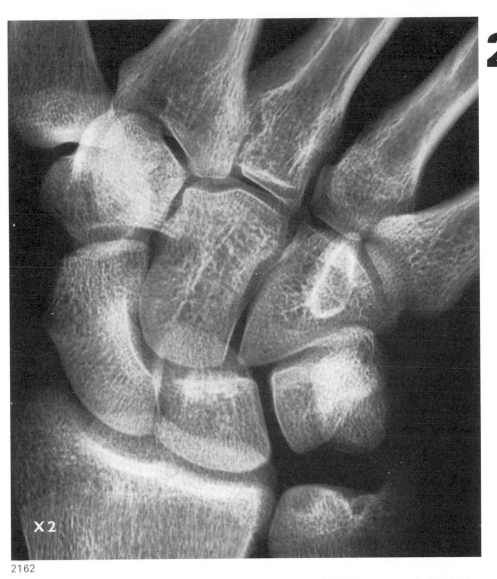

X2

2162

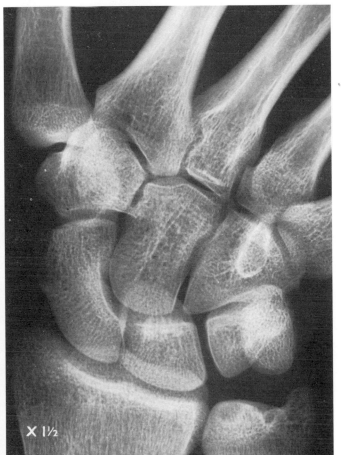

X 1½

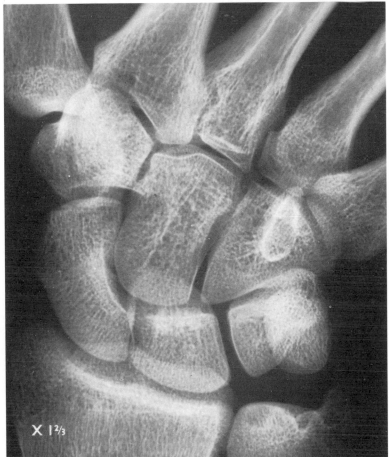

X 1⅔

2164

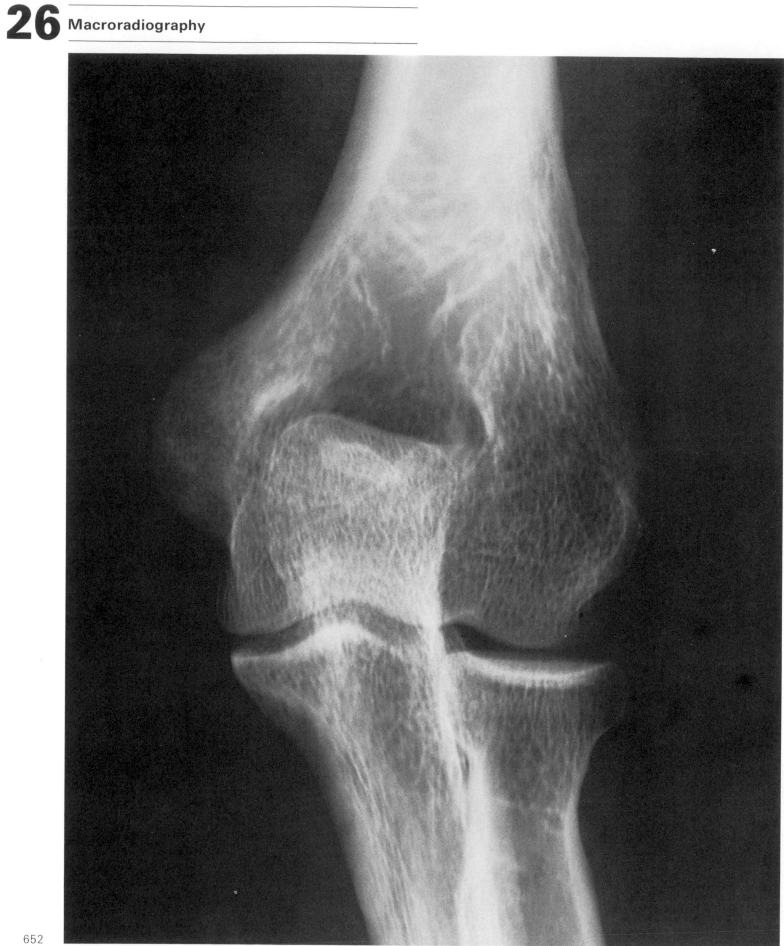

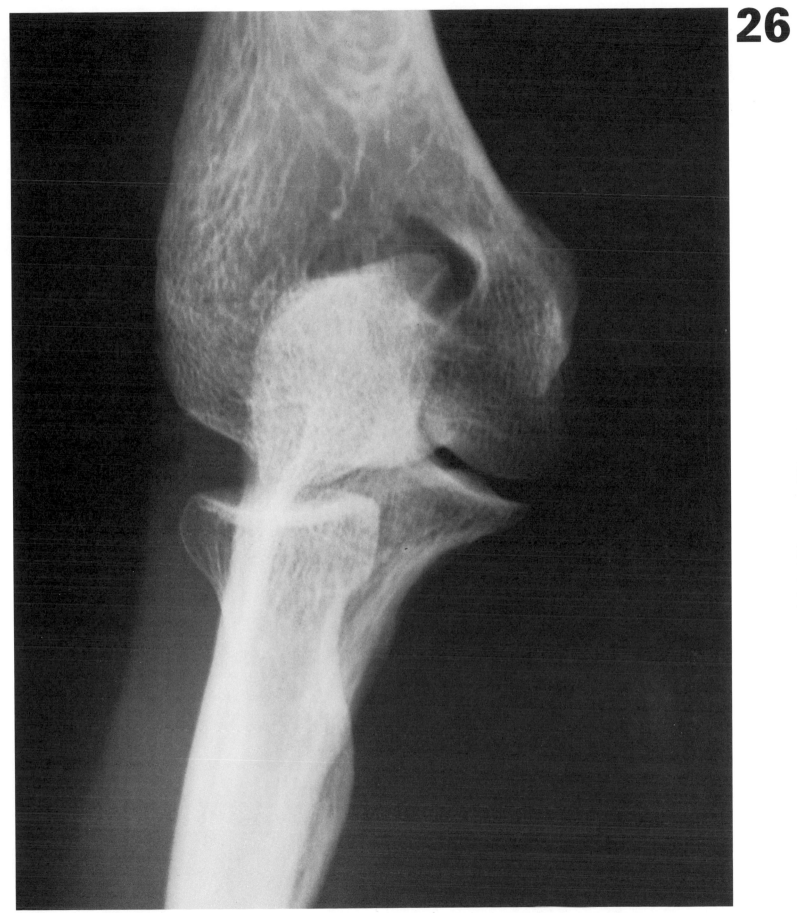

2165b

Petrous temporal

The skull unit is ideal for macroradiography as it has a small focal spot size, the grid can be removed, the table top is transparent and the film can be positioned on the inferior arc of the C-arm, (2166). Contact radiographs and macroradiographs are compared (2167, 2168, 2169, 2170, 2171) having been obtained with 0·3 mm tube focus to produce × 2 enlargement.

For (2167a, b) a lateral view with 25° caudal tube angulation was used, and for (2168, 2170) an occipito-frontal with the patient prone, the OMBL at 90° centring in the midline over the external occipital protuberance. In the macroradiograph the semi-circular canals, cochleae and internal auditory meatuses are clearly defined as they lie within the orbital margins.

For the half axial projection the tube was angled 25° for the macroradiograph (2171) and 35° for the conventional contact radiograph.

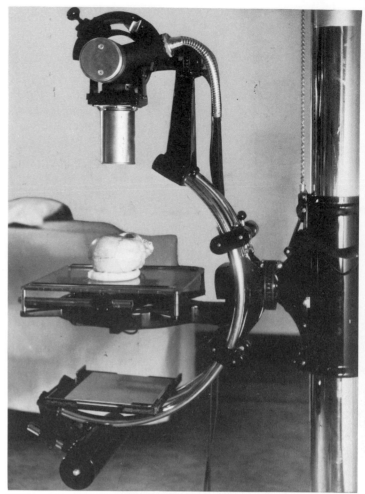

2166

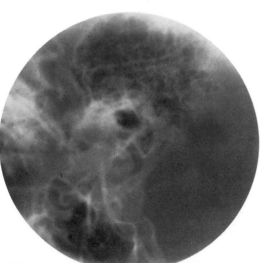

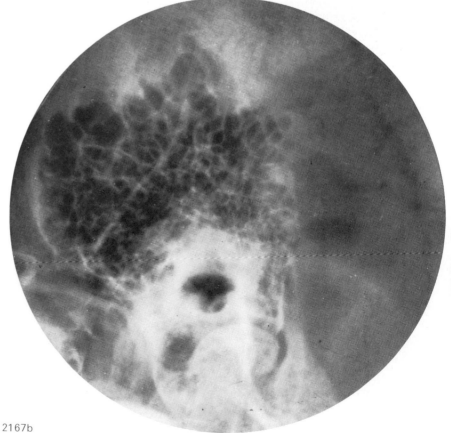

2167a

2167b

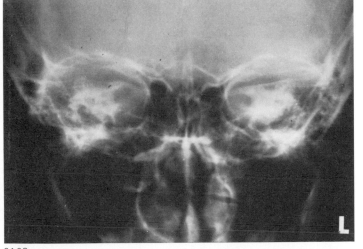 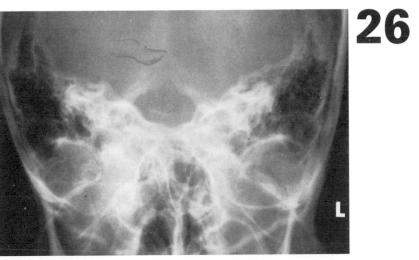

2168   2169

2170 2171

Lungs

For macroradiography of the lungs the thorax is divided into 4 zones on a 35 × 44 cm (14 × 17 ins) film for × 2 enlargement of each section as shown on the preliminary contact chest radiograph (2172). The upper zones (1) and (2) are at the level of the spines of the scapulae and the lower zones (3) and (4) at the inferior angles of the scapulae, centring 7·5–8 cm (3–3½ ins) from the midline. The centring points should be marked on the skin as a guide for the macroradiographs.

A macrograph of a lung quadrant (3) on (2172) shows the right lower zone.

The contact radiograph (2172) was taken with high definition intensifying screens and the macroradiograph (2175) with standard speed screens and fast film.

Exposure factors for macroradiographs

Upper zones   110 kVp 1·6 mAs at 25 mA
Lower zones   120 kVp 2·0 mAs at 25 mA

The chest support (2174) can be adjusted for enlargements up to × 2 and the patient is positioned against the 0·5 cm (¼ ins) perspex sheet. Routine contact radiography (2173) is shown at 152 cm (60 ins) and the macroradiograph is a × 2 enlargement for the same film-focal distance.

Because the air-gap reduces the effects of scatter, the kilovoltage can be increased to reduce the exposure time, thus reducing the loading on the small tube focus.

2172

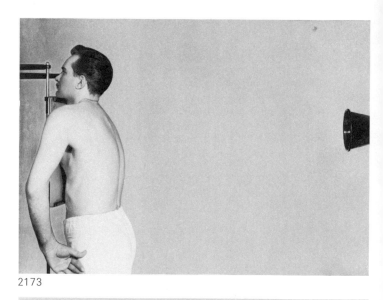

2173

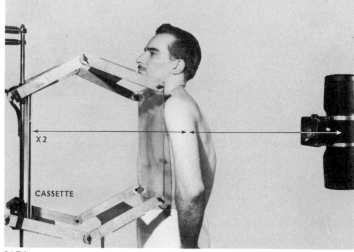

2174

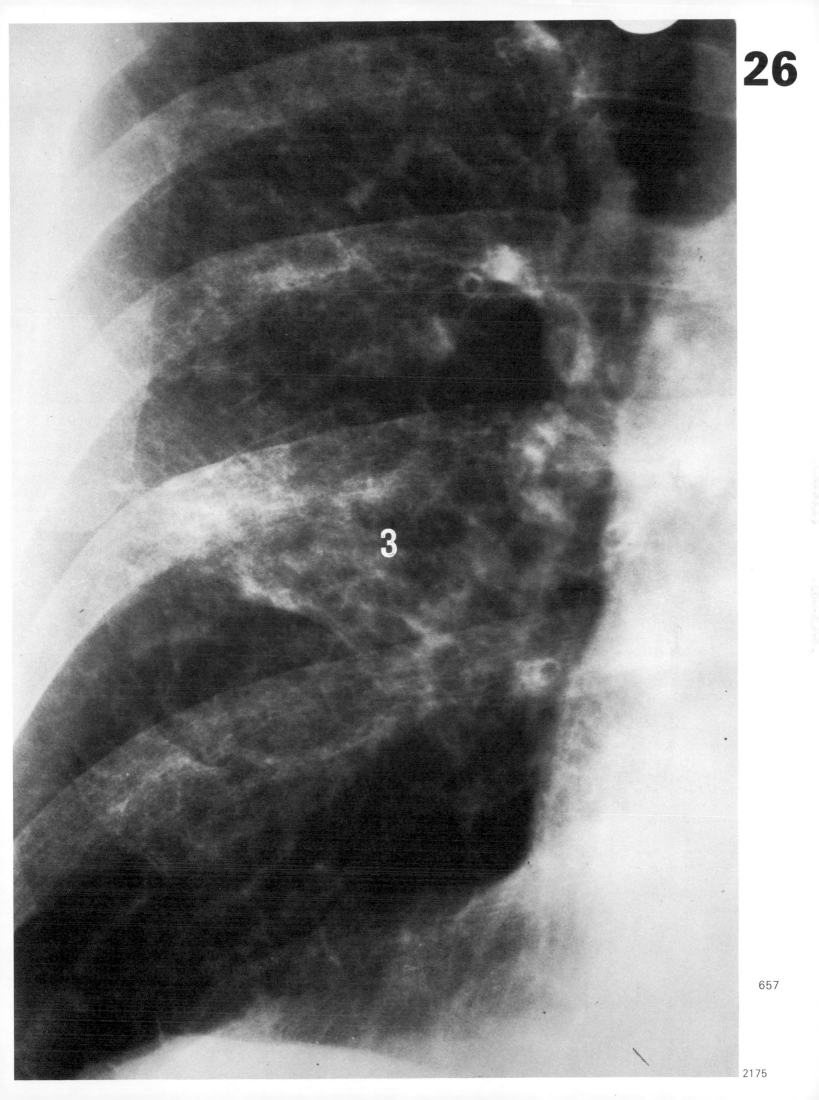

The Lacrimal System

The radiography of the lacrimal system is described in Section 20 page 521 and only the application of macroradiography follows.

A table adapted for macroradiography of the skull (2176) will allow enlargement up to $\times 2\frac{1}{2}$ and the photograph shows the relative positions of the tube, skull and film. The greater enlargement is obtained by moving the film further from the skull than the skull from the tube. Only the occipito-mental and not the fronto-occipital position should be used to limit the radiation dose to the lens of the eye. The OMBL is at 40° for this projection (2177).

Occipito-frontal and lateral macroradiographs of the lacrimal ducts shown with contrast are compared with contact radiographs in (2178, 2179, 2180).

Pubis

A tumour of the inferior rmaus of the pubis is shown in (2181).

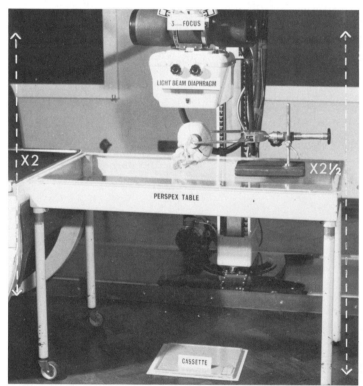

2176

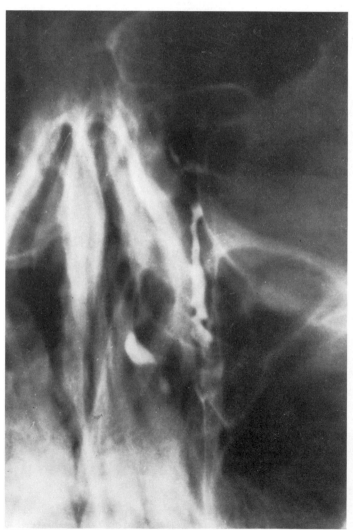

2177

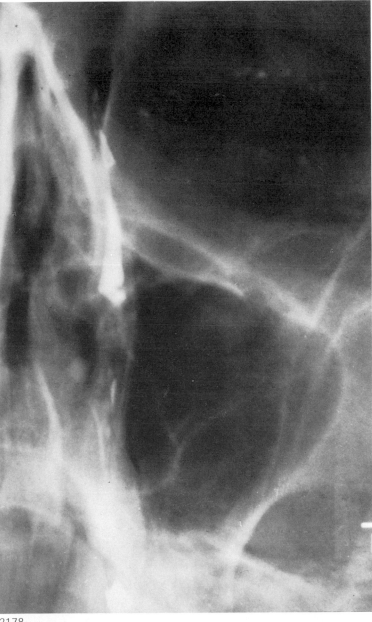

2178

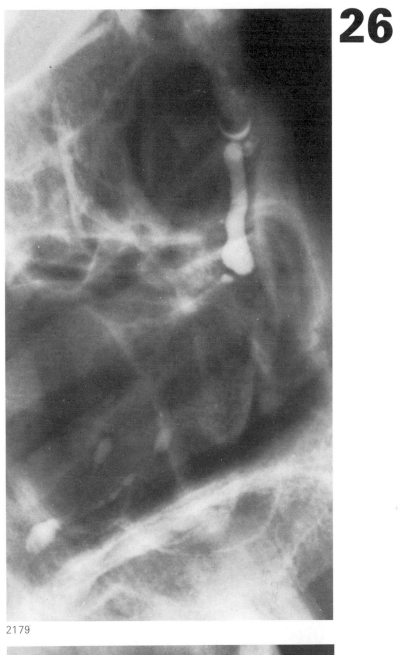

2179

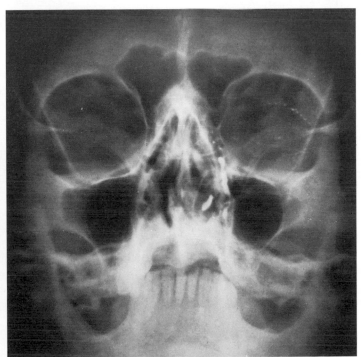

2180a

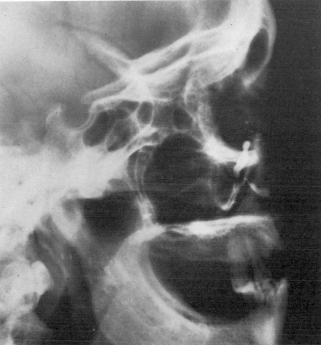

2180b

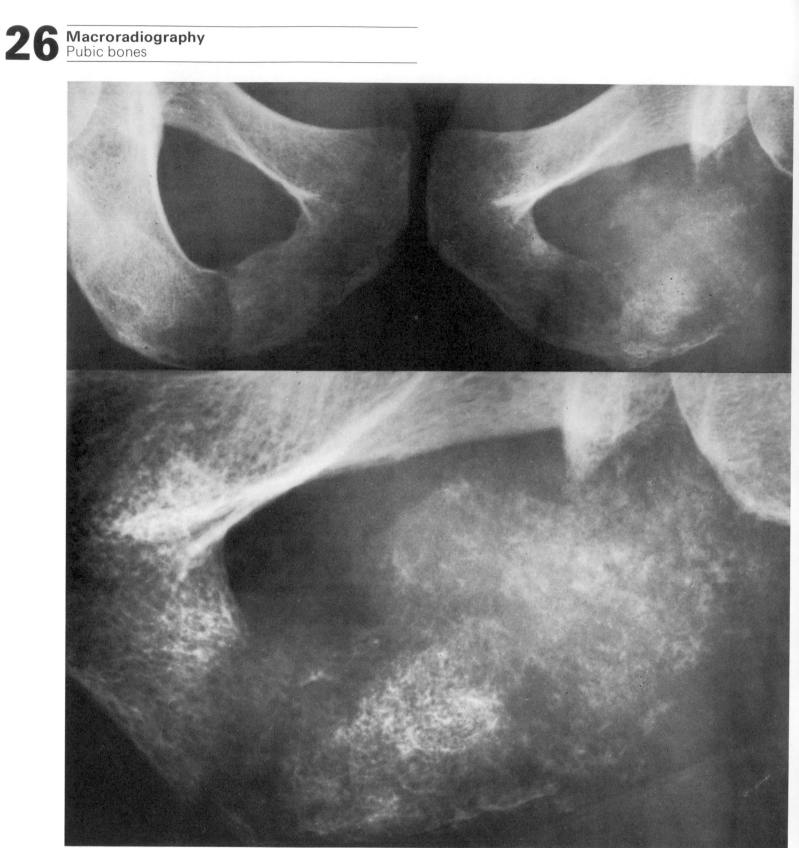

2181a   2181b

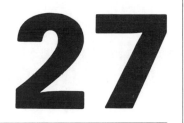

27

MULTIPLE RADIOGRAPHY

27 SECTION 27

SIMULTANEOUS MULTIPLE-FILM RADIOGRAPHY

There are many applications for the technique of simultaneously radiographing two films with one exposure. Two pairs of conventional intensifying screens are selected from the currently available range which include High Definition, Standard and Fast Tungstate and placed in a single cassette (2182). A single film is loaded in between each pair of screens which are then exposed together. The fastest pair of screens are placed close to the tube, with the slower pair behind, producing quite different degrees of exposure on each film (2183, 2184). The film nearer the tube in the faster screens are exposed to show bone (a) while the film behind is relatively underexposed for soft tissues (b). However, if the screens are reversed, the absorption of photons by the front pair of screens and the greater intensification by the rear pair of screen equalises the exposure on the two films.

Irrespective of the way the screens are arranged, the correct exposures for the region being examined is that required for the film in the front pair of screens.

Wide density range radiography

Where there is a wide range of radio density in the region being examined the fast screen must be nearest the tube to show the dense parts and the far screens are slow for the transradiant tissues.

In the neck (2183a, 2183b) and dorsal spine region (2184a, 2184b) the exposure on the film can be effectively halved to show bone on the front film (2183a, 2184a) and soft tissue on the rear film (2183b, 2184b).

Where the density range is even greater as in the frontal view of a sialogram, a non-screen film is placed on the front of the cassette and both exposed simultaneously to show the superficial parotid gland on the non-screen film as well as the parotid duct superimposed on the mandible on the screen film.

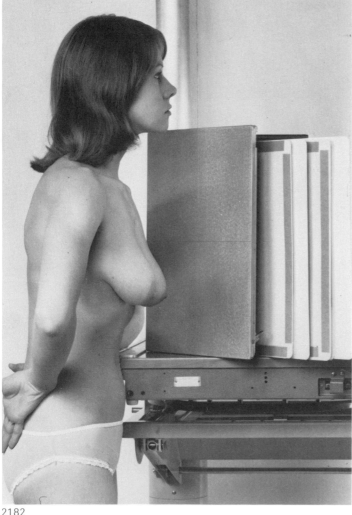

662 2182

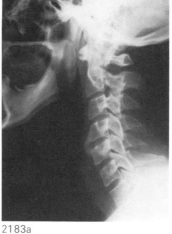

2183a

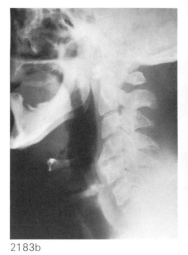

2183b

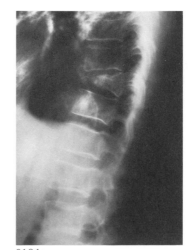

2184a

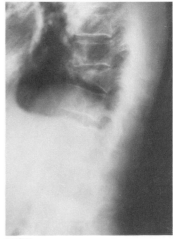

2184b

Recommended combination

For a moderate range of radiodensity differences a pair of fast tungstate screens nearer the tube and a pair of standard screens further from the tube is appropriate but for large differences in density a pair of fast tungstate nearer the tube is used in conjunction with a pair of high definition screens further from the tube (2185, 2186).

In (2186) the trachea and bifurcation are not visible but the peripheral bronchi are well shown, whereas in (2185) the dilated bronchi behind the heart and the trachea become visible.

Advantages of simultaneous multiple film radiography

1. Radiography is greatly simplified to produce films of diagnostic quality.
2. The exposure is that of the fast pair of screens, reducing the patient's radiation dose.
3. The contrast and definition is superior to that obtained with a high kilovoltage technique to show both bone and soft tissue.
4. There is greater latitude for unfamiliar examinations ensuring a successful result.

The main disadvantage of this technique is the expense of the extra film required in each examination. However, this technique can be applied to most areas of the body where both soft tissues and bone are to be visualised.

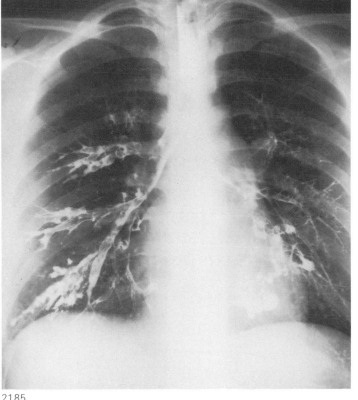

2185

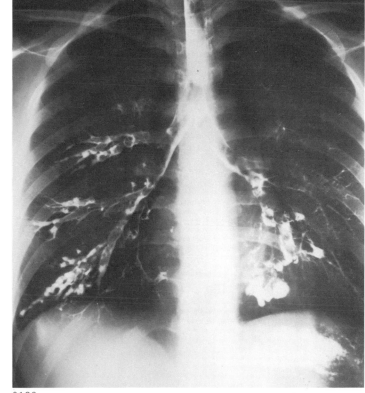

2186

Duplication

Two similar films can be obtained with two pairs of screens with the slower screen pair nearer the tube and the faster pair further away, as for example a pair of standard screens in front and a pair of fast tungstate screens behind. The exposure on each film is then comparable because the photon absorption of the front pair of screens balances the faster screens behind. This method has a limited application and is used mainly to produce films for the departmental film museum for teaching, without increasing the radiation to the patient.

The cassette

The cassette needed for two sets of screens must be sufficiently deep, as for example a grid cassette, with the thickness of the second pair of screens replacing the grid.

Often old cassettes with poor contact can hold two pairs of screens which then make good contact. However the screen contact must be tested for both sets of screens before using the system in practice.

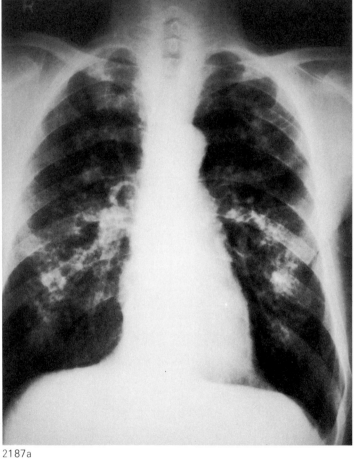

2187a

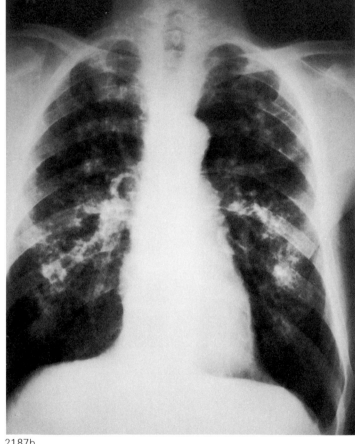

2187b

Simultaneous Contact radiography and Macroradiography

Contact radiography can be combined with macroradiography as a further variation of multiple radiography. For thinner regions a non-screen film is used for the contact radiograph and a pair of high definition screens with matching film for the $\times 2$ enlargement. The contact film and enlargement are exposed simultaneously and by using intensifying screens for the enlargement film and a non-screen film in the contact position, the exposures on the two films are comparable (2188a, b).

In thicker regions where intensifying screens are necessary for the contact radiograph the back of the cassette must be completely transradiant with the lead backing and all metal parts removed. The speed of the screens in the contact cassette must be considerably less than the enlargement film and a workable combination is high definition screens for the contact film and fast tungstate screens for the enlargement.

The skull unit with the grid removed (2166) is ideal for simultaneous contact and enlargement exposures for examinations such as macro-dacryocystography.

The advantages of this technique is that there is less radiation dose to the patient as both films are exposed simultaneously and the enlargement is comparable in every way without any change in the patient's position or the phase of the contrast injection.

Contact radiographs (2188a, 2189a) and macroradiographs (2188b, 2189b) were exposed simultaneously. In (2188) a fracture of the head of the radius is clearly demonstrated and an area of narrowing in the popliteal artery in (2189).

Multisection Tomography

Another form of multiple radiography is multisection tomography (Section 28, page 693). A number of cassettes are superimposed (2238) or in thin section tomography a number of screens of varying intensity. Tomograms at different levels are then taken simultaneously (2239).

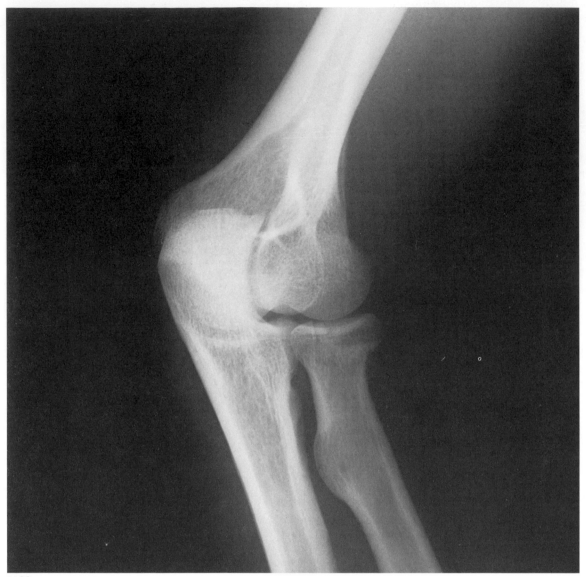

2188a

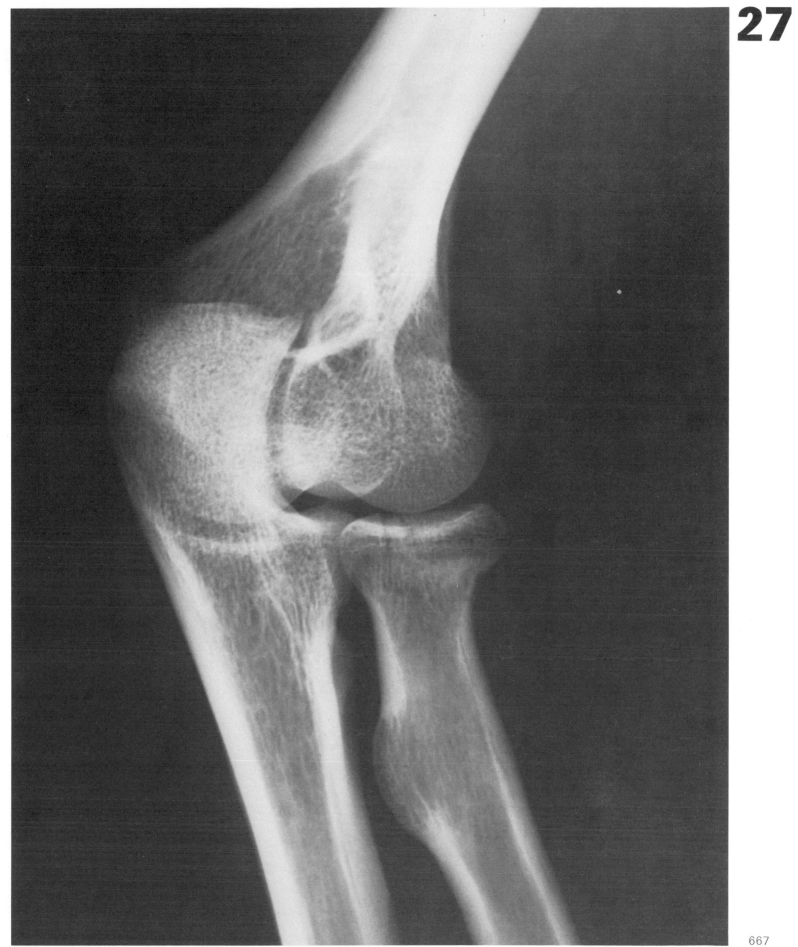

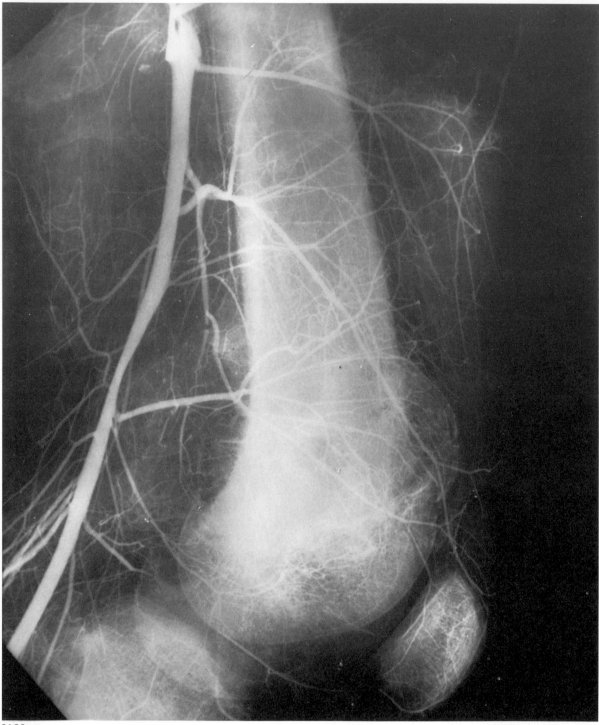

2189a

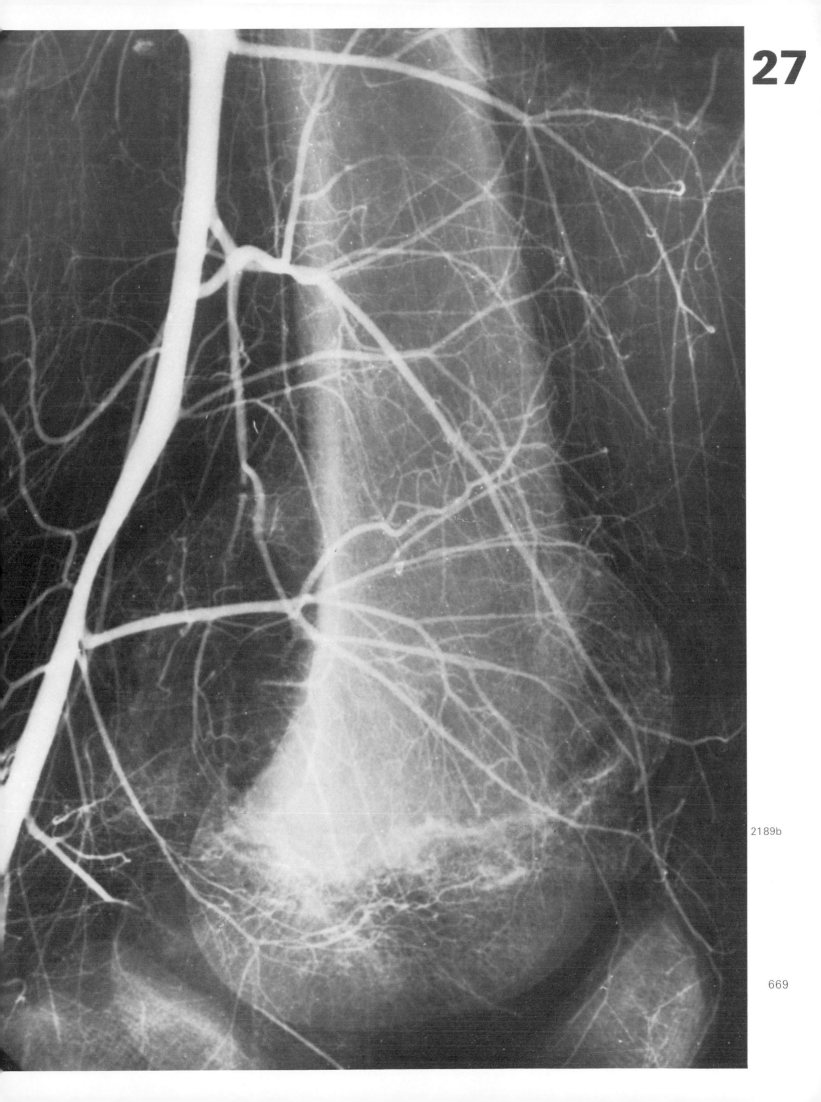

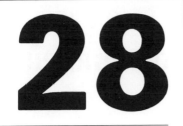

TOMOGRAPHY

28 SECTION 28

TOMOGRAPHY

In tomography, only a thin section of the body is in focus on the radiograph and the structures above and below this section are blurred out by movement. There are a number of different systems, using apparatus modified in various ways, each with a different name but tomograms is the generic term for the body-section radiographs produced by all these systems.

Principles

Conventional radiographs are two dimensional images of the full thickness of the region lying within the X-ray beam and contains information of structures both above and below the lesion or organ being demonstrated. The superimposition of the unwanted shadows will to a greater or lesser degree inevitably obscure detail required for diagnosis.

Overlying shadows can be blurred out simply by keeping the region to be examined quite still while the superimposed structures are blurred out by movement. Lateral radiographs of the dorsal spine taken with a long exposure during quiet breathing blur out the overlying ribs and lungs. The short distance technique of the sternum is another method of blurring out unwanted superimposed shadows. With tomography the superimposed structures are blurred out by the movement of the tube keeping a thin section in focus to produce a clear image. Thus if two of the three components, the tube, body and film, forming a radiographic image are moved, keeping the third stationary a particular section in the body can be freed of superimposed shadows. In tomography the tube and film move and the body remains stationary.

Plane of the Object

The plane of the object is the section in focus and occurs at the level of the fulcrum of the opposing movements of tube and film.

As a basic principle in tomography, the plane of the object and the plane of the film are always parallel. If the structure being examined lies obliquely in the body as is the case with the trachea or sacro-iliac joints, either the body or the film must be tilted to bring the structure and film parallel to each other.

Apparatus. Basically a rigid metal bar connects the X-ray tube and Potter-Bucky diaphragm which move in opposite directions pivoting about an adjustable axis or fulcrum. The X-ray tube is thus automatically centred to the Potter-Bucky diaphragm and the level or fulcrum about which the tube and film pivot, corresponds to the level of the tomographic section. The position of the fulcrum (2190) can be adjusted on a graduated centimetre scale to the height of the required section above the table top.

In most systems the distance from the tube to the table top remains constant but the traverse of the tube is variable covering angles from 5°–60°, and the angle though which the tube moves is directly proportional to the distance travelled by the tube. The wider the angle of tube traverse the narrower the tomographic section and vice versa, the narrower the angle the thicker the sections. Thick section tomography is used especially for the kidneys and is called zonography.

For ultra-thin sections of 0·5 and 1 mm the length of traverse of the tube is increased by circular, hypocycloidal or spiral movements (2208).

The angle chosen for each examination is preset which then adjusts the positions of the "on-off" contacts (2191) actuated by the lever as it passes through the required angle. Usually the angle during which the tube is exposed is symmetrical about the midline but can be confined to one or other side for an asymmetrical exposure angle.

The tube movement is powered by an electric motor although originally a traction spring was used and for a smooth action the force is transmitted at table top height. A moving grid, efficient for all kilovoltages, is used for all exposures and equally important, close collimation of the beam to diminish scattered radiation is essential for high quality films.

Essential Requirements. The movement of the tube and Potter-Bucky diaphragm must be smooth and stable without any vibrations and the tube must be constantly centred to the film without any slack in the reciprocal tube and film movement.

Exposure Factors. The exposure for a tomogram is approximately 30% greater than for a standard film.

Multisection Tomography. Multiple tomographic sections can be taken simultaneously if the film carrier has multiple cassettes (2238) or in ultra-thin section tomography, multiple screens.

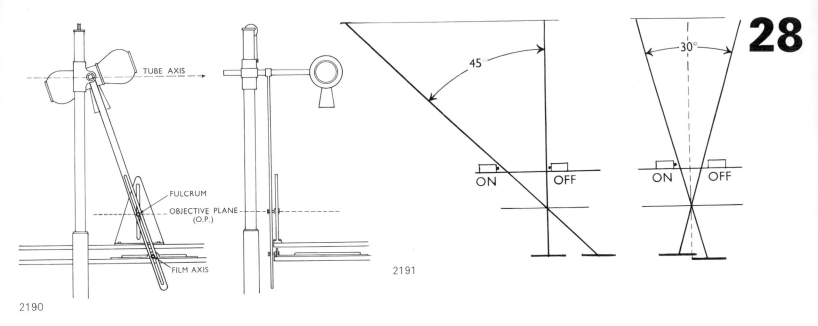

TUBE AXIS

FULCRUM

OBJECTIVE PLANE
(O.P.)

FILM AXIS

2190

2191

45°

30°

ON   OFF

ON   OFF

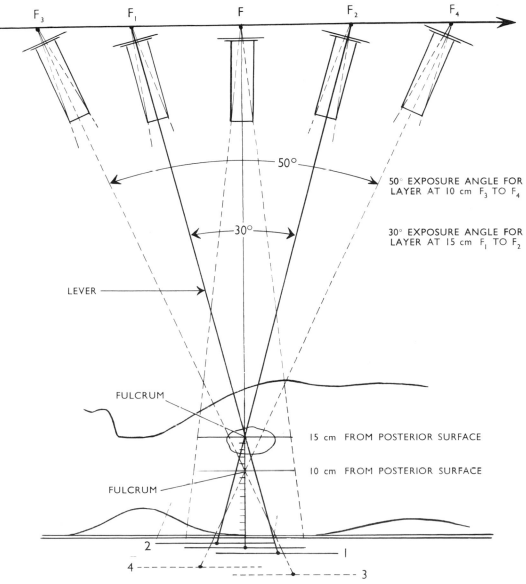

F_3 F_1 F F_2 F_4

50°

50° EXPOSURE ANGLE FOR
LAYER AT 10 cm F_3 TO F_4

30°

30° EXPOSURE ANGLE FOR
LAYER AT 15 cm F_1 TO F_2

LEVER

FULCRUM

15 cm FROM POSTERIOR SURFACE

10 cm FROM POSTERIOR SURFACE

FULCRUM

2

4

I

3

2192

Line to Line Movement (Parallel planes)

The tube and film move in straight lines, in opposite directions, and therefore in this system there is a constant ratio between the focus-object and object-film distances throughout the movement. The plane of the tomographic section is parallel to the film and the tube and is at the selected level corresponding to the fulcrum. The X-ray tube remains centred to the film by rotation through the axis of the focal spot.

However, the focal-film distance and photon absorption with the varying beam length in the body is greater at the ends of the tube traverse than in the centre. Theoretically therefore the tube movement should accelerate and decelerate to maintain a uniform exposure through all angles.

The difference in exposure between the centre and the periphery is acceptable in thin individuals or regions but with wide angles or large subjects the periphery will be under-exposed. The tomographic technique must then be suitably modified by using a smaller angle which will give a thicker tomographic section.

With modern equipment the exposure is modified automatically to produce a uniform distribution of the radiation beam using only effective angles.

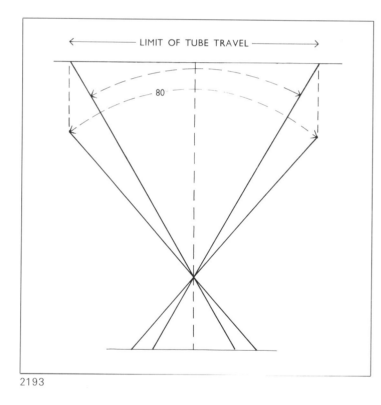

2193

Arc to Arc Movement

The tube and the film move through universely related opposing arcs centred on the fulcrum or pivoting point (2194). The film is kept parallel to the plane of section although the centre of the film moves through an arc. The focus-film distance, the focus-object distance and the object film ratio are constant and therefore the section selected at the level of the fulcrum is parallel to the film.

Arc to Line Movement

The tube in this system moves through an arc while the film moves in a straight line (2195). Although there is a slight variation in the magnification from the periphery to the centre of the tube traverse, the overall effect is marginal because the film is closer to the subject than with arc-to-arc movement.

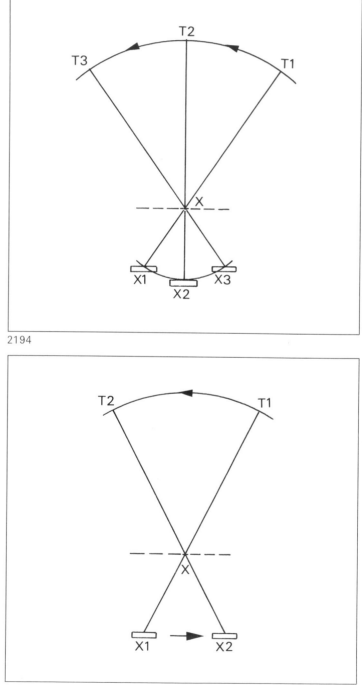

2194

2195

Confirmation of Depth and Exposure Angle. A standard test object made up of a series of steps (2196) or a 45° inclined ruler (2199) with lead markings is used to check the accuracy of the settings of the levels of the sections above the table top. The scale is marked with lead wires transversely from 0–21 cm and there is also a single longitudinal wire (2199). A tomogram of the test object with the movement at right angles to the longitudinal wire will show the height of the section above the table top by the numeral and line in focus (2197, 2198).

A discrepancy between the scale setting of the fulcrum and the test tomogram means the scale pointer needs adjustment either because the relative positions of the table top or the level of the film are incorrect. The scale pointer can be checked against the measured height of the fulcrum above the table.

If the scale is placed on a mattress and not on the table top there will obviously be a discrepancy. If on the other hand the scale pointer is correct for the test object on the table top, the cassette must be above or below the film axis. Small errors can be due to variations in cassette thicknesses and therefore the same cassettes must be used for the test and also for examinations. However, errors in the localisation of the levels of the tomographic sections do not affect the radiographic quality of the film.

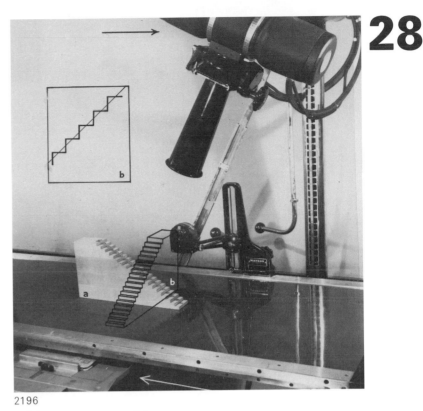
2196

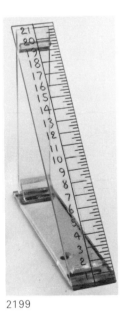
2199

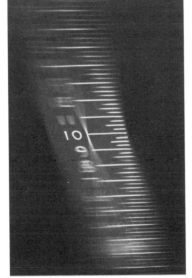
2200

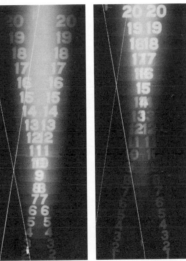
2197

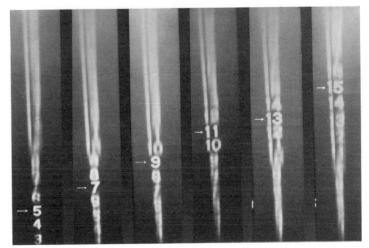
2198

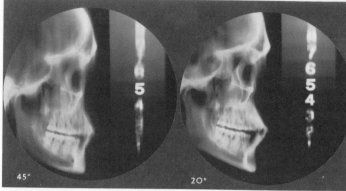

2201

Thickness of Tomographic Section

The thickness of tissue in focus on a tomographic section depends by and large on the exposure angle, the wider the exposure angle the thinner the section and vice versa the narrower the exposure angle the thicker the section (2201, 2202). Very thick sections done with narrow exposure angles of 5°–10° are called zonograms.

The choice of thin or thick sections depends on the region of the body being examined or on the size of the lesion being demonstrated. Renal outlines and calyces are best shown with zonograms but the middle ear ossicles with very thin sections of 1–2 mm.

For clear images with maximum detail and well defined margins the width of a tomographic section should be less than the diameter of the lesion.

The following relationships between the thickness of a section and the exposure angle can be used as a guide for linear movement tomography.

For a 10° arc the section is 2·0 cm thick
20° arc the section is 1·0 cm thick
30° arc the section is 0·5 cm thick
50° arc the section is 0·25 cm thick

As a general rule a 20° arc is used for lung tomography, and a 10° arc for renal tomography.

The initial tomograms of the spine or skull are done with a 20° arc but for further detail a 50° arc is used whereas for the petrous temporal the 'arc' needs to be so wide that hypocycloidal movements are used.

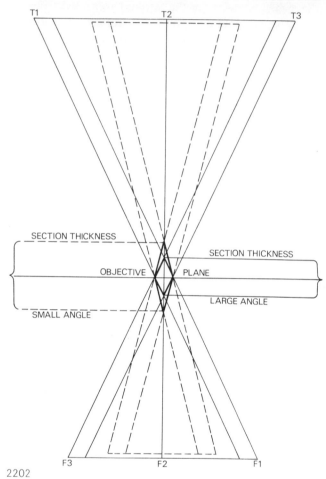

2202

The Tomographic Image

Sharpness and Contrast

The quality of a tomographic image depends on both sharpness and contrast. The sharpness of the image or spatial resolution is particularly related to the thickness of the section, the size of the lesion or structure being demonstrated and whether it is at the level of the tomographic section. For maximum sharpness the section must be thinner than the lesion and wholly within it, whereas if the section is only adjacent to the lesion there will be considerable blurring of the image. However in thin sections contrast is diminished. Therefore the thickness of the section depends on a balance between spatial resolution and contrast resolution.

There are a number of factors which influence the quality of the image on tomography including

(a) the sharpness and contrast of the lesion
(b) accurate localisation and efficient blurring
(c) the exposure angle
(d) minimising radiographic unsharpness
(e) suitable and accurate tube and film movement

The precise engineering of modern tomographic equipment and its efficient installation plays a major role in reducing unsharpness due to non-synchronous movement of the tube and Potter-Bucky diaphragm, nevertheless there is the possibility of vibration with large exposure angles.

Exposure Time. In tomography the film is being exposed while the tube moves through the required angle necessitating a long exposure time which is determined by the tube movement and unlikely to be less than 0·25 sec. Movement blurring is therefore more of a problem than routine radiography particularly for organs affected by cardiac pulsation.

The heart itself and larger vessels will obviously be affected but also adjacent structures such as the liver in contact with the heart or contrast filled lymph nodes adjacent to the aorta.

Inherent movements are particularly important with thin section radiography when a wide angle and long tube traverse is being used. However, ultra-thin sections are especially applicable to the middle ear where there is little or no inherent movement.

Immobilisation. Quite clearly with exposure times greater than 0·25 sec. immobilisation of the area being examined is imperative. The patient must hold his breath throughout the exposure and must be told before each exposure and in good time when to stop breathing and when to start again. Compression bands are extremely helpful and in middle ear tomography with the long exposure times needed, immobilisation is essential. There must not only be no movement during each individual tomographic section but no change of position throughout one projection. The great advantage of a multisection system is in allowing a rapid examination with less chance of the patient changing position.

Geometrical Unsharpness (Focal Spot Size). Because of the lowered contrast resolution with tomography and the inherent tendency for unsharpness due to the tube-film movement any further unsharpness must be minimised. In particular, geometric unsharpness must be limited by using focal spot sizes of under 1 mm. In arc-to-arc movement where there is also magnification of about × 1·3, a focal spot size of less than 0·6 mm is required and with hypocycloidal movements which produce a magnification of × 1·6, the focal spot size must be less than 0·3 mm.

Screen and Film Combination. The wider the angle and greater duration of its exposure the more screen unsharpness occurs and is particularly detrimental for demonstrating fine detail and small structures because of parallex. In these circumstances a single fast screen can be used as a back screen. Otherwise high definition screens can be used or new rare earth screens with high definition film. Rare earth screens are particularly important in single film tomography in the abdomen to reduce the radiation dose to the patient.

Direction of Linear Tomography. Overlying shadows lying parallel to the direction of movement of the tube are accentuated in tomography. Thus in tomography of the spine the lines of the apophyseal joints and spinous processes are accentuated whereas the lines adjacent to the intervertebral discs tend to be blurred out. This effect does not occur with a hypocycloidal movement.

With linear tomography, therefore, to obtain maximum visualisation of the lesion with maximum blurring of overlying structures the tube movement must be at right angles to the line of overlying structures.

Border or Marginal Sharpness. The lesion will be more clearly visualised the more rapid the contrast change or sharper the contrast border. Furthermore the borders lying parallel to the tube movement will be demonstrated most clearly.

The ideal situation for linear tomography is therefore to have the tube movement at right angles to overlying structures but parallel to the lesion being demonstrated and is particularly important when there is only slight differential contrast.

It is however not always possible to obtain the optimum orientation for a particular region because the long axis of the tube and table top are parallel and the patient cannot be positioned at right angles to the tube movement.

With complex circular or hypocycloidal tube movements edge accentuation of overlying structures or of the lesion is inconsequential.

Efficient Blurring. There are two distinct and mutually exclusive aspects in tomography, overlying shadows are removed by being blurred out and structures within the plane of the section are shown clearly by being in focus. Efficient blurring of overlying structures is thus an integral part of tomography and depends on a number of factors.

(a) **The distance of unwanted shadows from the plane of section.** A large angle of tube traverse will blur out shadows close to the plane of section but for more distant shadows a narrower tube swing is sufficient.

(b) **Direction of linear tube movement.** Tube movement will accentuate overlying shadows parallel to the tube movement and minimise those at right angles to tube movement.

(c) **Shadows above or below the plane in focus.** Blurring of unwanted shadows below the tomographic section in focus is less than shadows at a similar level above, and therefore a greater tube angle is needed to blur out shadows below than above the plane in focus.

(d) **Radio-opacity of overlying shadows.** The angle of tube movement needs to be greater to blur out shadows which are more opaque. However, where shadows close to the tomographic section are greater than the lesion to be shown circular or hypocycloidal movements are needed to effectively blur out the unwanted opacities.

Tomographic Contrast

Tomographic contrast is usually less than the contrast in routine radiographs, but contrast is greater in thicker section tomographs taken with a smaller angle than in thin section tomography with a larger angle. This is because only part of the total exposure produces the tomographic image while the rest is used to blur out unwanted shadows. The blurring density produces a veiling effect on the tomographic image diminishing contrast. Similarly, scattered radiation also lowers contrast and therefore the lowest kilovoltage to produce effective penetration should be used in tomography.

Subject contrast. The inherent contrast of the organ being examined is the limiting factor in obtaining thin section tomography. Where there is marked adjacent contrast as in the middle and inner ear, sections of 1–2 mm can be used with success but in soft tissue with little variation in contrast, sections of 0·5–1 cm are needed to obtain the necessary contrast.

Symmetric-Asymmetrical Movements

The angle of movement is usually equal about the perpendicular centring point. There are however a number of instances where it is an advantage to confine the exposure angle to one side of the perpendicular point producing an asymmetrical tube swing (2203).

This method is useful in

(a) Managing steep differences in opacity in adjoining areas.

(b) Projecting peripheral dense structures clear of the central area.

(c) Reducing exposure and radiation absorption (2203, 2204, 2206).

The following are illustrative examples

 (i) Tomography with a caudal asymmetrical angle of the base of the lung minimises radiation to the upper abdomen.

(ii) In examining the larynx (2204) a cephalic asymmetrical angle projects the mandible away from the vestibule, vocal cords and trachea.

(iii) In the cervico-thoracic region in a lateral projection (2206) a caudal asymmetrical movement avoids the dense superimposed shoulders.

Asymmetrical exposure angles can be obtained either by adjusting the positions of the contactor switches or the *total* angle should be set for one side and the timer set to terminate the exposure just prior to the tube reaching the perpendicular position (2203).

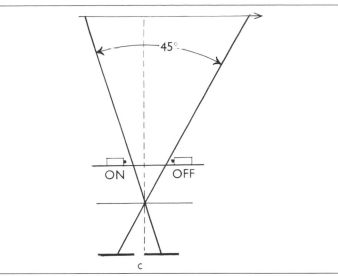

2203

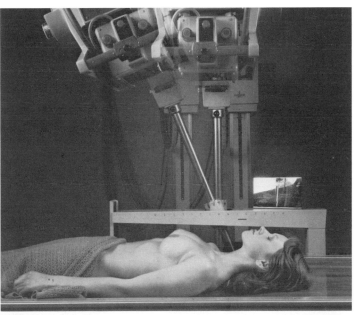

2204

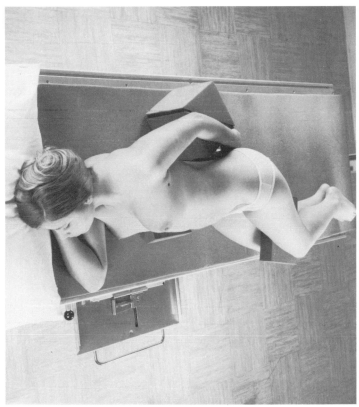

2206

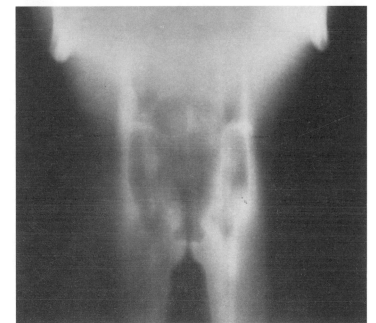

2205

Zonography

Thick tomographic sections of 2–3 cm are produced by exposure angles of 5°–10° and used for "thick" organs such as the kidney and gall-bladder, to blurr out gas shadows which are often some distance away (2207). Zonography is particularly useful for large soft tissue structures with little inherent contrast, as a preliminary for localising joint spaces at the shoulder and hip and in the lumbo-sacral region.

Linear Tomography

In rectilinear tomography the tube exposes throughout the traverse of the designated angle and is thus a continuum of exposures through all the angles from zero to the maximum.

Radiographs (2207). Zonography showing gallstones at the lower end of the common bile duct (arrows).

Multidirectional Movements

There are various tube movements in tomography (2208), the more complex increase the distance travelled by the tube making ultra thin sections possible.

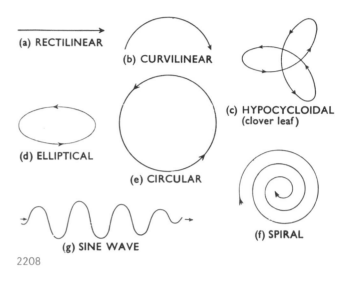

(a) RECTILINEAR
(b) CURVILINEAR
(c) HYPOCYCLOIDAL (clover leaf)
(d) ELLIPTICAL
(e) CIRCULAR
(f) SPIRAL
(g) SINE WAVE

2208

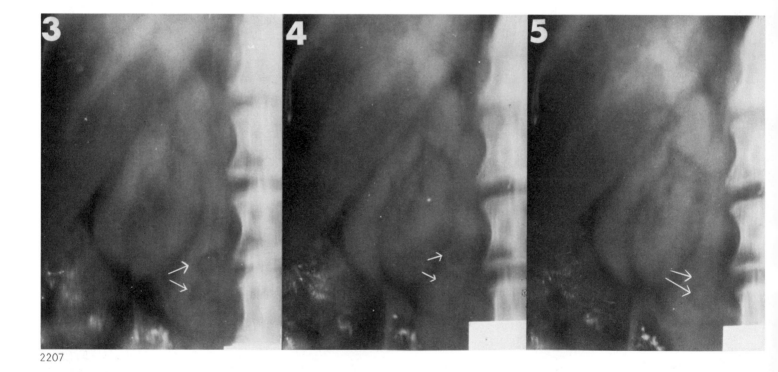

2207

Circular Movement

There are two main factors in blurring out unwanted shadows:

(a) the length of tube travel and therefore the length of travel of the unwanted shadows relative to the film.

(b) the direction of the structure and of the overlying shadows relative to the tube movement.

More complex movements increase effective blurring not only because of the greater tube travel but also because more of the tube travel is at the maximum angle especially when using a circular path and furthermore, the tube travels across anatomical lines rather than parallel to them. Circular movements are particularly useful in eliminating overlying spinal shadows for hilar tomography, however for circular objects such as the cochleas, circular striations tend to occur (2209) resulting in a less sharp image.

In tomography of structures with a low inherent contrast, circular movements may produce disappointing results due to the long tube travel which further reduces the contrast on the film. However if the circle is narrowed to reduce the tube traverse, contrast is enhanced and the results will compare favourably with linear tomography.

CIRCULAR

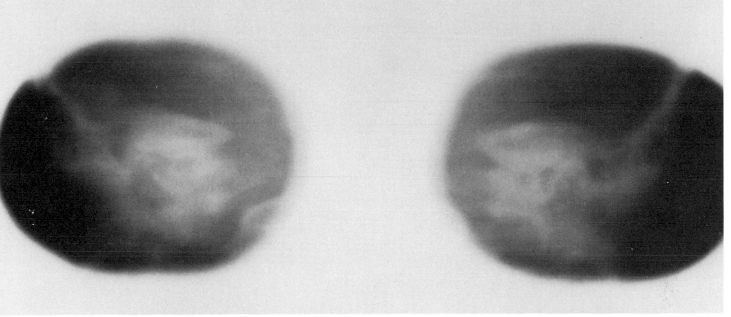

2209a

LINEAR

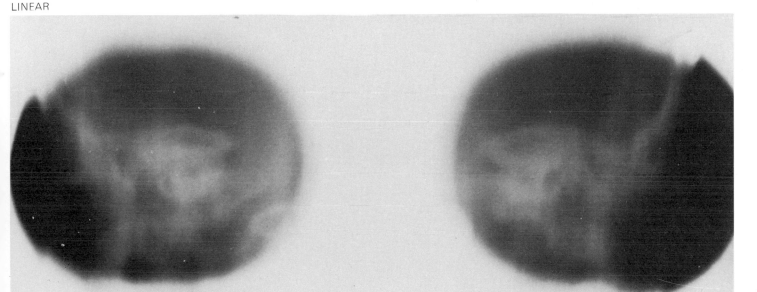

2209b

Hypocycloidal Movement (Clover Leaf)

The more complex hypocycloidal movements still further increases the homogenous diffusion of unwanted shadows by increasing the length of tube traverse and by more effectively cutting across anatomical lines. (2210a)

At a nominal angle of 48° a hypocycloidal movement can effectively produce tomographic sections of 1 mm. Due to the longer exposure time immobilisation is extremely important and the use of hypocycloidal tomography is limited to structures with good inherent contrast requiring high definition.

Petrous Bone

Hypocycloidal tomography produces ×1·6 magnification and an 0·3 mm focal spot is essential to maintain acceptable definition. Close collimation with a 1·5 cm tube aperture and an air-gap technique will prevent unnecessary scatter. The air-gap technique replaces the synchronous grid and can be further complemented with selective filtration.

Optimum contrast is maintained with a kilovoltage of 70–75 kVp using the air-gap technique, and is preferred to 120 kVp with a synchronous grid. The radiation dose can be further reduced by using rare earth screens.

HYPOCYCLOIDAL

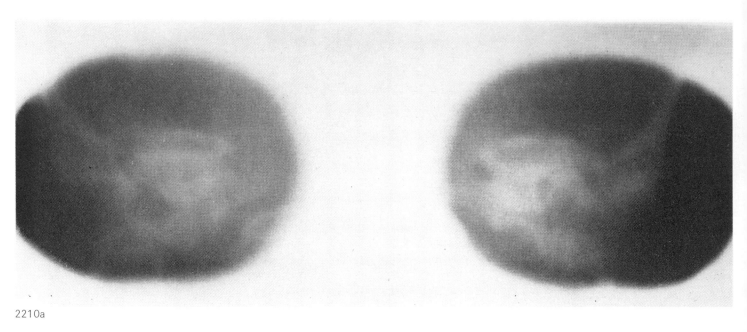

2210a

LINEAR

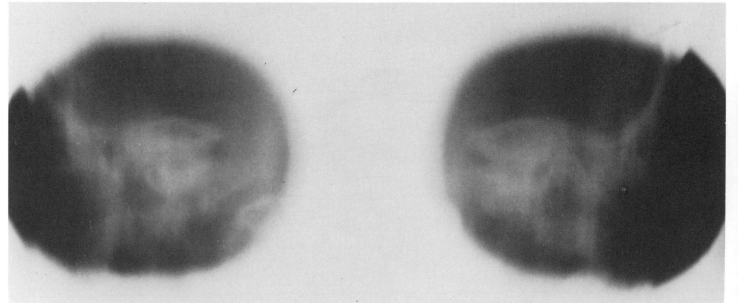

2210b

Thorax

Localisation

Preliminary chest films are essential in pulmonary tomography. Not infrequently the shadow seen on the original examination is no longer present on the preliminary film and proves to be an inflammatory lesion or infarct mimicking a tumour. Occasionally a nodule on the skin or in the subcutaneous tissue may appear to be in the lung on a frontal view but by examining the patient's skin or on fluoroscopy the nodule can be localised, dispensing with tomography.

Preliminary chest films also serve to localise the lesion within the lung fields as shown on postero-anterior and lateral (2212) views indicating the levels of the sections and the area to be covered. Sometimes comparing antero-posterior and postero-anterior films the relative position of the nodule can be deduced particularly if a short film-focal distance is used. If the nodule appears to move upwards on the antero-posterior view it is situated posteriorly (2211a, b) while an apparent change in size and definition of a nodule lying in the middle and lower lobes will also indicate its position. However, if the lesion is visible on the lateral view as well as on the postero-anterior, no other preliminary films are necessary (2211, 2212).

In most cases the required level of the tomographic section can be determined by measuring the position of the lesion on the preliminary films and also by relating it to the trachea which in an average sized patient in the supine position is 10 cm above the table top.

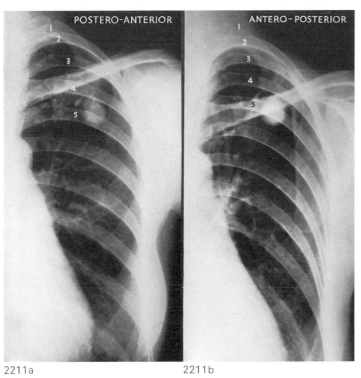

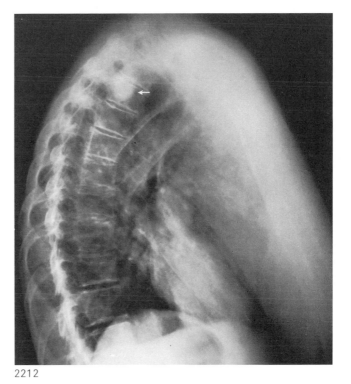

2211a   2211b   2212

Once the position of the lesion has been shown on two films at right angles to each other, the size and number of films and the interval between sections can be determined. Sections are then taken through the lesion as well as on either side till no longer visible.

For a discrete nodular lesion four to five 0·5–1 cm sections will usually be sufficient to cover the pathology but for lobar involvement 2 cm sections are more appropriate. However, if a carcinoma is suspected then the hilar regions must be included to assess metastatic spread to the regional lymph nodes.

If the level of the lesion cannot be determined before tomography, preliminary thick antero-posterior sections with the patient supine (2213) and exposure angles of 10° should be done for localisation.

Positioning the Patient

Tomography is generally done either in the frontal or lateral planes and the patient is positioned to bring the lesion close to the film. Thus where the lesion lies posteriorly the patient is supine but when anteriorly the patient is prone. Bringing the region close to the film increases the definition obtained. In (2214) the sternoclavicular joints were examined supine (8 cm) and prone (4 cm), the latter film showing greater definition. However, the region being examined must be at least 4 cm away from the table top to achieve the necessary tomographic effect.

For maximum blurring with a rectilinear tube movement the anatomical lines must be at right angles to the tube and for an adequate view on tomography the structure must lie parallel to the plane of section.

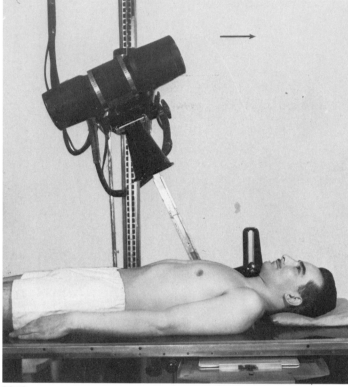

2213

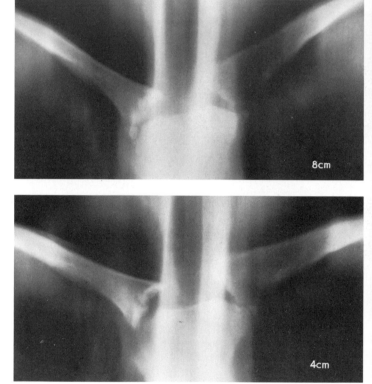

2214

For some areas more efficient blurring can be obtained with the patient lying obliquely, as shown in two positions for the sternum (2215, 2216).

In the first position the patient is in the right anterior oblique projection to throw the shadow of the spine away from the sternum. In the second position the sternum lies across the midline of the table with the line of the tube traverse running across the line of the sternum.

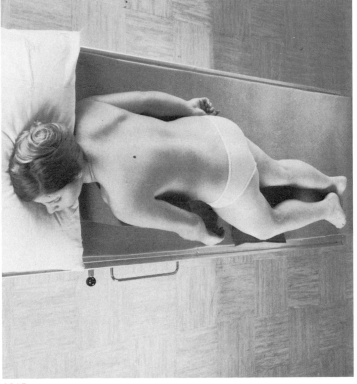

2215

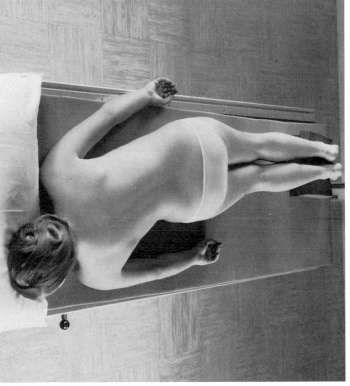

2216

The Trachea, Major Bronchi and Hilar Regions

The trachea lies obliquely in the chest being more anterior at the root of the neck and more posterior at its bifurcation. To show the whole trachea on a tomogram, its long axis must be parallel to the film. In the supine position sponge pads are used to lift the lower thorax off the table bringing the trachea (2217) parallel to the film while in the prone position the upper part of the chest is raised off the table (2218).

The correct exposure for the trachea and bronchi is 10–15 kVp more than for the lungs and hilar vessels. Tomography for the trachea and lungs therefore requires separate exposures; the trachea will not be adequately shown on tomography done for the lung parenchyma and vice versa (2219).

Oblique

With the patient supine, in the posterior oblique position the tube is centred to the side nearest the film and in the anterior oblique the tube is centred to the raised side. Oblique tomography is particularly valuable to show the carinal region (2219b) below the bifurcation of the trachea.

Where a sequence of single exposures are taken for lung tomography, each film must be exposed in the same phase of respiration and requires a careful explanation to the patient.

With the patient supine for lesions lying posteriorly in the chest near the diaphragm, the trunk should be raised with a large pad under the buttocks (2220). Using a caudal asymmetrical tube traverse prevents unnecessary radiation to the abdomen.

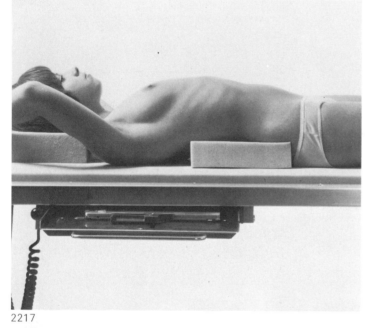

2217

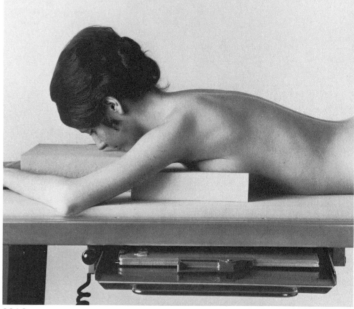

2218

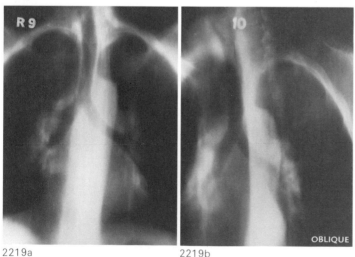

2219a   2219b

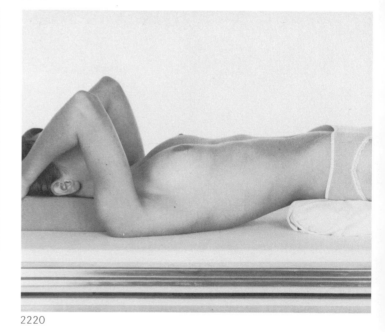

2220

Lateral

For lateral tomography the patient is turned onto the affected side to bring the lesion as close as possible to the film for maximum definition. A cephalic asymmetrical tube traverse is recommended for the upper lobes, with the patient's arms held above the head. An anomalous pulmonary vessel is shown on frontal and lateral tomography in (2226, 2227).

35° Posterior Oblique. The side to be examined is in contact with the table top and the opposite side raised 35° to the film. In this position the major bronchi at the bifurcation lie parallel to the film (2221a).

55° Posterior Oblique. The patient is rotated backwards from the lateral position till the sagittal plane forms an angle of 55° with the table top (2221b).

In this position the upper lobe, pulmonary vessels and apex of the lower lobe are all well shown.

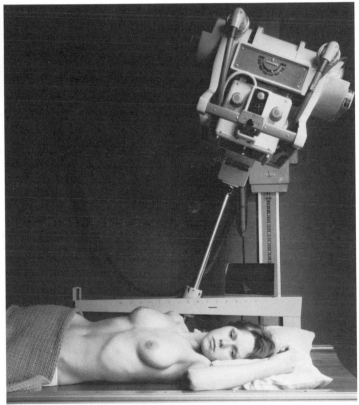

2221a

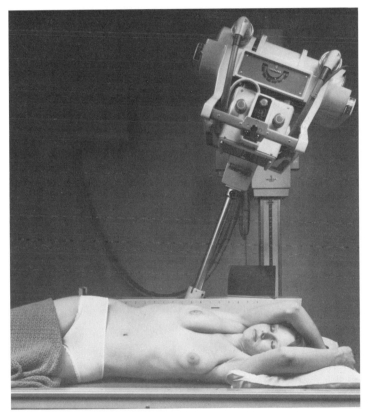

2221b

Planned Procedure

Tomography should be carefully planned before the examination starts and the patient should receive a full explanation of the procedure.

Read and Understand the Request

The previous film of the region should be viewed and an antero-posterior and lateral film taken for comparison. The lesion may have disappeared or may be visible in only one view because it is on the skin surface or lying subcutaneously.

If tomography has been done previously, the examination should aim to be technically similar and at the same levels as the films which showed the pathology.

For new patients the plane of the sections should be assessed and consequently the required position of the patient. The position and levels of the sections are then determined which will show the pathology. Thereafter the angle of tube traverse can be selected which will produce sections narrower than the size of the lesion.

Exposed and unexposed cassettes must be kept in quite separate positions to avoid any possibility of double exposures and lead numbers corresponding to the range of levels must be available to tape onto each cassette.

Whole Lung Tomography

The detection of pulmonary metastases is critical in staging malignant disease and routine whole lung tomography is carried out for this purpose. The whole thorax in antero-posterior view from apex to base is included at 1 cm intervals and where possible on 35×35 cm (14×14 ins) films. The tomograms must be exposed as for the lung fields using 65–70 kVp for maximum contrast. A preliminary chest film is imperative and must be carefully inspected for possible nodular shadows. It is however now recognised that computed tomography of the thorax is considerably more sensitive in the detection of small pulmonary metastases.

Procedure

Position the patient to bring the lesion as close as possible to the film and then

Set exposure angle
Set pivoting height
Fix number on cassette
Insert cassette
Take 3 exploratory sections
  (i) at the estimated level
  (ii) at 1–2 cm interval below the level
  (iii) at 1–2 cm interval above the level

The distance between sections will depend on the size of the lesion and the size of the region being examined.

After viewing the first three films it should be clear whether to proceed to levels above, below or between the exploratory films and how to adjust the exposure for optimum contrast. Sufficient films should be taken to fully cover the lesion and its disappearance on either side.

Processing

Automatic processing is now almost universal and a 90 sec. cycle is a great advantage. Rapid automatic processing which allows the viewing of dry films is essential for quality control in procedures using multiple films.

The major advantage is that automatic processing produces a uniform predictable result and the exposures can be standardised.

Radiographs

(2222) Multisection tomographs taken on a deep cassette producing sections at 0.25 cm intervals showing the optic foramen.

(2223, 2224) Tumour of the right side of the larynx shown on linear tomography.

(2225) Prone tomography of the sternoclavicular joints at 0.5 cm intervals obtained with a 30 arc.

(2226) Supine tomography showing an arteriovenous malformation on the A-P view.

(2227) The arteriovenous malformation is shown on lateral tomography.

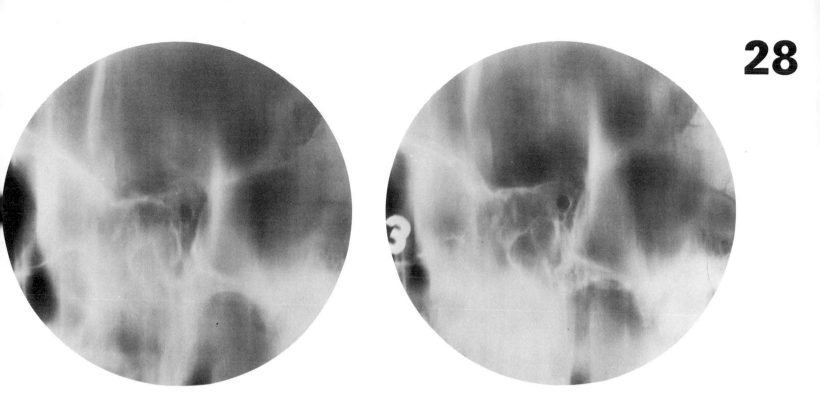

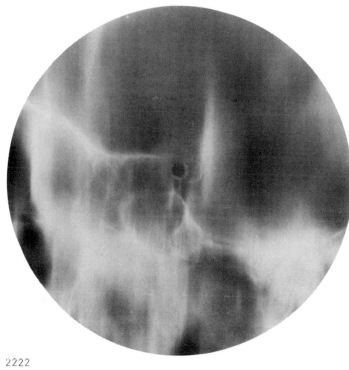

2222

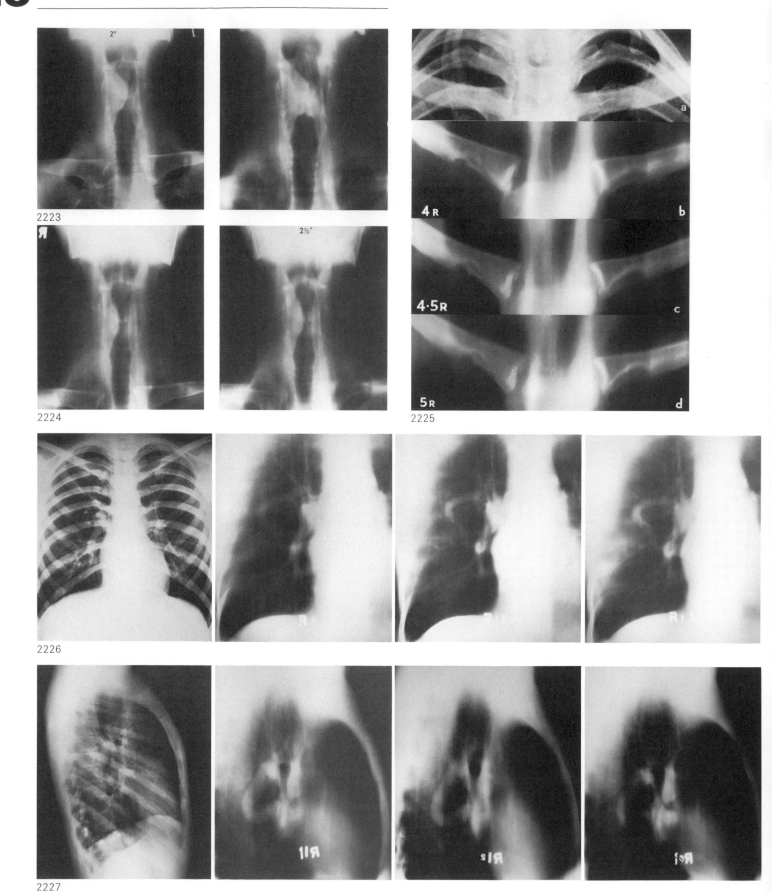

2223

2224

2225

2226

2227

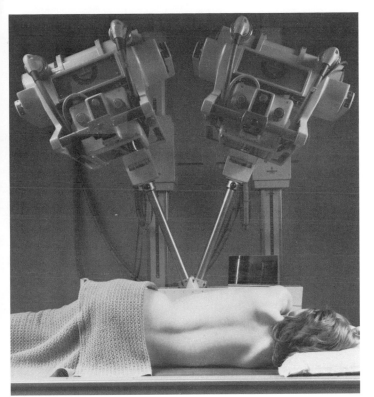

2228

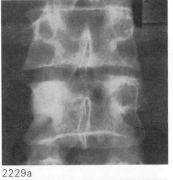

2229a

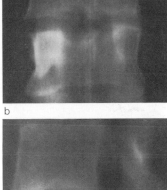

b

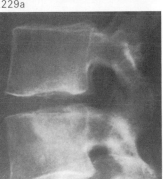

2230a

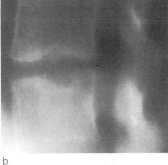

b

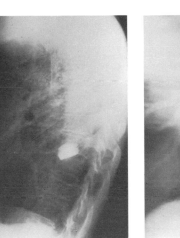

2232

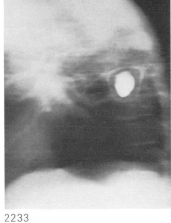

2233

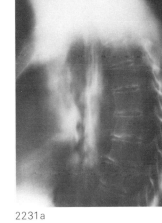

2231a

b

Radiographs (a-plain film, b-tomograph)
(2229) Anterior view tomograph of a lumbar vertebral body showing a sclerotic lesion at the base of the right pedicle.

(2230) A lateral tomograph shows the sclerotic lesion is in the posterior part of the vertebral body.

(2231) Lateral tomograph showing an enlarged intervertebral foramen.

(2232, 2233) Plain film and tomograph (lateral) of a bullet in the lung.

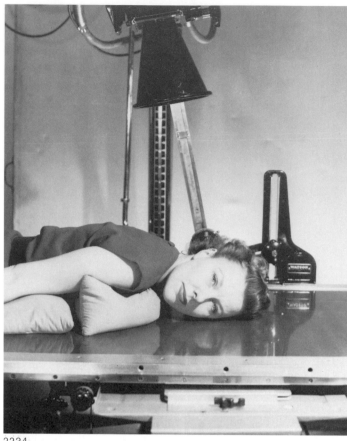

2234

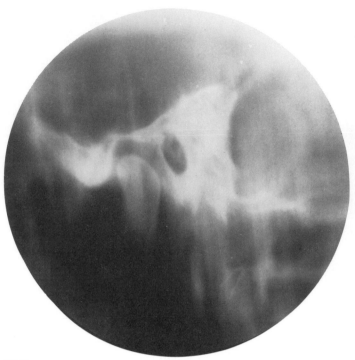

2235

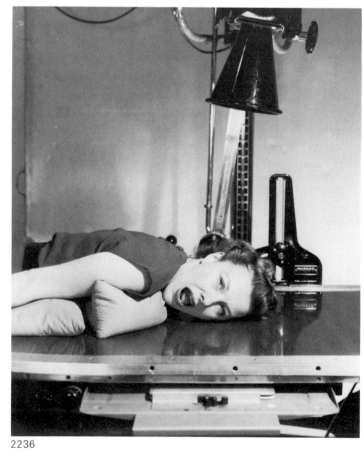

2236

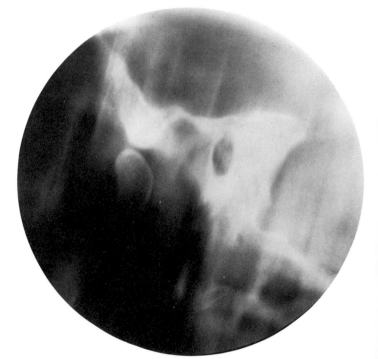

2237

Simultaneous Multisection Tomography

Tomography, Multitomography

In multisection tomography, multiple adjacent levels are tomographed simultaneously with a considerable saving in time and radiation. Furthermore the films are taken in the same respiratory phase and are therefore more comparable than sequential films.

Multitomography magazines are essentially light-tight boxes containing from 3 to 7 pairs of screens 0·3–1 cm apart, separated by equal thicknesses of transradiant material such as polyester foam (2238). A compression block is included for adequate screen contact. A modified Bucky diaphragm with a central aperture supports the multi-section box and the normal film tray is removed so that the top film in the box is at the normal film level.

Uniform Exposures

To compensate for the attenuation of the X-ray beam by the successive screens and by the increased distance where the inverse square law operates, graduated screens decreasing in speed from above downwards are required. For instance for three pairs of screens

(i) a standard screen with a high definition screen
(ii) a standard screen with a fast tungstate screen
(iii) a pair of fast tungstate screens

and for five pairs of screens

(i) a pair of high definition screens
(ii) a high definition screen with a fast tungstate screen
(iii) a pair of standard screens
(iv) a standard screen and a fast tungstate screen
(v) a pair of fast tungstate screens.

Note—The screens must be kept in the recommended sequence to produce uniform exposures. A centimetre wedge scale placed alongside a skull shows how the film separation provides 1 cm interval sections on multi-tomographic films (2239).

Radiographs

(2235) Lateral tomograph of the temporo-mandibular joint with the mouth closed (2234).

(2237) Same view with the mouth open (2236) showing forward movement of the condyle of the mandible.

Spacing Intervals

Due to magnification the spacing between films is greater than the distance between body sections and can be calculated by

$$Fl = Bl\left(1 + \frac{d}{D}\right)$$

where Fl = film spacing in magazine
Bl = distance between body sections
d = distance of fulcrum to top-film
D = distance of focus to fulcrum

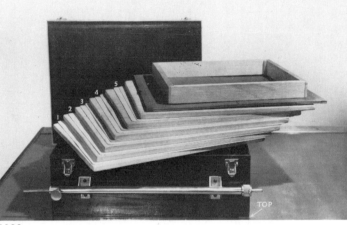

2238

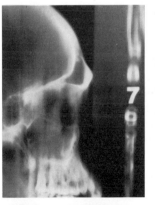
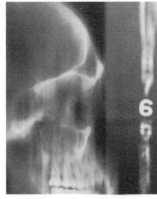

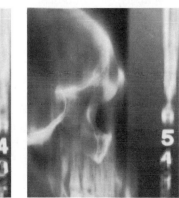

2239

Quality: If the film-screen combinations are correctly chosen there is little if any loss of definition using multisection tomography provided not too many simultaneous sections are attempted, and there is good film-screen contact throughout. Nevertheless the quality of two sets of three screen units is definitely better than a single six pair unit.

Other very important factors in maintaining quality in multisection tomography include the absence of movement of the multisection box in the Bucky diaphragm and strict collimation of the X-ray beam.

Operating Angle relative to Body Intervals

The width of the body section is approximately related to the angle of tube traverse as follows

10° arc produces a 2 cm section
20° arc produces a 1 cm section
30° arc produces a 0·5 cm section
50° arc produces a 0·25 cm section

Therefore if the multisection box has a film spacing of 0·5 cm a 30° arc will produce adjacent sections. However if the arc is 10° the section widths of 2 cm will overlap on successive films and for a 50° arc many 0·25 cm sections will fall on each film.

Exposure. The exposure for all the films in multisection tomography is essentially that for the uppermost pair of screens. Any saving in radiation dose is the difference between a series of sections with faster screens and the single exposure for the slower top screens of the multisection box. The saving in radiation is therefore not a simple addition of each extra sequential exposure.

Kilovoltage. To maintain good contrast with a multisection cassette compared with sequential films, approximately 5 kVp must be added for a 3 screen box and 7 kVp for a 5 screen box to ensure adequate penetration of each screen assembly.

The kilovoltage range within which comparable exposures can be obtained with multisection tomograms is 70–90 kVp. Below this level the top film will have the greatest exposure and conversely with a kVp above this level the bottom film will have the greatest exposure.

Operating Angle: For uniform exposure of all films with 0·5–1 cm spacing 30° should be the maximum angle of tube traverse.

Sequence of Body Intervals. The top film generally corresponds to the level set for the fulcrum. Where sections are required both above and below a particular level in the body, the top film should accordingly be moved upwards.

Note—For safety in identifying the correct screen sequence and the correct anatomical level the screens should be clearly numbered from below upwards and the corresponding number should show on each film.

Methods of Identification

A **Phantom Scale** adjacent to the patient and included in the collimated beam provides each film with its own numbered level and checks the accuracy of the fulcrum setting. However, it has the disadvantage that the X-ray beam must be opened to include the phantom. (2239)

Printed Height Identification

Each film has its own identification with the appropriate number (1–15 cm) adjacent to the name, date and hospital number. The number can be written on each film separately prior to being processed.

Deep Cassette Multisection Radiography

A deep cassette which can hold a 4 film screen combination spaced at 0·25 cm intervals provides a maximum interval of 1·5 cm between top and bottom film and has the advantage that it can be held rigidly in the normal cassette position (2242). This is the ideal system when narrow section cuts, as for optic foramina (2222) are required and can also be used to complement tomography of the gall bladder (2207) and kidney.

Using maximum linear and circular angles, films should not be separated by less than 0·25 cm to obtain adjacent anatomical sections but for hypocycloidal tube movements the film separation can be as little as 0·1 cm (2244).

Radiographs

(2240) Pulmonary cavity shown on the frontal view-multisection tomographs.

(2241) On the lateral tomograph, the pulmonary cavity lies posteriorly in the subapical segment of the right lower lobe.

(2243) Adjacent multisection tomograms at 0·1 cm intervals at the base of the skull.

(2244) Hypocycloidal multisection tomographs of the middle ear at 0·1 cm film separation.

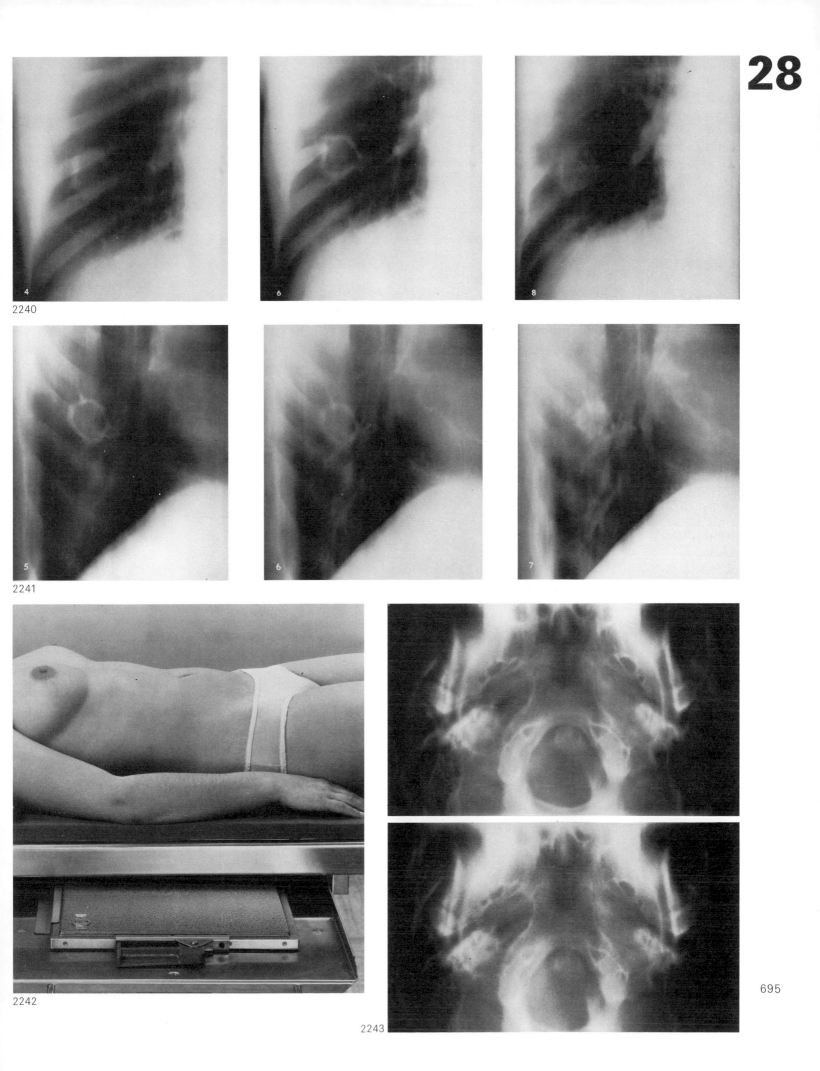

2240

2241

2242

2243

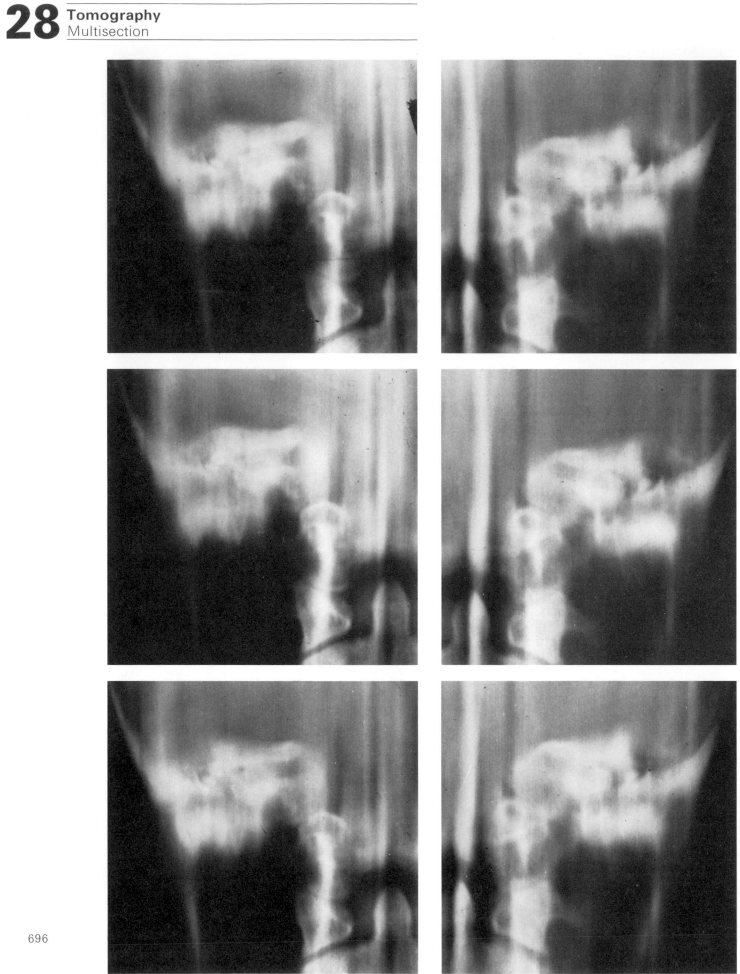

2244

Positioning for suitable orientation of lung structure

Right Lung	Position
R. Main Bronchus	Patient Prone
R. Middle Lobe	55° R. Posterior oblique
Anterior Segmental Bronchus	65° R. Posterior oblique
Apical Segmental Bronchus	Supine
Posterior Segmental Bronchus	20° L. Posterior oblique
R. Lower Lobe Lateral Segmental Bronchus	Supine Position
Posterior Segmental Bronchus	15° L. Posterior oblique
Anterior Basal Segment	15° L. Posterior oblique

Left Lung	Position
Main Bronchus, Upper Lobe Bronchus	35° L. Posterior oblique
Anterior Segmental Bronchus	55° L. Posterior oblique
Posterior Segmental Bronchus	15° R. Posterior oblique
Lower Lobe—Lateral Basal Segmental Bronchus	10° R. Posterior oblique
Anterior Basal Segmental Bronchus	20° L. Posterior oblique
Posterior Basal Segment	Supine raised 10°

28 Approximate Levels

Routine positioning is used and when the head needs to be rotated or adjusted accordingly, it must be immobilised in the appropriate position. The levels quoted are based on an average patient and measured from the table top.

Skull Approximate Levels

Part	Position	Level
Petrous both sides	A.P. baseline 90°	Measured distance to centre EAM
Internal auditory canal Petrous (Single)	A.P. baseline 90° A.P. 10–20° rotation away from affected side	Anterior rim of EAM 2·5 cm (1 in) below EAM on affected side
Optic Foramen	A.P. (35° × 35°) Chin raised to bring base-line 35° beyond perpendicular. Rotate head 35° away from affected side	Measured distance on affected side to centre of EAM
Sella Turcica	Lateral	Measured distance to nasion
Antra (facial bones) Frontal Sinuses Upper Orbital Margin	P.A. baseline 70°	6 cm (2·5 ins)
Lower Orbital Margin fracture	A.P. baseline 20° beyond perpendicular (Raised chin)	Measured distance to lower orbital margin
Ethmoidal Sinuses	P.A. 45° rotation Baseline 30°	5 cm (2 ins)

Respiratory Tract—(Approximate levels)

Part	Position	Level
Larynx	A.P.	1 cm below Thyroid cartilage—14 cm Cephalad tube movement—asymmetrical exposure
Apical Region	A.P.	4, 6, 8 cm ($1\frac{5}{8}$, $2\frac{3}{8}$, $3\frac{1}{4}$ ins) Routine chest kilovoltages plus 7–10 kVp
Hilar Region	Preferably Prone Supine	P.A. 5, 7, 9 cm (2, $2\frac{3}{4}$, $3\frac{5}{8}$ ins) A.P. 8, 10, 12 cm ($3\frac{1}{4}$, 4, $4\frac{3}{4}$ ins)
Trachea and Bifurcation	Preferably P.A. A.P.—Partial oblique Lateral	P.A. 7, 9, 11 cm ($2\frac{3}{4}$, $3\frac{5}{8}$, $4\frac{3}{8}$ ins) A.P. 9, 11, 13 cm ($3\frac{5}{8}$, $4\frac{3}{8}$, $5\frac{1}{8}$ ins)
Lesions at diaphragm level	A.P. Lateral	Caudal tube movement—asymmetrical exposure
Peripheral lesions	A.P.—Partial oblique P.A.—Partial oblique	
Lateral Upper Zones	Lateral	Cephalad tube movement—asymmetrical exposure
R. Mid-zone	A.P. or P.A. Lateral 35°R. Posterior oblique 55° R. Posterior oblique	9–14 cm ($3\frac{5}{8}$–$5\frac{5}{8}$ ins) 10–16 cm (4–$6\frac{3}{8}$ ins)
L. Mid-zone	A.P. or P.A. Lateral 35° L. Posterior oblique 55° L. Posterior oblique	9–14 cm ($3\frac{5}{8}$–$5\frac{5}{8}$ ins) 10–16 cm (4–$6\frac{3}{8}$ ins)
General for Vascular pattern	R. Posterior oblique 55°	2 cm sections ($\frac{3}{4}$ ins) 8–16 cm ($3\frac{1}{4}$–$6\frac{3}{8}$ ins)
1 cm 0·5 cm	Subject intervals Subject intervals	20° operational angle (approximate) 30° operational angle (approximate)

28 Spine—Approximate Levels

Part	Position	Level
Atlas-Axis	A.P.	10 cm (4 ins) or 2·5 cm (1 in) below angle of jaw
Cervical Spine	A.P.	2 cm ($\frac{3}{4}$ in) below Thyroid cartilage
Thoracic Spine	A.P.	3–4 cm ($1\frac{1}{4}$–$1\frac{3}{4}$ ins)
Thoracic Spine	Lateral	Measured distance to spinous process
Lumbar Spine	A.P.	7 cm ($2\frac{3}{4}$ ins)
Lumbar Spine	Lateral	Measured distance to spinous process
Sacro-Illiac Joints	A.P.	6 cm ($2\frac{1}{2}$ ins)

Additional Subjects

Sternum	Modified R. Anterior oblique	5 cm (2 ins)
Kidneys	A.P.	8 cm ($3\frac{1}{4}$ ins)
	20° L. & R. Posterior oblique	9 cm ($3\frac{3}{4}$ ins)
Gallbladder	P.A.	8 cm ($3\frac{1}{4}$ ins)
	A.P.	13 cm ($5\frac{1}{8}$ ins)
	20° L. Anterior oblique	10 cm (4 ins)
	20° R. Posterior oblique	15 cm (6 ins)

General multisection recommendations

3–4 screen unit
Linear movement–operational angles
1 cm spacing   20° angle (approximate)
0·5 cm spacing   30° angle (approximate)
2·5 mm spacing   40°–50° angle (approximate)

Technique

Exposure to suit speed of film and top screen
Kilovoltage—For subject thickness plus 5–7 kVp

Transverse Axial Tomography

The simplest method of obtaining axial sections is now by computed axial tomography, however conventional radiographic equipment can also be adapted to provide axial sections but the definition is vastly superior on computed tomography (2247a vs 2247b).

For conventional axial tomography the film is on a turntable and linked to the rotating pedestal of the patient. The patient and film rotate synchronously through 360° during an exposure from a tube at 3 metres angled downwards at 30° (2255). The level of the section is obtained by raising or lowering the patient.

A bronchial carcinoma is shown on conventional axial tomography (2248–2251) and on computed tomography (2252–2254) for comparison of the definition possible with the two different methods. Previously conventional transverse axial tomography was used largely for radiotherapy planning (2248–2251) and has now been replaced by computed tomography (CT) (2252–2254).

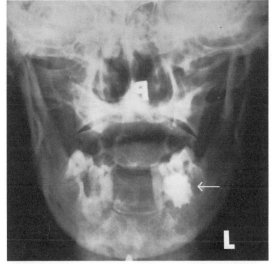

2245

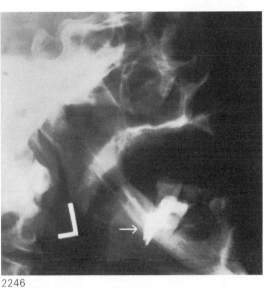

2246

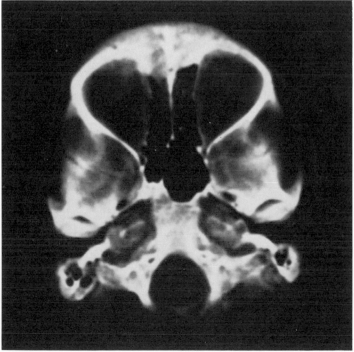

2247b

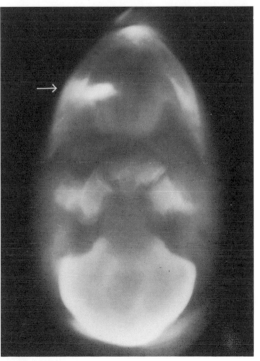

2247a

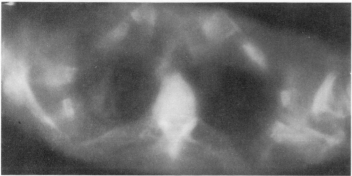

2248

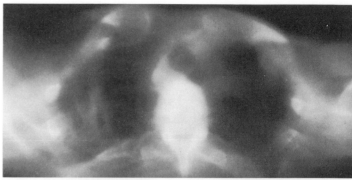

2249

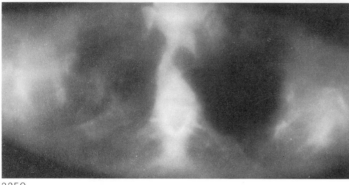

2250

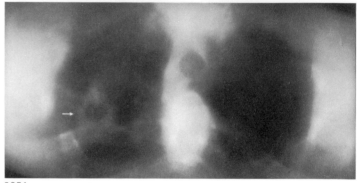

2251

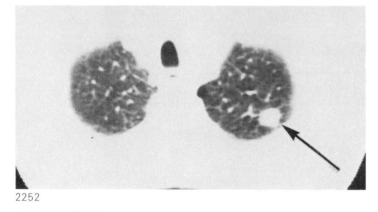

2252

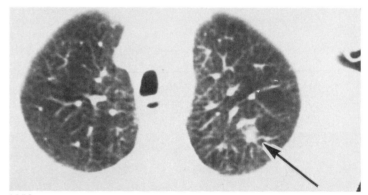

2253

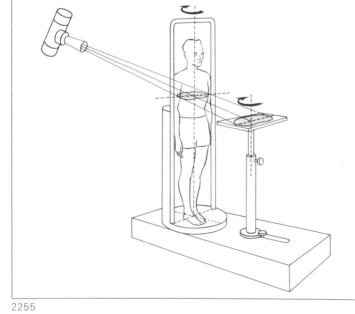

2255

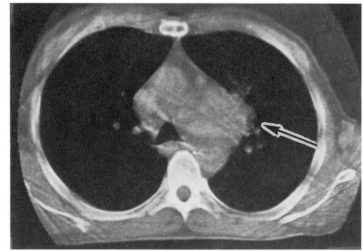

2254

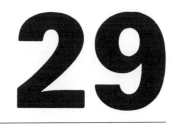

STEREOGRAPHY

STEREOGRAPHY

A three dimensional view giving the appearance of depth can be obtained from two radiographs taken sequentially with a change in the position of the tube but no change in the position of the subject or the two cassettes (2256). The method is similar to obtaining an image on each eye which is then combined in the brain as an aid to depth perception.

The two radiographs obtained after "tube-shift" are viewed in such a way as to be superimposed and then produce an impression of depth.

Procedure

The patient is immobilised and the first exposure is made in the usual way. The film/cassette is changed and the tube is shifted 6 cm (2½ ins) laterally and the exposure repeated without any change in the position of the patient. In the frontal plane the first exposure should be 3 cm (1¼ ins) from the midline and the second exposure on the contralateral side again 3 cm (1¼ ins) from the midline. A tube shift of 6 cm matches the average interpupillary distance, but for an ideal stereoscopic effect the focus-film distance should be ten times the tube shift distance which would produce a focal-film distance of only 60 cm (25 ins) resulting in a high radiation dose and therefore a tube shift of 8–10 cm is more usual.

The tube shift should be at right angles to the predominant anatomical lines. In the legs it should be across from left to right as with the spine but for the chest it should be cranio-caudal at right angles to the lie of the ribs.

The films taken must have identical processing. Different degrees of radiographic density will nullify the stereoscopic effect.

In general radiography, particularly of the skeleton, the patient can be sufficiently immobilised to allow time to move the tube by hand and change the cassette. But for chest radiography the two exposures must be taken in the same phase of respiration. The tube shift and cassette change must be automated or two assistants will be needed.

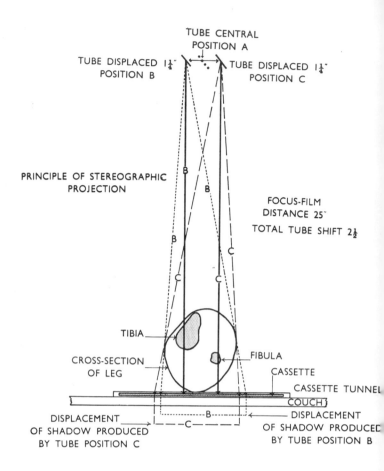

PRINCIPLE OF STEREOGRAPHIC PROJECTION

2256

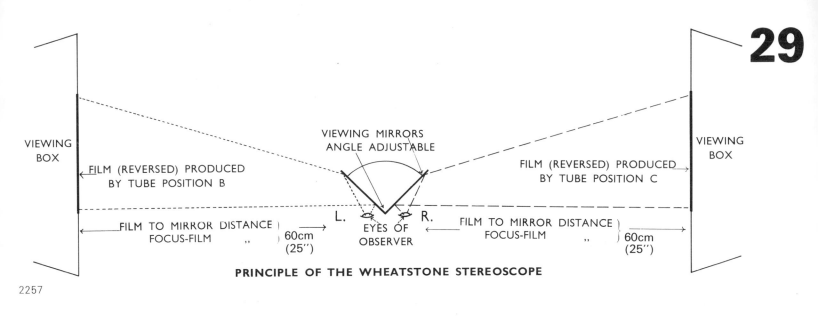

VIEWING
BOX

VIEWING MIRRORS
ANGLE ADJUSTABLE

VIEWING
BOX

FILM (REVERSED) PRODUCED
BY TUBE POSITION B

FILM (REVERSED) PRODUCED
BY TUBE POSITION C

L.

R.

EYES OF
OBSERVER

FILM TO MIRROR DISTANCE
FOCUS-FILM   „   } 60cm
                                        (25″)

FILM TO MIRROR DISTANCE
FOCUS-FILM   „   } 60cm
                                        (25″)

PRINCIPLE OF THE WHEATSTONE STEREOSCOPE

2257

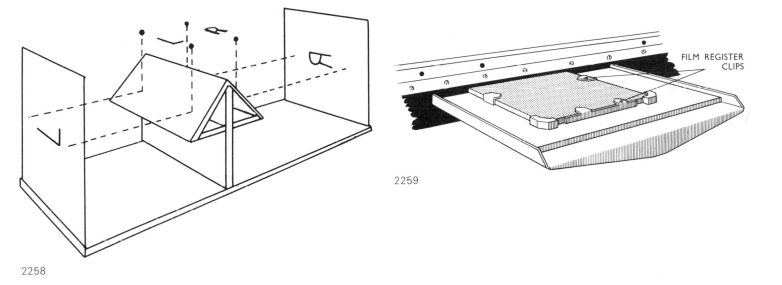

2258

FILM REGISTER
CLIPS

2259

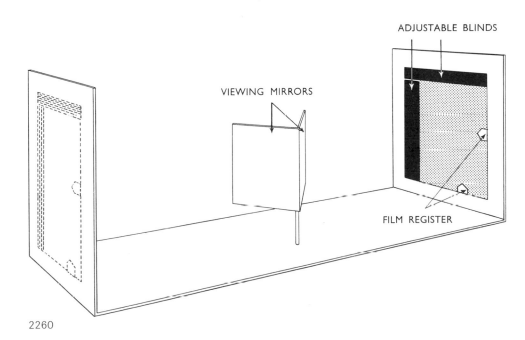

ADJUSTABLE BLINDS

VIEWING MIRRORS

FILM REGISTER

2260

Markers

By labelling each stereoscopic film with two letters either RR or RL the first letter indicates the side of the patient and the second letter the viewers eye for which the film is intended. Correct stereoscopic viewing is then possible, the nearside of the 3-dimensional view corresponding with the tube side of the patient, the orthoscopic view. However, if the films are viewed "about-face" the in depth view will be reversed as though viewing is towards the tube side of the patient, the pseudo-scopic view.

To determine the correct method of viewing a pair of stereoscopic films when there is only one letter indicating the right or left side of the patient, the films should be superimposed edge-to-edge and the images will then be slightly out of alignment. The image projected towards the left will have been produced by the right tube shift and vice versa (2261, 2262).

The images will be reversed if the films are mounted incorrectly on the illuminators or incorrectly lettered on the film, allowing the left eye to view the right shift image. The in depth view will be seen from the opposite side to that radiographed and the sides will be reversed. Reversing the individual films will reverse the aspect, from which the image is being viewed but right and left sides would still be wrong.

Serious errors in interpretation of the films can be caused by faulty labelling and viewing of the films which therefore requires the utmost care and attention.

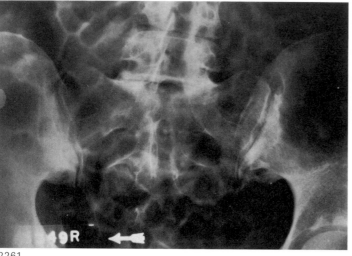

2261

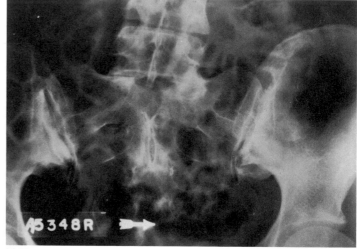

2262

Viewing

The apparatus used for stereoscopic viewing is either a Wheatstone unit or Stereo Binoculars. It is however also possible, after considerable practice, to view stereoscopically with "naked eyes" by squinting till the retinal images are superimposed.

The Wheatstone unit has a pair of mirrors at right angles to each other midway between illuminators (2257). The angle of the mirrors can be varied to suit the viewer and can also be moved up and down and across the line of the illuminators to bring the films into view and the distance between illuminators can be adjusted. Distances in the film can be measured accurately if the ratios of FFD to stereo-shift and viewing distance to film are the same.

Prismatic binoculars are a convenient method for a stereoscopic viewing. The films are placed side by side in a rectangular illuminator with the right stereo film to the right and the left stereo to the left. Each eye views its own film through its own prismatic eyepiece and with proper adjustment the two images are merged into a single 3-dimensional view.

A mirror image is obtained with both systems which can be corrected by turning the films over for the tube side of the film to face the illuminators. The letters which if correctly positioned towards the tube side will then read ЛЯ (on left viewing box) ЯЯ (on right viewing box).

A dual stereoscope (2258) allows simultaneous viewing by two observers. Both see the image from the same aspect but appears upside down to one viewer.

Direct-measuring Stereoscope

Internal measurements can be determined precisely with the direct measuring stereoscope which is particularly valuable for the pelvis. However, the measurement will only be accurate if the cassettes are fitted into identical positions on the Bucky tray (2259) and then the films marked accordingly are in corresponding identical positions on the illuminators (2260). In addition a rigid opaque marker such as two metal arrowheads exactly 10 cm (or 4 ins) apart in a plastic mount, is placed on the skin surface parallel to the film symmetrically about the midline, in the line of the tube shift. The tube shift must be exactly the same as the distance between the markers when the stereographs are viewed in the precision stereoscope. The 10 cm (4 ins) distance between the markers can be used to measure pelvic diameters accurately on a 3-dimensional image. On the direct measuring stereoscope the pelvic diameters can be read off on an attached scale which can be positioned to read each diameter in turn because the mirrors are transparent and the scale appears to lie within the radiographic image (2263).

By applying simple formulae as for localising foreign bodies in Section 32, the pelvic diameters can be calculated from measurements on the radiographs without using the direct-measuring stereoscope.

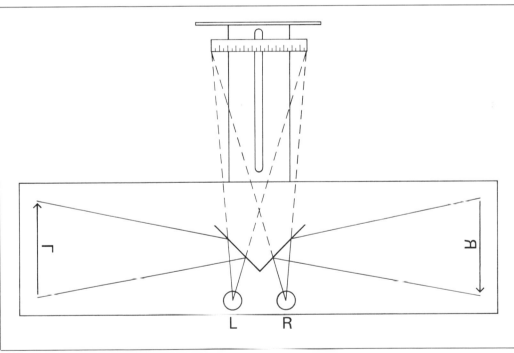

2263

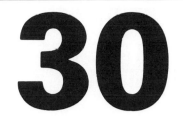

FEMALE
REPRODUCTIVE
SYSTEM

FEMALE REPRODUCTIVE SYSTEM

Imaging methods in obstetrics and gynaecology have changed completely since the introduction of ultrasonography producing a marked reduction in radiation to the fetus and ovaries and a considerable gain in diagnostic information. The early detection of pregnancy, the accurate assessment of growth and development of the fetus, the localization of the placenta and the demonstration of mass lesions in the pelvis can now be achieved without ionizing radiation. Conventional radiography has become out moded for most abnormalities and obstetric assessments for which it was previously considered essential, and its indications are now much more limited. Hysterosalpinography for showing the fallopian tubes is still essential, but gynaecography for showing the uterus and ovaries has been replaced by ultrasonography, and where efficient ultrasonography is available, radiography in pregnancy becomes strictly limited.

The normal anatomy

The female genital or reproductive system consists of the ovaries, uterine or fallopian tubes, uterus, vagina (2264) and external genitals or vulva. The uterus is a thick walled muscular organ with a "T"-shaped cavity communicating with the vagina below and the fallopian tubes above and lies between the bladder and rectum in the midline (2265). It is normally in close contact with the superior margin of the bladder causing a visible indentation on the bladder shadow as seen during urography.

There are three parts to the uterus, the cervix or neck, the narrow lower part of the body and the expanded fundus. The nulliparous uterus is 7·5 cm (3 in) long and 5 cm (2 in) wide but expands up to 35 cm (14 in) in length and 25 cm (10 in) in width during pregnancy.

The uterus is relatively mobile, usually being anteverted with the cavity facing backwards and downwards towards the fornices of the vagina which are formed around the cervix. The vaginal cavity however, tends to pass forwards and downwards (2265).

The ovaries or reproductive organs producing the ova, lie one on each side of the pelvis, but are somewhat variable in position and may lie anywhere from just below the posterolateral brim of the pelvis in the ovarian fossae, to close to the side of the uterus. In relation to the surface of the body, they lie beneath a point midway between the antero-superior iliac spine and the symphysis pubis.

Each fallopian or uterine tube connects the lateral margin of the fundus of the uterus with the ovary and is about 10 cm (4 ins) long. The cavity of the uterus is continuous with the medial end of the fallopian tube but expands and opens laterally into the peritoneal cavity. The lateral expanded opening of the tube is not actually in contact with the ovary but is fringed with finger-like processes called fimbriae and one fimbriated strand is attached to the ovary (2264). The

uppermost part of the vagina encircles the cervix and extends downwards and forwards to the external genitalia or vulva (2264, 2265). Thus while the vagina is directed upward and backwards, the uterus is usually anteverted and anteflexed lying on the superior surface of the bladder.

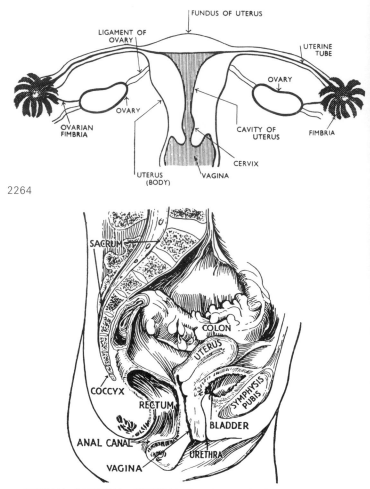

2264

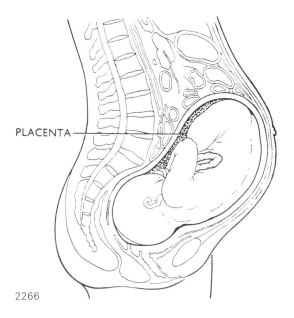

A MEDIAN SAGITTAL SECTION THROUGH THE FEMALE PELVIS
2265

2266

Pelvis

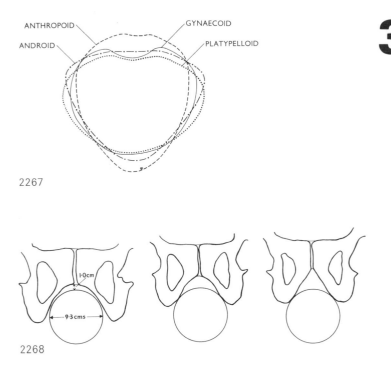

2267

There is a marked difference in shape between the male and female pelvis. The male pelvis tends to be long and narrow, whereas the female pelvis is broad and deep but even the female pelvis may show marked variations (2267). In the gynecoid type the pelvic brim is large and circular, in the anthrapoid type it is elongated and narrow or oval, in the platypelloid it is broad and shallow with a wide subpubic arch and in the android type almost triangular with a narrow subpubic arch. Over and above these recognized types the pelvis may be congenitally deformed or deformed by diseases such as rickets or following trauma.

The shape of the pubic arch also varies and may be wide or narrow but obstetrically is divided into 3 groups (2268). If a circle with a diameter of 9·3 cm is placed under the pubic arch, there is a gap between the pubis and the circle which is called the "Waste-space of Morris", and is normally less than 1 cm. The variable capacity of the pelvis is also associated with different sacral cruves (2269a) and can be demonstrated and measured on lateral radiographs.

2268

Range of examinations

The placenta and fetus are now almost exclusively assessed with ultrasonography (2269b). However, after the 34th week of pregnancy a radiograph for fetal maturity is often still required. A film to elucidate the cause of non-engagement of the head should only be done after "non-engagement" has been checked with the patient standing erect.

Patency of the fallopian tubes and the appearance of the uterine cavity is determined by hysterosalpingography but the size, shape and position of the uterus and ovaries is now invariably shown by ultrasonography, and not as previously by gynaecography.

After fetal death has been diagnosed by ultrasonography, radiography of the fetus can also be of value to show the nature of any bone deformity.

A full range of projections in pregnancy is provided, but must be strictly limited to one or at the most two views to minimize radiation to the fetus and mother. There are now virtually no indications for radiography up to 30 weeks of pregnancy; ultrasonography is used exclusively in this period.

Radiography in obstetrics, when essential for the well being of either the mother or fetus is limited to one projection, often a prone oblique for the fetus or one of the four basic projections for the mother, namely antero-posterior, postero-anterior, erect-lateral or horizontal lateral.

To further limit radiation in obstetric radiography, fast rare earth screens must be used, repeat examinations avoided and pelvimetry should by and large only be done following childbirth.

Ultrasonograph (2269b) shows a posterior placenta with an overlying limb casting an acoustic shadow.

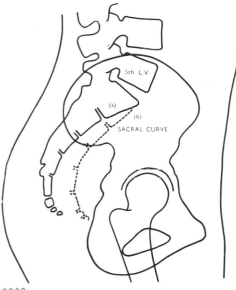

2269a

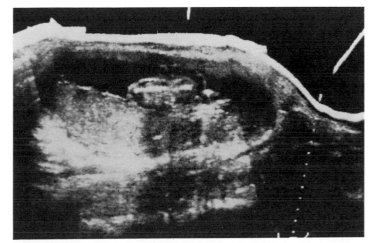

2269b

Care of the patient

A warm outer gown should be provided for each patient while waiting for the examination. During the procedure the patient wears a large three quarter length gown fastened only behind the neck which can be easily adjusted so as not to hinder the examination. Before the examination the bladder, and if possible, the bowel must be emptied.

The patient should be as comfortable as possible, although some of the projections are difficult especially if compression is used. With the necessary encouragement and assistance a satisfactory examination can be achieved. When compression is acceptable the band should be broad enough for uniform pressure because satisfactory compression produces an overall even radiodensity with good immobilization and a reduction in exposure. For clarity in the illustrations, the linen band has been replaced by a plastic band.

All the information needed by the radiologist must be carefully recorded and the radiograph accurately labelled with the date, name and hospital number.

Exposure conditions

Fast intensifying screens preferably rare earth screens and an efficient grid is essential and for certain projections a moving grid is combined with sheet tin as a selective filter for added absorption of the scattered radiation. Careful collimation with a light beam diaphragm for each examination to cover only the film also limits the radiation and scatter. The conventional 2 mm aluminium filter at the tube aperture reduces radiation to the patient by 50%. The focus-film distance varies from 100–120 cm (40–48 in) and movement blurring especially of the fetus, is avoided by using a high output transformer and tube and fast screens. The exposure can be made with the breath held on either inspiration or expiration. High kilovoltage exposures markedly reduce exposure times, but the contrast is more acceptable at medium kilovoltages and two sets of exposure factors for selected positions are given in the table on page 738.

Radiation protection

Unnecessary radiation to the mother and fetus is best avoided by having comprehensive ultrasonography available. However, when radiography is essential fast films and intensifying screens must be used and repeat examinations avoided. The genetic hazard to the fetus and possible complication to the child of malignancy such as leukemia after many years, must be borne in mind.

Chest radiography of the mother to exclude tuberculosis must be confined to the last four weeks of pregnancy and preferably done after childbirth.

Hysterosalpingography

Contrast medium injected through the cervix fills the uterine cavity and can then demonstrate the uterine tubes. The examination is used largely in infertility to show whether the uterine tubes are patent, to demonstrate the cause of any obstruction, to show abnormalities in the uterine cavity and the efficacy of ligation of the tubes for contraception.

Early pregnancy must be excluded and the examination is done immediately after menstruation, but before ovulation which is related to the midcycle. A non-irritant water soluble contrast agent is used.

Radiation is reduced to a minimum by careful collimation, fast intensifying screens and by image amplication if fluoroscopy is being used. Two films taken supine are usually quite sufficient to demonstrate the uterine tubes and peritoneal spill.

The patient

A worried and nervous patient should be reassured, creating a feeling of friendly understanding by carefully explaining the procedure before the examination starts. The bladder and rectum must be evacuated and some patients will need premedication.

Technique

With the patient in the lithotomy position a small Foley's balloon catheter, a special uterine bulbous backed cannula (2270) or a vacuum attached catheter is inserted into the cervix. The patient's legs are then lowered.

With minimal fluoroscopy using image amplification, a television monitor and close collimation, 3–4 ml of contrast is injected. A film is taken as the tubes fill out to the periphery (2271). If there is any hold up of contrast medium particularly at the utero-tubal junction (2272) an intravenous injection of a myo-relaxant such as 0·25 mgm of Glucagon or 20 mgm Buscopan is given. A further 3–4 ml of contrast may be needed and both a film of the tubes filling to the periphery (2273a) and of the subsequent peritoneal spill three to five minutes later (2273b) should be taken.

Hysterosalpingography can be performed without fluoroscopy. Films are taken with an overhead tube accurately centred and collimated to the pelvic cavity (2270).

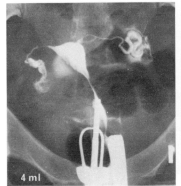

PROTECTION

2270

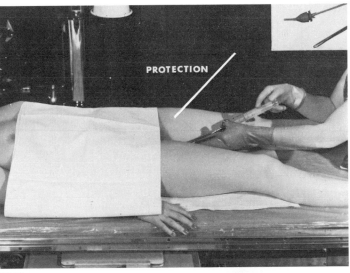

4 ml

2273a

8 ml

2273b

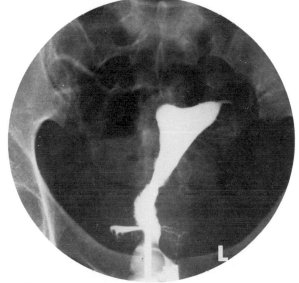

IMMEDIATE · L

2271

L

2272

The uterus, broad ligaments, ovaries and lateral pelvic walls can be well demonstrated following a diagnostic pneumoperitoneum and the patient suitably positioned to fill the pelvic cavity with the gas.

The patient empties her bladder and rectum, and after premedication lies supine on the radiographic couch. Following local anaesthesia, a pneumoperitoneum is induced using 300–400 ml of air or oxygen. Considerably more gas is required if carbon dioxide is used because it is rapidly absorbed, and therefore 2 litres are injected at the rate of 300 ml per min. The patient is then turned prone and tilted head down approximately 28–30° and the tube angled 10° towards the head and centred on the coccyx (2274). The Bucky film must be suitably displaced to be centred to the tube angulation associated with the head down tilt. The exposure factors are given on page 738.

When ultrasonography is not available gynaecography can demonstrate enlarged polycystic ovaries (2275b), ovarian tumours, agenesis (2275c) and endometriosis. Unquestionably, however, this is another radiological procedure which will shortly be out-moded with the introduction of ultrasonography.

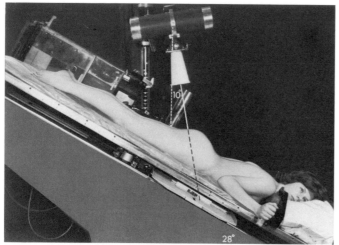

2274

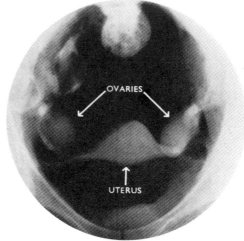

2275(a)

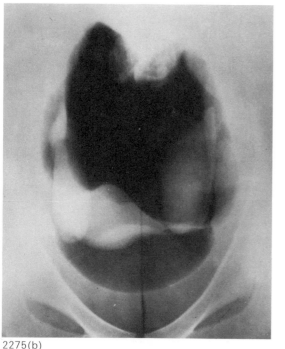

2275(b)

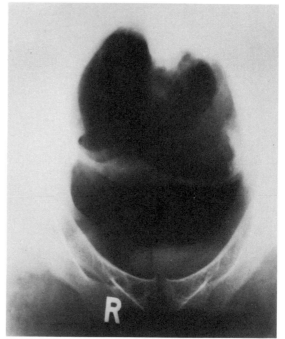

2275(c)

Advanced pregnancy

Postero-anterior
There are now no indications for radiography in early pregnancy only contraindications. The "ten day" rule is specifically directed towards ensuring that an early pregnancy is not inadvertently irradiated. By and large obstetric patients up to 36 weeks pregnant are investigated by ultrasonography (2277, 2278).

Advanced pregnancy
During late pregnancy good definition is required to show fetal maturity, possible fetal abnormalities, multiplicity, fetal presentation and extended limbs. However, most fetal abnormalities such as anencephaly and hydrocephalus are diagnosed by ultrasonography in or before the second trimester.

For pelvic abnormalities unassociated with pregnancy a clear view of the pelvic cavity is obtained with the patient prone and the tube angled 15–25° towards the head (2276).

The patient is prone in the centre of the couch with support under the ankles and a broad Bucky band is firmly applied for immobilization.

■ Centre below the coccyx with the tube angled approximately 25° towards the head to project the sacrum above any abnormal opacity (2276).

Ultrasonograph (2277) shows midline echoes of the fetal head and (2278) a twin pregnancy at 4–6 weeks.

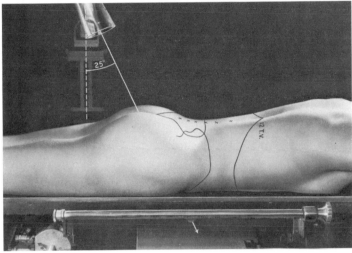

2276

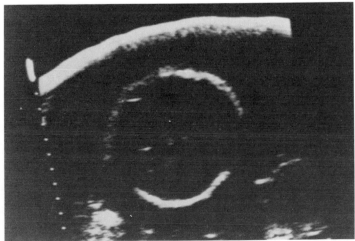

2277

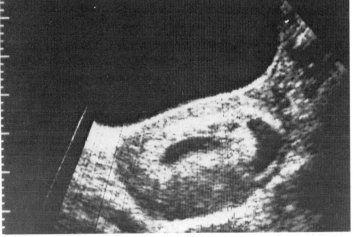

2278

Antero-posterior (Basic)

The patient is supine, central to the x-ray table with the hands clasped over the upper chest and a small sandbag under the knees (2279). The 40 cm (16 ins) broad linen immobilizing band is applied gradually and compression must stop before the patient feels uncomfortable with a final firm adjustment just before the exposure (2280) when the patient holds her breath. Following the exposure the immobilizing band is slowly and carefully released. Compression limits the movement of the mother and fetus and the radiodensity becomes more uniform to produce a radiograph with maximum definition, detail and contrast.

■ Centre to the apex of the abdominal curve approximately at the level of the fourth and fifth lumbar vertebrae to include the symphysis pubis and the diaphragm collimated to a rectangle to cover a 35 × 44 cm (14 × 17 ins) film (2281–2282). The exposure factors are given on page 738.

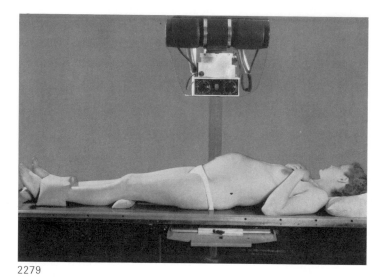

2279

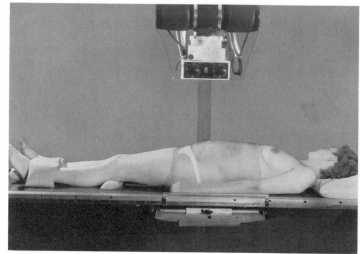

2280

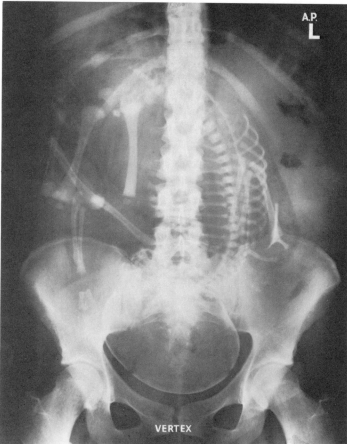

2281

VERTEX

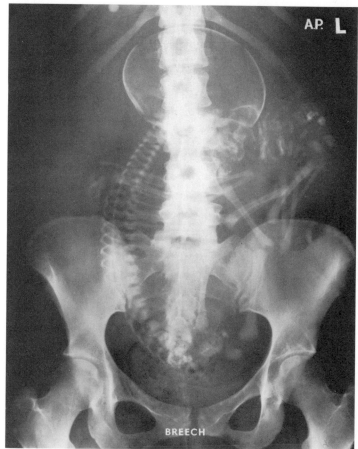

2282

BREECH

Postero-anterior

Assist the patient in turning prone and central to the X-ray couch. The head is turned to one side with a sandbag under the ankles. Without the compression band the arms are adjacent to the head to slightly support the patient (2283). If more compression is possible the arms hang over the couch (2284) but for minimal compression, plastic foam supports are positioned under the chest and pelvis (2287).

■ Centre to approximately the level of the fourth and fifth lumbar vertebrae with the diaphragm collimated to cover a 35 × 44 cm (14 × 17 ins) film and expose while the patient holds her breath (2283, 2284, 2285, 2286, 2287).

The fetus, particularly the fetal head, is well defined in this position because it is nearer to the film and the radiation dose to the fetus is less. However, the prone position is more uncomfortable for the mother.

Radiographs (2281 and 2285), show the fetus in a vertex presentation taken supine and prone, and in (2282 and 2286) the fetus is in a breech presentation, again with the patient supine and another prone for comparison.

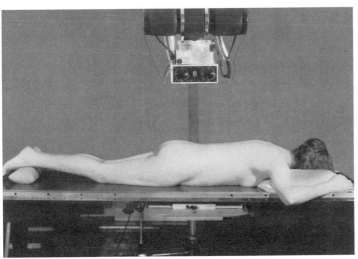

2283

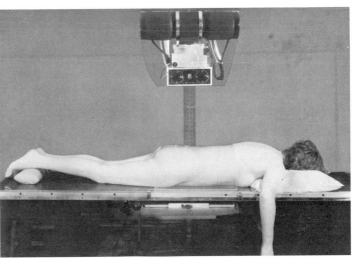

2284

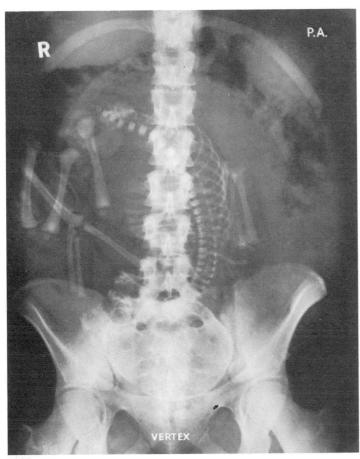

2285

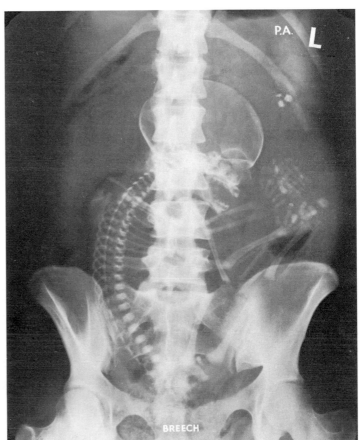

2286

Lateral (Basic)

The patient turns onto the side towards which the fetal spine is lying as judged by palpation and is supported with the legs extended so as not to obscure the pelvis (2288). The limbs are raised at the ankles, symmetrically to the pelvis to prevent rotation with plastic sponge pads between the knees and ankles. The upper arm is raised over the head and the patient clasps the end of the couch for support. A compression band will also help in steadying the patient.

■ Centre at the level of the apex of the abdominal curve midway between the spine and the anterior margin of the abdomen. A 35 × 44 cm (14 × 17 ins) cassette is positioned to include the symphysis pubis and during the exposure the patient stops breathing. The exposure factors are given on page 738. Radiograph (2289) is of a fetus in vertex presentation and in (2290) the fetus is in a breech presentation.

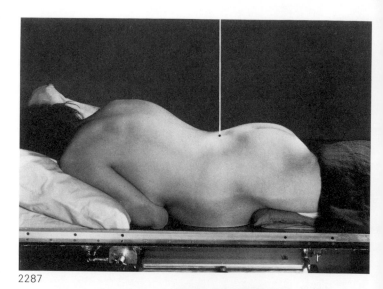

2287

2288

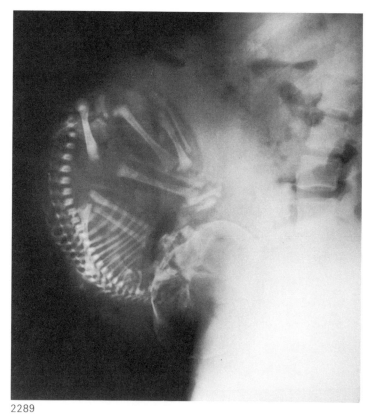

2289

2290

Lateral-supine (1)

The lateral view can also be taken with a horizontal ray with the patient supine. The tube is lowered for the horizontal projection and the pedestal type Bucky-diaphragm is in the vertical position. The patient is moved towards the Bucky to be in contact with it (2291).

■ Centre with the tube in horizontal position either (a) for the whole fetus at the level of the apex of the abdominal curve midway between the anterior abdominal wall and the spine or (b) for the fetal head in the pelvis.

Lateral-supine (2)

The X-ray couch is at an angle of 25–40° with the feet down. The fetal head may be in the "engaged" position. The trunk is raised on a plastic sponge pillow to include the posterior margin of the pelvis on the film (2293), and the vertical cassette and stationary grid are supported against the side of the trunk.

■ Centre with the tube lowered for a horizontal ray to cover the fetal head in the pelvis using a 25 × 30 cm (10 × 12 ins) film (2293, 2294).

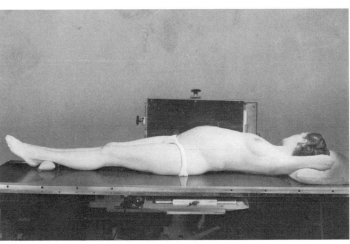

2291

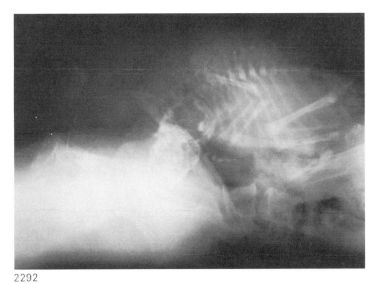

2292

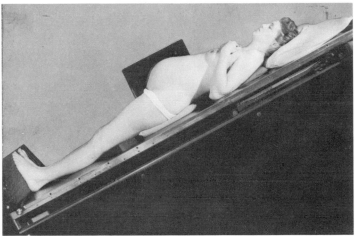

2293

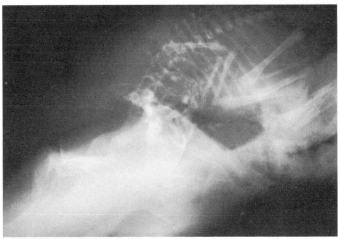

2294

Lateral erect (basic)

When the patient is erect, the fetal head in a vertex presentation moves well down into the maternal pelvis and for pelvimetry measurements, a true lateral projection is essential. With the patient erect and in the true lateral position, the hip is against the Bucky, and to be well balanced the feet are separated. When viewed from the side, front and back, the position is carefully adjusted to avoid tilting or rotation of the pelvis (2296 a, b, 2297) and the patient is steadied with the immobilization band (2298).

The prominence of the greater trochanter should be 6 cm (2½ ins) below the centre of the grid and a 25 × 30 cm (10 × 12 ins) film placed transversely (2298). The distance between the film and median plane of the pelvis must be recorded as well as the film focus distance for subsequent pelvimetry calculations.

■ Centre 6 cm (2½ ins) above the prominence of the greater trochanter, central to the film. In a satisfactory lateral film, the femoral heads coincide (2295).

On page 731 the measurements required in pelvimetry on a lateral view are shown on (2326). However, for a general lateral view, although the patient is positioned similarly (2298), a 35 × 44 cm (14 × 17 ins) cassette is required. The position of the placenta is now shown by ultrasonography but previously many different radiographic techniques were recommended, including the erect lateral view for the posterior placenta previa (2299). The horizontal view (2300) was considered inadequate.

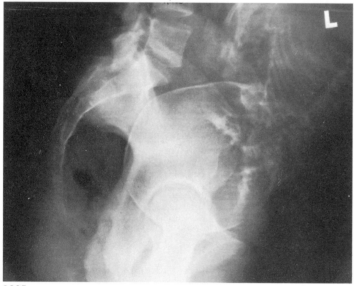

2295

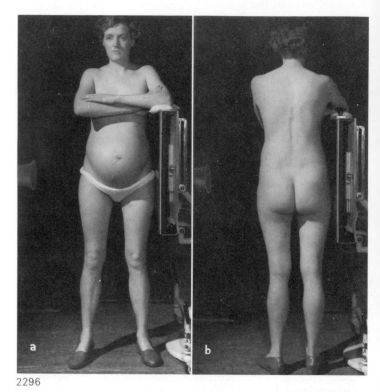

2296

· 2297   2298

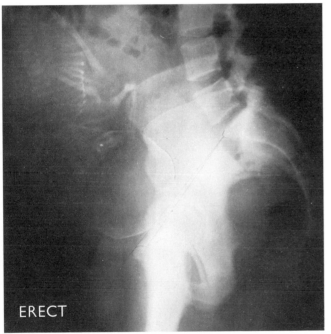

ERECT

2299

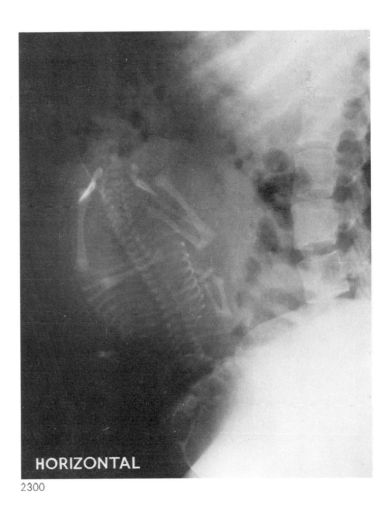

HORIZONTAL

2300

Right or left posterior oblique

The fetus is usually seen more clearly on the oblique view. The position of the fetal spine is determined by palpation or ultrasonography and the patient is lateral with the spine of the fetus towards the X-ray couch. The patient is then rotated backwards by 45° with the legs extended, supported by plastic sponge blocks under the raised hip, shoulder and leg (2302), and a compression band assists immobilization. The left posterior oblique projection is shown in (2302) and the right posterior oblique in (2303).

■ Centre to the side nearest the film at the estimated midpoint of the fetal spine to include the whole fetus. The 35 × 44 cm (14 × 17 ins) film is positioned to include the symphysis pubis (2301, 2302, 2303).

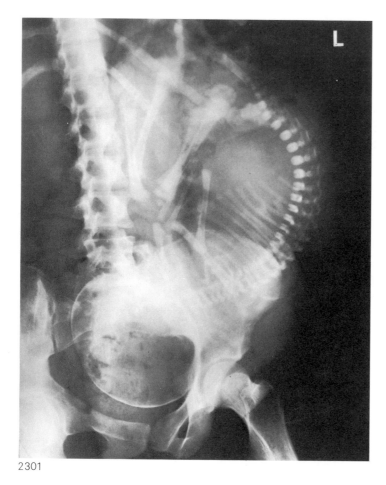

2301

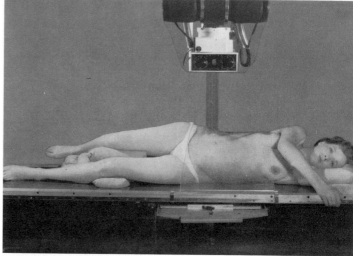

2302

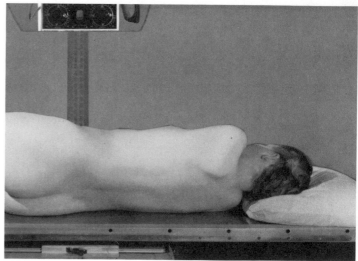

2303

Supero-inferior for pelvic inlet

This view is now rarely used during pregnancy, because of the high radiation dose to the fetus but is included to show the relationship of the fetal head to the pelvic inlet.

With the patient sitting on a grid, the back support at an angle of 55°, and the feet resting on the floor, the central ray is directed vertically through the centre of the pelvic inlet. A back rest may be fitted onto the X-ray couch, with the knees flexed over the end to achieve the same position. The brim of the pelvis or pelvic inlet lies parallel to the film when the superior margin of the pubis and the space between the fourth and fifth lumbar spinous processes are at the same distance above the film (2304).

■ Centre between the antero-superior iliac spines, approximately 5 cm (2 ins) behind the symphysis pubis using a 25 × 30 cm (10 × 12 ins) film. A high kilovoltage is needed to show the whole pelvic brim (2304, 2305, 2306); for exposure factors see page 738.

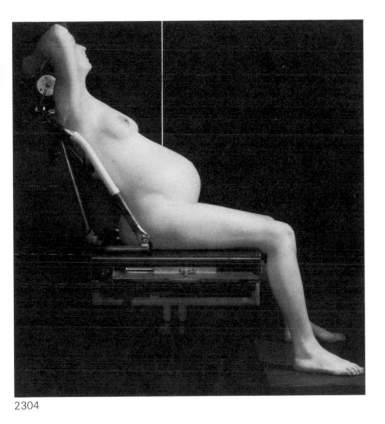

2304

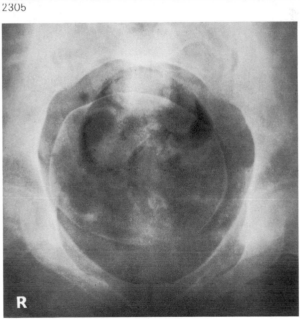

2305

2306

When a patient has had a difficult labour and pelvic measurements are required the radiographs are taken in the postpartum period.

The obturator foramina are a good guide for the degree of inclination of the back rest to bring the pelvic brim parallel to the film. If the obturator foramina appear shallow on the frontal radiograph, the patient must lean back further with a small angle between the back rest and couch (2308), but if the obturator foramina appear large, then the patient will need to be almost upright (2307). However, quite considerable movement of the trunk occurs before the position of the pelvis is changed and it may be necessary to lower the back rest by 10° to avoid projecting the breast shadows over the posterior border of the pelvic brim.

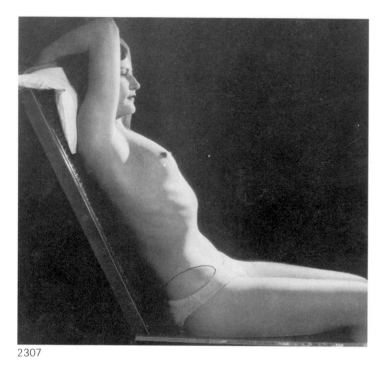

2307

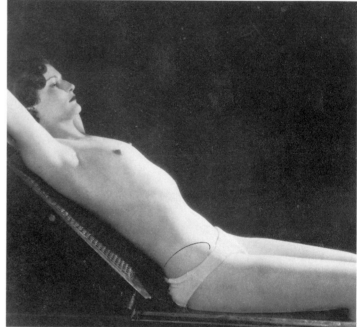

2308

Supero-inferior for pelvic outlet and subpubic arch

In this projection there is again a high radiation dose to the fetus and is no longer used in pregnancy but it is interesting to see the relationship between the fetus and pelvis on old films.

While seated on a pelvimetry Bucky or on the end of the couch with the feet widely separated and resting on the floor, the patient leans gently forwards, flexing at the hips to bring the abdomen between the thighs. The subpubic arch should lie parallel to the film. Usually the hands rest on the floor (2309) rather than holding a support.

■ Centre over the pubic arch with a vertical central ray (2309, 2310, 2311) unless the patient cannot bend sufficiently far forward then the tube should be tilted 5–10° towards the head. A film in this projection can be taken with a stationary grid on a 20 × 25 cm (8 × 10 ins) cassette (2311).

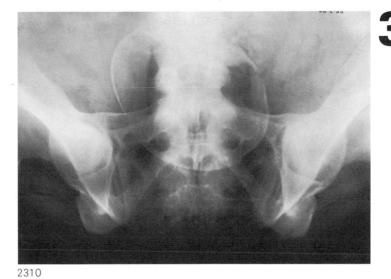

2310

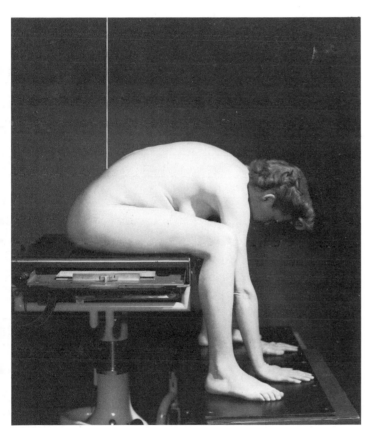

2309

2311

Radiograph (2314) shows calcification in a placenta taken after parturition.

Ultrasonograph (2313) shows a placenta praevia and part of the placenta is hidden by shadowing of the body of the fetus.

Placentography

The radiographic demonstration of the placenta is now only of historical interest. The methods included the plain film (2312), cystography and angiography, and for a while isotope scanning was in vogue. At present ultrasonography is used exclusively.

In placenta praevia, the placenta encroaches on the cervical os to a varying degree causing antepartum haemorrhage at about the 30th week of pregnancy. With complete placenta praevia the internal os is completely covered but more commonly there is a partial placenta praevia.

In early pregnancy the placenta is often low in position suggesting the possibility of placenta praevia, but as the uterus enlarges the placenta is carried away from the region of the internal os. It is therefore, extremely difficult to diagnose a placenta praevia before the 30th week of pregnancy. The anterior placenta is much more easily and accurately localized than the posterior placenta even with ultrasonography because the acoustic shadowing caused by the fetus itself tends to hide part of the placenta. (2313).

The placenta can be examined for abnormalities such as calcifications after being passed following parturition. (2314).

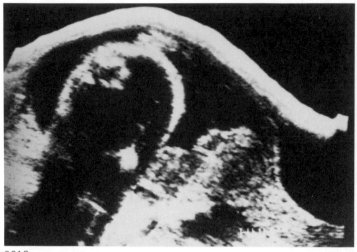

2313

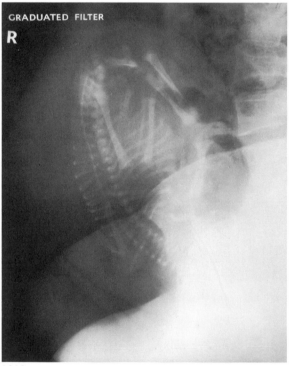

2312

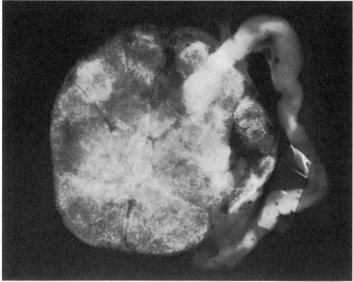

2314

Fetal maturity

Fetal maturity is now only estimated radiographically after the 34th week of pregnancy and is used especially in cases of post-maturity. Before the 34th week ultrasonography is used for estimating fetal maturity.

Good quality radiographs with satisfactory definition, density and contrast are needed to see the fetal epiphyses. A short exposure time is essential and complete immobilization to avoid movement blurring.

The lower femoral epiphyses are visible at 36 weeks and the upper tibial epiphyses become visible at 38 weeks, but appear large and well defined at term and then the fetus has well defined subcutaneous fatty tissue as shown on the radiograph (2314), of a fetus in a breech presentation with extended legs.

Fetal death

There are a number of radiographic signs associated with fetal death including overlapping of cranial bones (2315), known as Spalding's sign, gas in the cardiovascular system (2316), small size of the fetus, collapse of the fetus and hyperextension of the fetal spine. However, the diagnosis of fetal death is now usually made by the absence of fetal cardiac movements on ultrasonography.

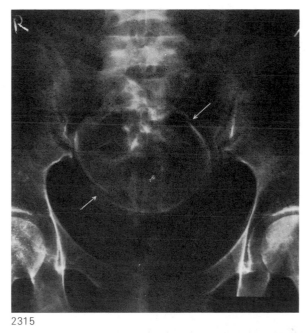

2315

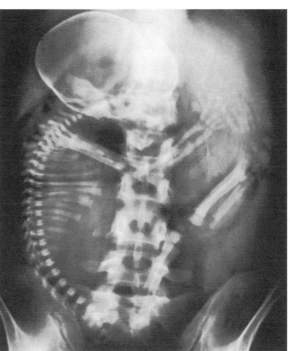

2314

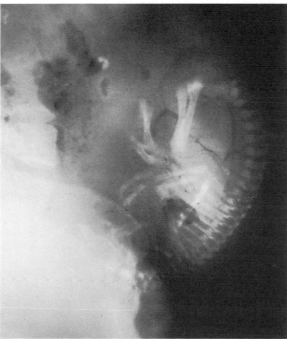

2316

The stillborn fetus

In many hospitals, stillborn fetuses are now radiographed routinely and the films form part of the case record. An antero-posterior and a lateral view should be taken. Radiographs at 15 weeks (2317), 24 to 35 weeks (2318) and 35 weeks (2319) indicate the change in size and appearance as the fetus matures.

There will be a marked variation in the exposure not only because of the size of the fetus but also because of the different film and screens that can be used. The table below should act merely as a guide for the various exposures.

Age	kVp	mAS	FFD	Film ILFORD	Screens ILFORD	Grid
15 weeks	44	100	106 cm (42″)	Rapid R (NS)	—	—
24/25 weeks	65	55	106 cm (42″)	Rapid R	HD	Grid
35 weeks	65	80	106 cm (42″)	Rapid R	HD	Grid

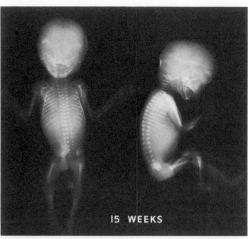

15 WEEKS

2317

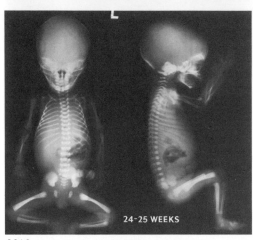

24-25 WEEKS

2318

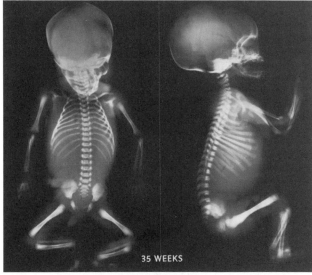

35 WEEKS

2319

Urography in pregnancy

Urography is only very occasionally needed in pregnancy and then only, one or at the most, two films are taken using fast film and rare earth screens to reduce fetal irradiation to a minimum.

In pregnancy the pelvicalyceal systems and ureters are normally dilated (2320) and remain so well into the post-partum period.

An antero-posterior film is taken approximately 15 to 20 minutes after the intravenous contrast medium has been injected.

Amniography

Rarely, after some amniotic fluid has been aspirated a water soluble contrast medium such as diatrizoate (Hypaque or Renografin) is injected and outlines the margin of the fetus and placenta. The contrast medium also shows the fetal gastrointestinal tract due to the fetus swallowing the contrast medium (2321).

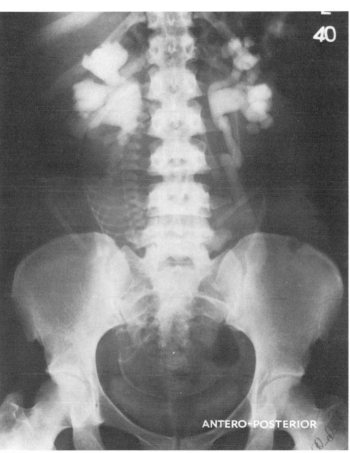

2320

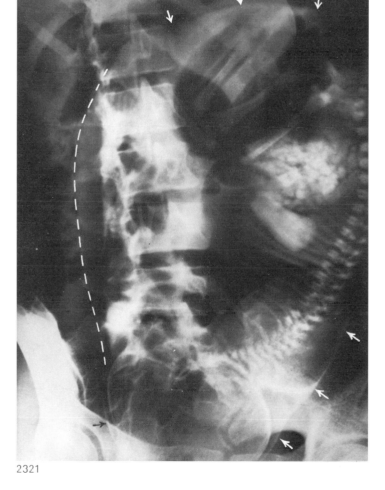

2321

Pelvimetry

A small pelvis causing difficulties in labour due to disproportion between the fetal head and the pelvis can be determined by pelvimetry, but if there are difficulties in labour the baby will be delivered by Caesarian section, that is, through an incision in the abdominal and uterine walls. Pelvimetry is then performed later.

Just prior to labour a radiograph may be needed because the fetal head fails to engage in the pelvic inlet. However, such a diagnosis should only be entertained if descent of the fetal head is tested with the patient erect and with an empty bladder.

The illustrative radiographs (2322, 2323, 2328) have been retained because of their historical interest, and because they show the relationship between the fetal head and the pelvic diameters. Several methods of pelvimetry are used but basically the measurements must be determined in both the frontal and lateral planes. Two basic projections

(a) antero-posterior with the patient supine (2322)
(b) lateral with the patient erect (2326).

are therefore described.

Because the X-ray beam diverges from its source there is some enlargement with the focal-film distances used and varies with the distance of the subject from the film. In pelvimetry the measurement of the subject-film distance is essential, must be done for every patient and recorded on the request/report form for subsequent calculations.

On the antero-posterior radiograph (2322)
(1) The transverse diameter of the pelvic inlet and,
(2) the bi-ischial spinous diameter can be measured.

On the lateral radiograph (2326, 2327)
(1) The true conjugate; from the upper inner border of the symphysis pubis to the sacral promontory.
(2) The antero-posterior midplane; from the middle of the symphysis pubis to the middle of the third sacral segment.
(3) The outlet; from the lower inner border of the symphysis pubis to the last fixed coccygeal segment can be measured.

In the very occasional case radiographed, when the fetal head is fully engaged the biparietal diameter can be measured from the lateral and frontal views (2323, 2326) providing a clear view of the relationship between the fetal head and maternal pelvis. Although the supero-inferior view is no longer used in pregnancy (2323, 2324, 2325) because of the excessive fetal irradiation, it clearly shows the important diameters and their relationship to the fetal head as indicated.

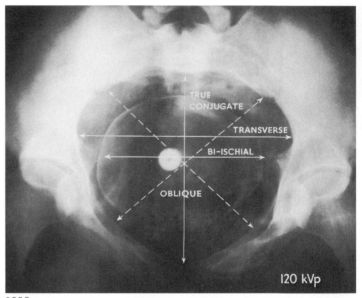

2323

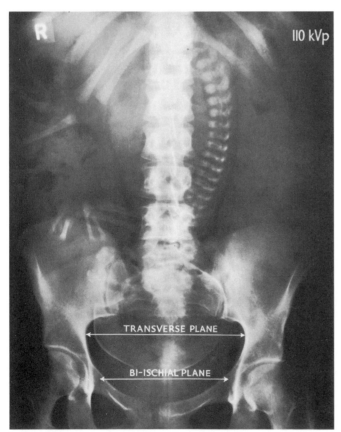

2322

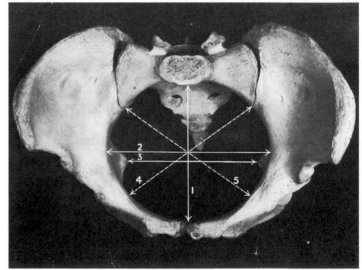

2324

(1) The transverse diameter; from side to side at the widest points of the brim.

(2) The interspinous diameter between the ischial spines.

(3) The true conjugate from the inner margin of the symphysis pubis to the sacral promontory.

(4) The oblique diameters from the ilio-pubic eminence on one side to the sacroiliac joint at the brim on the opposite side.

Similarly the supero-inferior view to show the pelvic outlet and subpubic arch is no longer permissible because of excessive fetal irradiation. The outlet plane to film height is variable but can be calculated particularly as the pubic arch is close to the film in the pelvic outlet and subpubic view (2328).

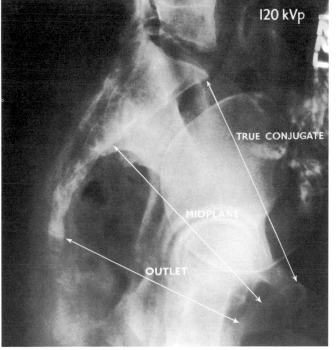

2326

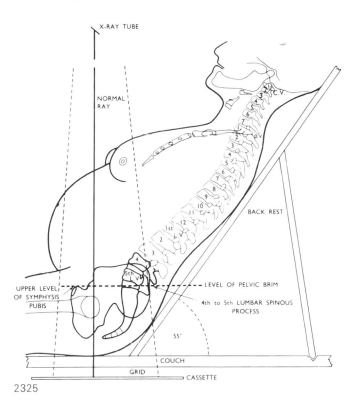

2325

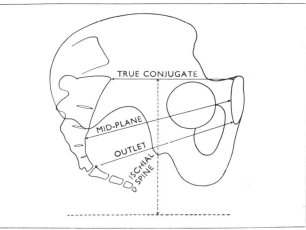

2327

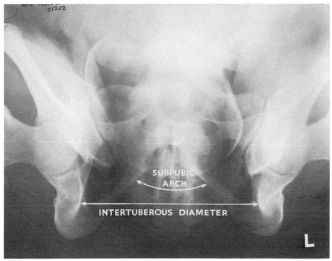

2328

Calculation of pelvic diameters

If the radiographs are taken correctly, the film-focal distance and the measured subject-film distance are known, then the pelvic diameters in the frontal and lateral planes can be calculated by

(a) Mathematical formula or,
(b) A geometrical correction scale or,
(c) Using a radiopaque ruler during radiography

(a) Mathematical formula

The required diameters are accurately measured on the radiograph and the true pelvic measurements calculated which is, for example, given for the transverse diameters.

True pelvic diameter

$$= \frac{\text{measured film diameter} \times \text{focus-symphysis distance}}{\text{focus-film distance}}$$

If the measured film diameter was 15 cm (6 ins), the focus-film distance 105 cm (42 ins) and the focus-symphysis distance 90 cm (36 ins) the symphysis to film distance being 12 cm (5 ins) then the actual pelvic transverse diameter is

$$\frac{15 \times 90 \text{ cm}}{105 \text{ cm}} \frac{(6 \times 36 \text{ ins})}{(42 \text{ ins})} = 12.9 \text{ cm (5·1 ins)}$$

and with pocket calculators the simple arithmetic presents no problem.

The distance of the ischial spine from the true conjugate can be calculated from the lateral view (2326, 2327), and the figure is then subtracted from the measured symphysis to film-distance (2329) to give the ischial spines to film distance. The bi-ischial spinous diameter can then be calculated in the same way as for the transverse diameter in the example given above.

Pelvimetry calipers are used to establish the levels of the pelvic diameters from the film. From experience, in the supine position, the transverse plane of the pelvic inlet is two thirds of the distance of the anterior margin of the symphysis pubis from the table top and the ischial spines at one third the distance. The thin flat base of the metal calipers slips under the patient from the side (2329) while the movable arm is slid down the vertical supporting strut onto the symphysis pubis, and the height read off on the vertical arm. The thickness of the base of the caliper must be allowed for in calculating the subject to film distance.

To establish the distance of the median plane of the body to the film for calculations on the lateral view, the width of the pelvis at the greater trochanter is measured (2330). The calipers are firmly compressed over the greater trochanters and one half this distance is the height of the midplane of the pelvis from the table top for calculations of the lateral projection.

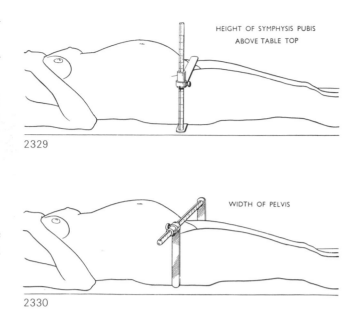

HEIGHT OF SYMPHYSIS PUBIS
ABOVE TABLE TOP

2329

WIDTH OF PELVIS

2330

(b) Geometrical correction scale

Some pelvic measurements can be obtained by using calipers (2329, 2330) together with a geometric scale and table of distances (2331).

The distance table gives a range of heights of the upper border of the symphysis pubis from the table top at $\frac{1}{4}$ inch spacings from $5\frac{1}{2}$–9 ins (13–23 cm), and the corresponding heights of the transverse and bi-spinous (ischial spines) diameter in separate columns as two-thirds and one-third of the symphysis to table top distance, respectively.

The geometrical correction scale is prepared by radiographing a steel ruler notched at $\frac{1}{4}$ inch intervals first at table top level and then at $7\frac{1}{2}$ ins from the table top. The two radiographs of the ruler are then placed on graph paper, $7\frac{1}{2}$ ins apart and parallel to each other, centralizing the 4 ins. points. The chart is completed by correcting the corresponding points and by adding the appropriate measurements (2331).

A glare free transparency of the table can then be prepared with the charts placed one above the other (2331) by exposing onto X-ray film and can be used directly on a radiograph.

To calculate the transverse planes from the antero-posterior projection, the true height is first determined from the table of distances. The required plane is then measured on the film and this measurement is then transferred onto the true height line, which in this case is 4 ins, and the true diameter read off on the corresponding scale.

To calculate the antero-posterior conjugates from the lateral projection the measured bi-trochanteric distance, say 13 ins, is halved to give the midplane to film distance of $6\frac{1}{2}$ ins. The conjugates are measured on the film, laid on the $6\frac{1}{2}$ in line on the scale and the true distances are then read off in turn.

(c) By radiopaque or perforated ruler

A radiopaque ruler positioned in the natal cleft in the midline parallel to the film is included in the exposure of the lateral projection. The scale on the ruler will have the same magnification as the mid-plane conjugates (2332).

Alternatively radiographs of the ruler taken at various distances from the film can be used. If the radiograph of the ruler with the same distance from the film as the mid-plane to film distance of the patient is used, the conjugate can be read off directly. (2333)

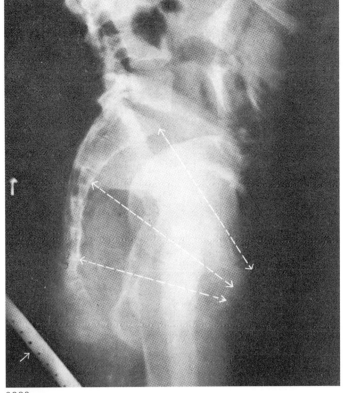

2332

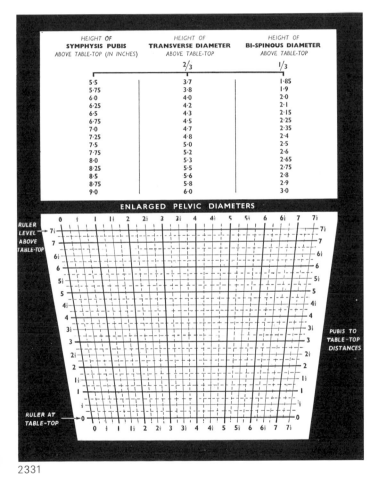

HEIGHT OF SYMPHYSIS PUBIS ABOVE TABLE-TOP (IN INCHES)	HEIGHT OF TRANSVERSE DIAMETER ABOVE TABLE-TOP 2/3	HEIGHT OF BI-SPINOUS DIAMETER ABOVE TABLE-TOP 1/3
5·5	3·7	1·85
5·75	3·8	1·9
6·0	4·0	2·0
6·25	4·2	2·1
6·5	4·3	2·15
6·75	4·5	2·25
7·0	4·7	2·35
7·25	4·8	2·4
7·5	5·0	2·5
7·75	5·2	2·6
8·0	5·3	2·65
8·25	5·5	2·75
8·5	5·6	2·8
8·75	5·8	2·9
9·0	6·0	3·0

ENLARGED PELVIC DIAMETERS

2331

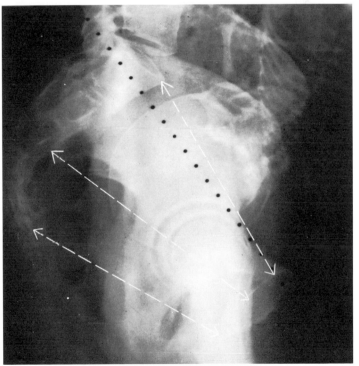

2333

Fetal head measurements

The radiation dose to the fetus is unacceptably high and radiographic methods for measuring the fetal head (2323) are no longer used. If required, fetal head measurements are obtained by ultrasonography.

The Angle of Pelvic inclination is the angle formed by the plane of the brim of the pelvis and the anterior margin of the fifth lumbar vertebral body (2334), varying from one person to another and with posture, changing considerably from extension (2334) to flexion (2335).

Ultrasonography is at present the major method for imaging of the fetus and pregnant uterus, having almost completely replaced radiography up to 34 weeks gestation and is particularly useful for the following:

1. Determination of gestational age by cephalometry and body measurements.
2. Diagnosing fetal "failure to thrive".
3. Placentography.
4. Multiple pregnancy.
5. Fetal abnormalities.
6. Amniocentesis.
7. Diagnosis of early pregnancy.
8. Blighted ovum.
9. Hydatidiform mole.
10. Fetal death.

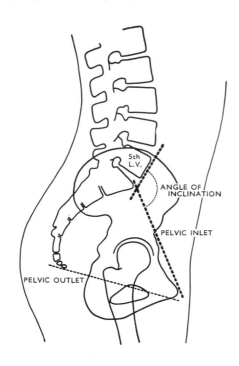

2334

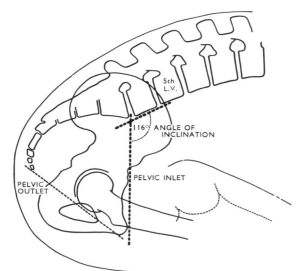

2335

Multiple pregnancy

There are now very few cases of multiple pregnancy coming for radiography that have not already been diagnosed by ultrasonography. Radiography is used only in cases of doubt and for confirmation. Twins (2336), quadruplets (2337, 2338), and even quintuplets (2339) may be shown and usually the oblique or lateral projection is more informative than the anteroposterior.

Conjoined or siamese twins (2340) may be attached in any part of their bodies; thoracic attachment being illustrated.

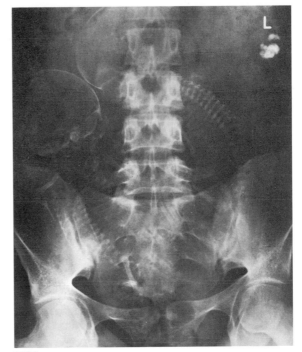

2336

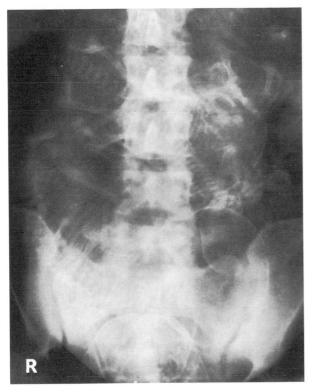

2337

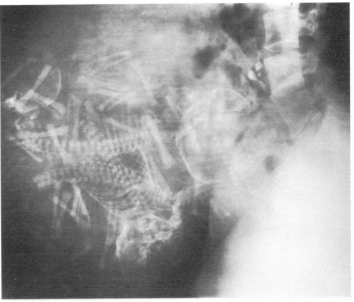

2339

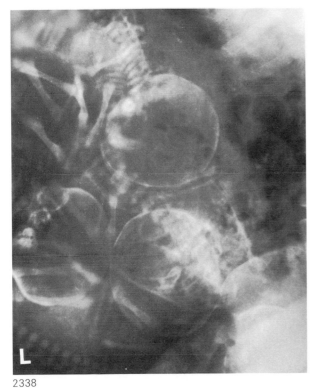

2338

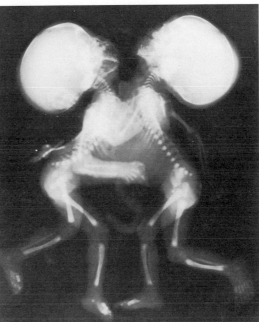

2340

735

Ultrasonography

Multiplicity is now reliably diagnosed on ultrasonography but for triplets, quadruplets or quintuplets a radiograph near term is taken for confirmation.

After 13–14 weeks more than one fetal head can be demonstrated but between 8 and 14 weeks multiple pregnancy is diagnosed by showing more than one gestation sac (2341).

Multiple serial longitudinal and transverse sections are used to explore the uterus. In late pregnancy a second fetal head may be missed deep in the pelvis, in the flanks or under the ribs. The fetal trunk must not be mistaken for a second head. The head remains round in two planes and contains a midline echo; the trunk is round in only one plane and contains the spine. If there is more than one head an oblique scanning plane is used to show both heads on the same scan to exclude a rapidly moving fetus mimicking twins (2342).

The exact number of fetuses is best determined on a radiograph taken after 34 weeks.

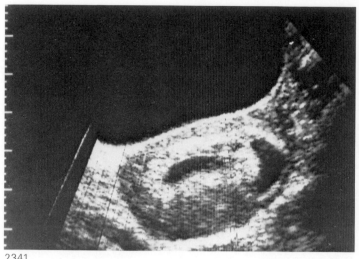

2341

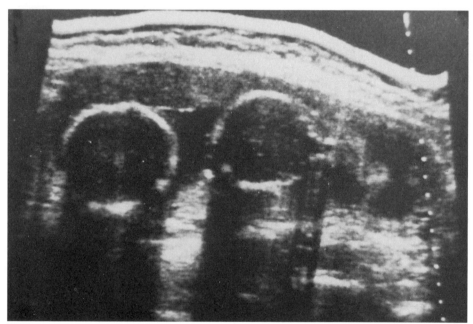

2342

The placenta

The placenta produces a diffuse speckled appearance with its fetal surface clearly outlined by the chorionic plate, (2343) but in late pregnancy the placenta may be difficult to visualize as it is hidden by the acoustic shadowing of the fetus (2344a).

In early pregnancy the placenta is large relative to the size of the uterus and appears to migrate towards the body and fundus as the lower segment expands.

Indications for placental localization

1. Vaginal bleeding usually in mid to late pregnancy. If a placenta praevia is excluded the patient can be discharged from hospital.
2. Unstable lie of the fetus near term.
3. Prior to amniocentesis to avoid the placenta
4. Prior to placentocentesis of the maternal side for the investigation of haemaglobinopathies—a highly specialized procedure for a limited number of centres.

Ultrasonographic technique

The bladder must be full to act as an acoustic window for the lower segment, internal os and vagina (2345). Multiple linear longitudinal and transverse scans are performed. The internal os may be well demonstrated otherwise its position is taken as lying at the junction of the bladder fundus and posterior wall of the moderately filled bladder.

Placenta praevia

A placenta praevia is confidently excluded when shown in its normal position in the fundus of the uterus (2343) and major degrees of praevia are readily diagnosed when the placenta covers the internal os (2345).

There are, however, difficulties in diagnosing minor degrees of placenta praevia. The placenta can be within a radius of 5 cm of the os before 30 weeks leading to a false positive diagnosis. As the lower segment grows the placental margin can move away from the region of the os. In marginal cases if the presenting part of the fetus can be pushed passed the placenta a normal delivery is likely.

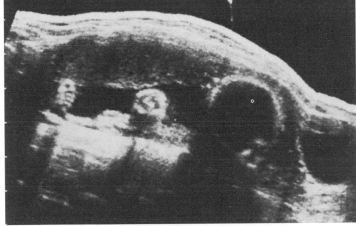

2343

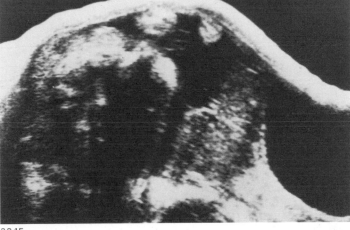

2345

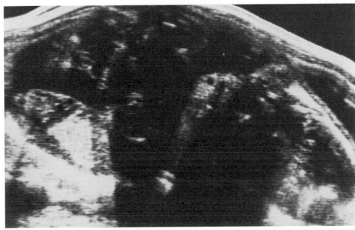

2344a

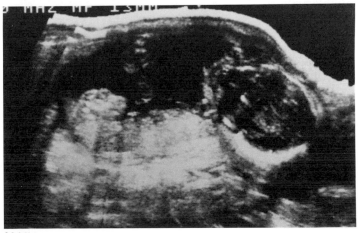

2344b

Difficulties in ultrasonographic diagnosis

1. The posterior placenta may be hidden by the fetus in the third trimester and should be suspected,if the space between the fetus and posterior uterine wall is increased.

The placenta may then be shown

(a) if the sensitivity is increased to fill in the placental echoes.

(b) by scanning laterally and at the fundus where the uterus is not covered by fetus. (2347a)

If the presenting fetal part is close to the sacrum (2344b) there is no praevia therefore the fetus is either pushed into the pelvis or the lower placenta may be shown by tilting the patient 15–20° head down to move the fetus towards the uterine fundus.

2. The anterior placenta may "disappear" if the time gain compensation (TGC) is too high.

3. A "false" placenta may appear due to reverberating echoes but a true picture can be obtained by altering the transducer angle.

4. It may be difficult to show the inferior edge of the anterior placenta. The chorionic plate should be identified and followed inferiorly with the transducer at right angles to the chorionic plate.

5. Do not diagnose placenta praevia before 30 weeks because of "migrating" placenta.

6. The lower segment or a fetal limb can be confused with the placenta. The true position of the placenta should obviate these difficulties.

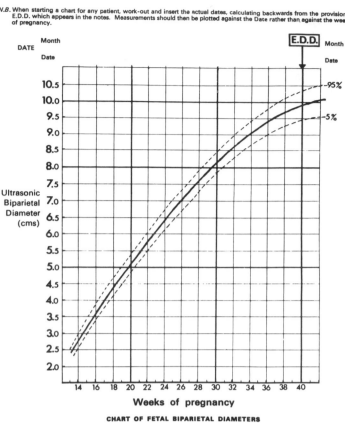

N.B. When starting a chart for any patient, work-out and insert the actual dates, calculating backwards from the provisional E.D.D. which appears in the notes. Measurements should then be plotted against the Date rather than against the weeks of pregnancy.

Weeks of pregnancy

CHART OF FETAL BIPARIETAL DIAMETERS
(Derived by Stuart Campbell, M.R.C.O.G., at Queen Charlotte's Hospital)
(J. Obstet. Gynaec. Brit. Cwlth. 1971, 78, 513)

2346a

A summary of exposure conditions for the Female reproductive system

Region and Position	kVp	mAS	FFD	Film ILFORD	Screens ILFORD	Grid
Hysterosalpingography Antero-posterior	65	44	90 cm (40")	Rapid R	FT	Grid
Gynaecography Postero-anterior	86	40	90 cm (40")	Rapid R	FT	Grid
Pregnancy-early Postero-anterior/antero-posterior	60	34	90 cm (40")	Rapid R	FT	Grid
Pregnancy—Full Term	62·5	65	90 cm (40")	Rapid R	FT	Grid
Antero-posterior-supine	120	18	90 cm (40")	Rapid R	FT	Grid
Postero-anterior-prone	62·5	55	90 cm (40")	Rapid R	FT	Grid
Lateral-horizontal	80	44	90 cm (40")	Rapid R	FT	Grid
Lateral-supine	80	55	90 cm (40")	Rapid R	FT	Grid
Lateral-tilted	80	44	90 cm (40")	Rapid R	FT	Grid
Lateral-erect	98	220	90 cm (40")	Rapid R	FT	Stationary Moving and
	120	80	90 cm (40")	Rapid R	FT	Stationary
Oblique-antero-posterior	70	55	90 cm (40")	Rapid R	FT	Grid
Supero-inferior-inlet	90	135	90 cm (40")	Rapid R	FT	Moving and
	120	44	90 cm (40")	Rapid R	FT	Stationary
	70	65	90 cm (40")	Rapid R	FT	Grid
Supero-inferior-outlet	120	14	90 cm (40")	Rapid R	FT	Grid

Cephalometry

Fetal maturity can be reliably assessed by measuring the biparietal diameter between 14 and 34 weeks gestation. Before 14 weeks the crown rump length is measured. The mean growth rate of the biparietal diameter (BPD) is 3·5 mm per week from 13–30 weeks and falls to 2·2 mm per week from 30–34 weeks. Thus single measurements of BPD are more reliable before 30 weeks but ideally at least 3 examinations should be done and plotted on Campbell's chart (2346a). Fetal body circumference measurements at the level of the fetal liver showing the umbilical vein is an even more reliable method of estimating placental insufficiency and failure to thrive in respect of the fetus.

Technique

The biparietal diameter is the distance between the fetal parietal eminences and is the widest diameter of the skull at right angles to the falx cerebri.

Initial longitudinal scans locate the fetal head which is usually occipito-transverse (OT) in a vertex presentation, with the head flexed laterally to a variable degree and the transverse scan must compensate for variable asynclitism (2346b) which displaces the echoes of the falx away from the midline (2346c).

To compensate for the angle of asynclitism

Having located the falx on the longitudinal scan the transducer is tilted so that the sound beam strikes the falx at right angles and the angle of tilt from the vertical equals the angle of asynclitism (2346c) which is measured.

Transverse scans are now made with the transducer tilted to the previously measured angle producing cross sections of the fetal head showing the falx as midline echoes. Several sections are then taken and the largest corresponds to the biparietal diameter. The margins of the parietal bones are then marked electronically and read off on the machine or a hard copy taken and the biparietal diameter measured on the hard copy.

An A-mode display with the transducer held at right angles to the falx at the maximum width of the fetal head can also be used to measure the biparietal diameter (2347b).

Sonogram (2347b) shows the measurement of the biparietal diameter on both B-mode and above it on an A-mode (BPD = 5·6 cm).

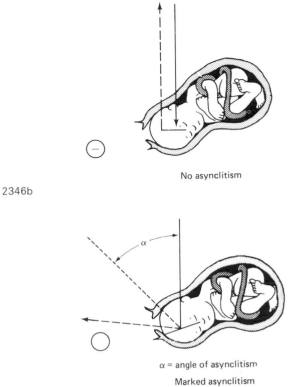

No asynclitism

2346b

α = angle of asynclitism
Marked asynclitism

2346c

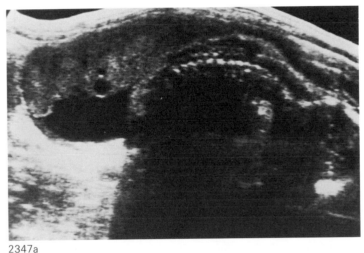

2347a

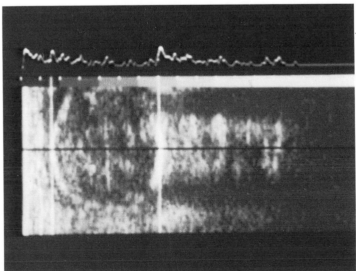

2347b

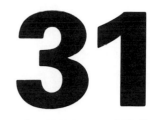

HIGH KILOVOLTAGE SELECTIVE FILTRATION

HIGH KILOVOLTAGE AND SELECTIVE FILTRATION

High Kilovoltage

Short exposure times in the millisecond range become possible with a high kilovoltage technique and avoids the movement unsharpness due to the cardiovascular system and to involuntary movements. In addition even greater sharpness is obtained by using small foci. High kilovoltage exposures also provide more penetrated films showing the structures in the denser areas, such as the mediastinum as well as showing the periphery of the lungs, and can also be used to penetrate contrast medium. However, inherent radiographic contrast is reduced and small soft tissue densities in the lung fields are not so easily visible.

In examinations such as angiography with multiple films taken in a rapid sequence short exposure times are essential, and the lower milliampere seconds is thus a great advantage.

The loss of contrast above 100 kVp severely limits its use in bone radiography and the increased scatter must be controlled by careful collimation of the X-ray beam and by using fine line stationary grids with ratios of 10:1 or 12:1. In chest radiography the air-gap technique with a long film-focus distance can be used to eliminate the unwanted scattered radiation.

The exposure factors become more critical and timing devices need to be more efficient in the millisecond range.

Applications

Chest radiography—The high kilovoltage technique is advantageous in chest radiography in showing the mediastinum and opacities otherwise hidden by ribs particularly in large patients.

Angiography—Short exposure times can be obtained for a rapid sequence of films within the tube rating.

Gastrointestinal tract—Dense barium can be penetrated and short exposure times avoid blurring due to involuntary bowel movements.

Radiation Hazard

There is less absorption with the increased penetration producing a lower skin and depth dose, but with the increased scattered radiation the gonadal dose will be higher with some examinations.

Exposure Factors

kVp	mAS	FFD	Film	Screens	Grid
Chest lateral (2348)					
140	6	150 cm (60″)	Rapid R	HD	Grid
Stomach and Duodenum (2349)					
140	5	90 cm (36″)	Rapid R	HD	Grid
Cholangiogram (2350)					
140	4	90 cm (36″)	Rapid	HD	Grid

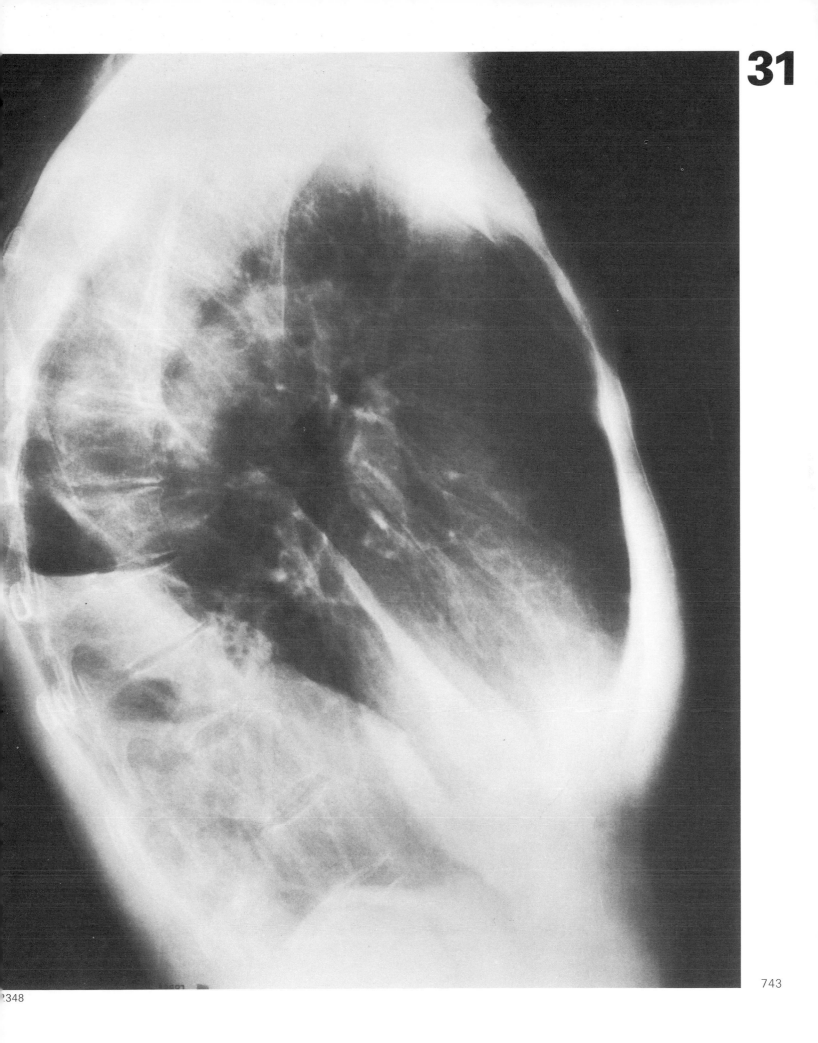

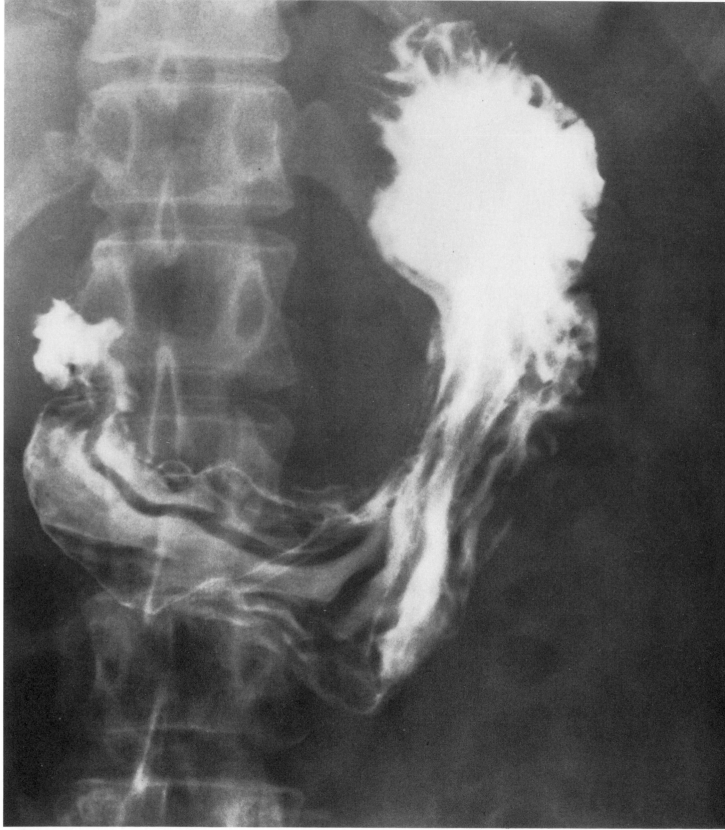

2349(a)

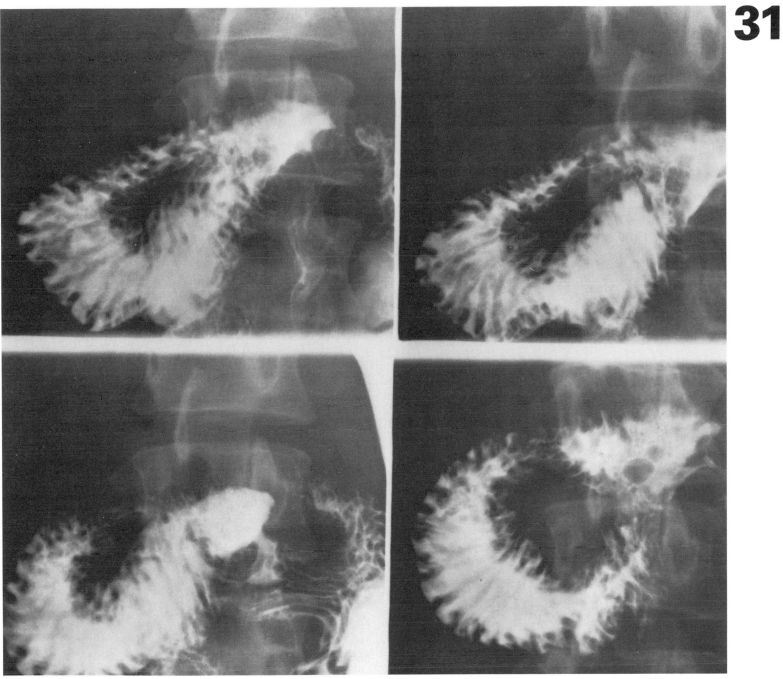

2349(b)

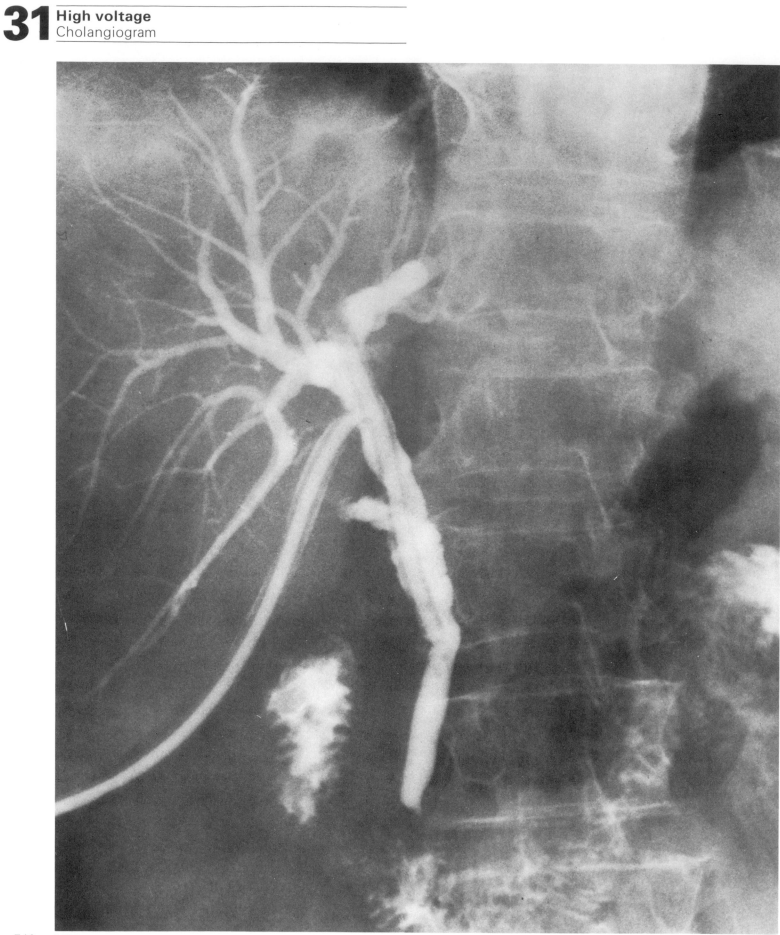

Selective Filtration

Thin metal sheets to reduce unwanted scatter can possibly be used (1) to replace grids (2) in conjunction with 8:1 or 10:1 ratio grids to both eliminate grid scatter and residual subject scatter and (3) in conjunction with air-gap technique, on the front of the cassette.

(1) To replace grids
Tin coated mild steel, 29 gauge 1/8000 ins (0·002 ins) thick industrial lead screens alone, are satisfactory for regions requiring a technique between screen and non-screen film. Such as:

(a) Knees and shoulders.
(b) Antero-posterior and oblique cervical spine.
(c) Localized mastoid and sinus views.
(d) The chest in thick set individuals.
(e) In the lateral view of the hip (2351) as in hip pinning, a lead screen 0·004 ins thick provides adequate contrast with less exposure compared with grids.

(2) Used in conjunction with a grid
Tin coated mild steel sheet or lead screens placed on top of the cassette in the Bucky tray, together with a 8:1 or 10:1 grid and kilovoltage of 90–150 kVp will improve definition by eliminating residual scatter. The results are comparable to those obtained with 16:1 grids, but with reduced exposure and considerably more latitude in centring.

Above 90 kVp no increase in exposure is needed. The evidence suggests that grid scatter is also eliminated, and in conjunction with a grid is particularly valuable in biplane angiography and in micturating cystography, where the direction and amount of scatter presents a problem. The filtration effect also produces a more uniform exposure when there is a wide range of adjacent radio-densities, and is therefore useful in the petrous mastoid or mediastinum at the bifurcations of the trachea and bronchi, where the lung fields can be shown on the same film.

(3) In the air-gap technique
A tin coated, mild steel filter is particularly useful for radiography of the middle ear with hypocycloidal tomography. When the grid in the Polytome is removed and replaced by a tin coated mild steel filter on the front of the cassette, low kilovoltages in the region of 70 kVp can be used which produces maximum contrast.

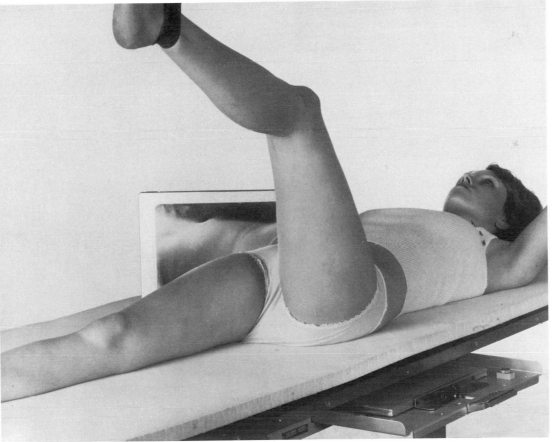

2351

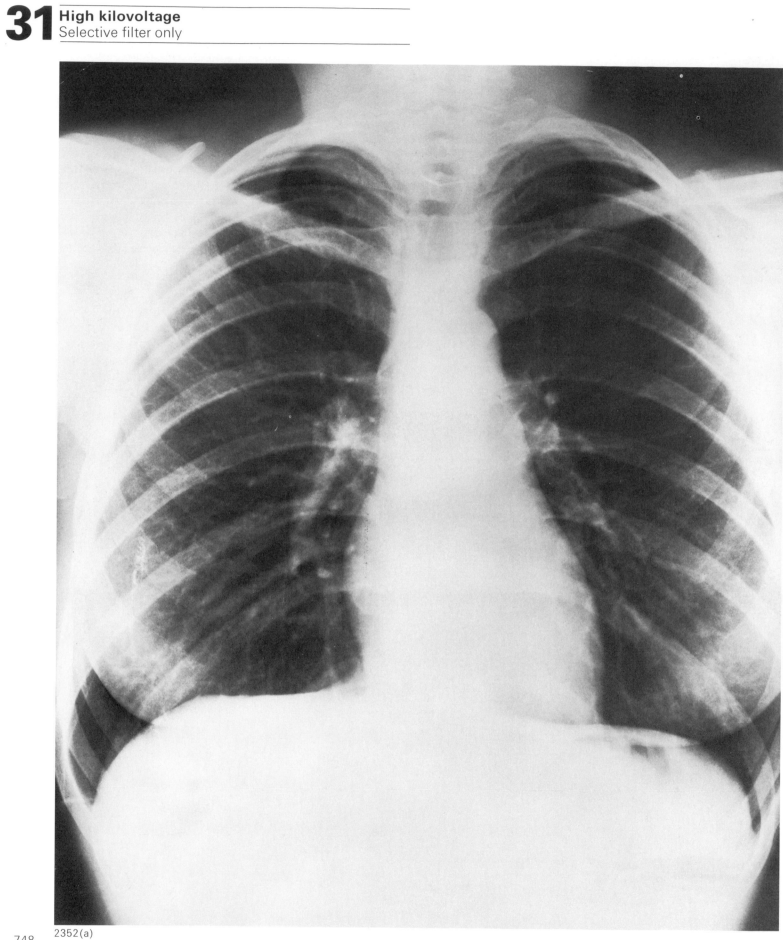

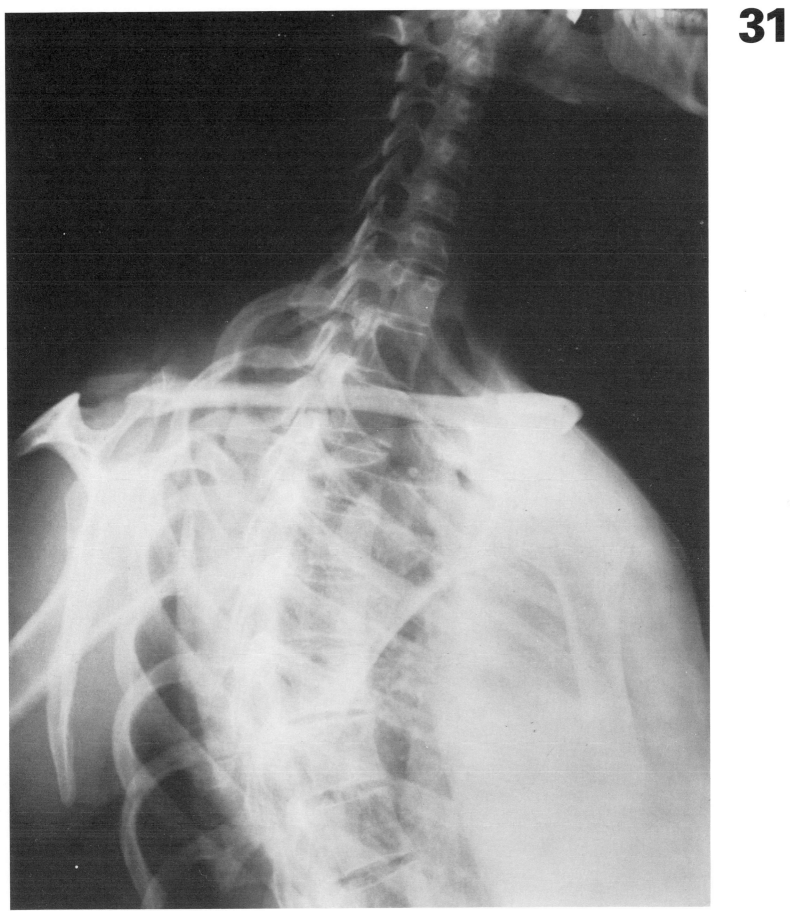

2352(b)

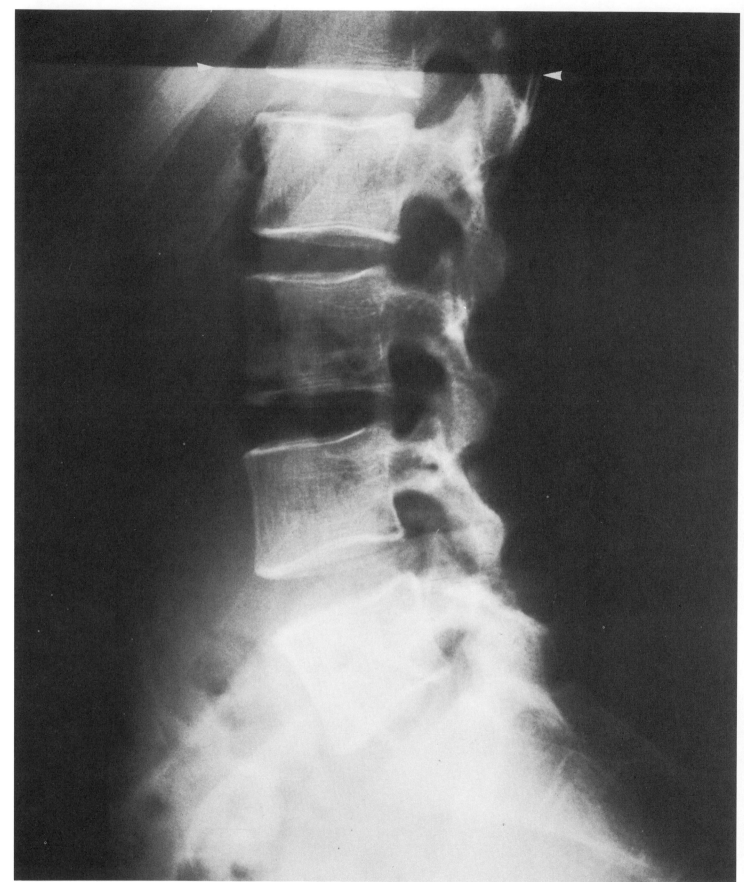

32

FOREIGN BODIES

FOREIGN BODIES

Many different objects may enter body tissues under a variety of circumstances, and if opaque, can be detected and localized radiographically. Radiopaque foreign bodies are commonly associated with industrial and motor accidents, war injuries and children inadvertently swallowing such objects as pins and coins. Swabs may be left in the body following surgery and now have lead strips included (2353) for their identification.

Foreign bodies may not only move down the gastrointestinal tract or along the trachea and bronchi, but also along muscle and fibrous tissue planes in the limbs, and may later appear in the heart. Needles which have been in tissues for some time have irregular, indistinct margins as the surface undergoes slow erosion.

Many foreign bodies, such as wood splinters and plastic are not visible on radiographs because they have the same radio-density as soft tissue, and some types of glass which contain lead are visible while others are not.

High velocity foreign bodies are not infrequently associated with gas in the soft tissues due to disruption of the skin and subcutaneous tissue. The gas tracks along the muscle planes appearing as transradiant or black bands in the soft tissues (2354).

Initial examination

Both antero-posterior and lateral projections should be taken for cases with foreign bodies, large fields used, and the entry wound on the skin clearly indicated with an opaque marker which will show on the radiograph. The routine projections for each area of the body has been described previously, and is also applicable in the detection of foreign bodies. The exposure must show both bone and soft tissue particularly for the less dense opacities such as non-lead containing glass. Xeroradiography accentuates the contrast by enhancing the edge effect and can be used in thin areas of the body, such as the hands and feet. The skin and subcutaneous wound may be visible on the radiograph as a soft tissue defect, and late films may be needed if gas gangrene is suspected or develops (2354b).

Most of the examinations for foreign bodies will be done in accident and emergency departments, and will be similar to those performed on other casualty patients. In wartime the conditions may well be primitive, with low output mobile equipment, and poor developing facilities.

Anatomical location

In simple terms an opaque foreign body can be located in the body from two radiographs, an antero-posterior and a lateral taken at right angles to each other, but it is more difficult to determine the internal organ in which the foreign body is lodged Further examinations, such as fluoroscopy, tomography, stereoscopy and scanning methods, such as ultrasonography and computed tomography are then required. Ultrasonography and computed tomography are particularly valuable for locating foreign bodies as they produce in depth body sections which clearly show the relationship of the internal organs to each other.

Precise depth localization is required prior to surgical removal of a foreign body. The position within the internal organ as well as the track of the foreign body may need demonstration.

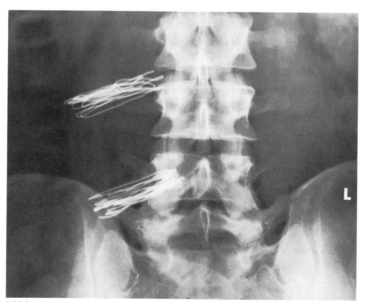

2353

Limbs

A frontal and a lateral view (2354a) are taken without changing the position of the limb between exposures. The entry wound must be clearly indicated with an opaque marker and if surgical removal of the foreign body is to follow, the relative position on the overlying skin (2354a) should be indicated preferably at fluoroscopy.

Oblique views (2355) are also required to show the relationship to bone and with multiple projections each foreign body can be shown separately from the adjacent bone. However, if a foreign body has been embedded in bone for some time, an area of bone resorption is produced showing a halo of lesser density around the foreign body.

Fluoroscopy can be extremely valuable in localizing a foreign body and in indicating its position on the overlying skin. Stereoscopic films can show its position in a 3-dimensional view.

The projections for each area of the limb have been described previously in the appropriate section and should be consulted.

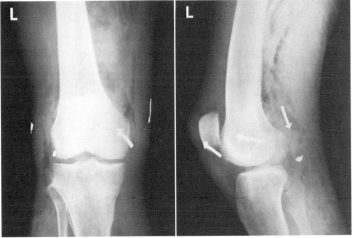

2354a

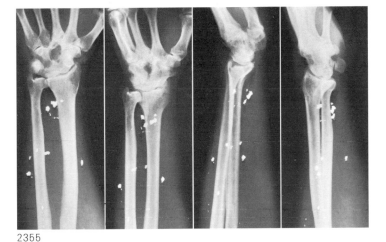

2355

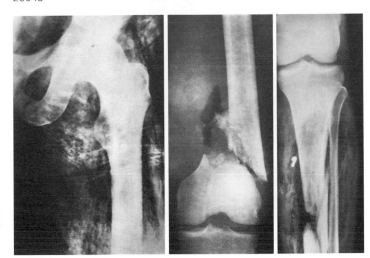

2354b

Head

The localization of foreign bodies in the head presents different problems in the various areas especially in the cranium and orbit, but even the nose, tongue and jaw will require special views. It is usually necessary to show both the bone and soft tissues and a high kilovoltage may be used which provides a wider range of radio-densities than a low kilovoltage exposure. However, soft tissue films in addition to bone films are obtained if a non-screen film is placed on the front of the cassette and both exposed together (2356). A fast and a slow film can be loaded into a single cassette with the fast film on the tube side. As described in the Section on Multiple Radiographs adequate bone and soft tissue films are especially important in the face to show all the opaque foreign bodies which may be present, more particularly in the nose and ears (2357). Multiple views of the face, including the occipito-frontal, occipito-mental, lateral and oblique will be needed to accurately locate foreign bodies in the face (2359, 2360). However, if computed tomography is available, precise identification and localization can be rapidly achieved particularly as an aid to plastic surgery.

For the tongue, exposures will be needed with the tongue resting in the mouth and if possible extended over a film outside the mouth for accurate localization.

The distinction between foreign bodies in the scalp, embedded in bone or within the cranium is essential and in addition to the routine projections a sky-line view may be necessary (2357, 2360). For stereoscopy, the head may be rotated in place of the more usual movement of the X-ray tube. Furthermore, the direction of tube shift can be in the median plane rather than transversely. If the opaque foreign body is intracranial tomography could help with localization, but there is little doubt that at present the best method is computed tomography in the axial and if possible also in the coronal plane. The axial sections should be taken parallel to the OMBL for more accurate localization.

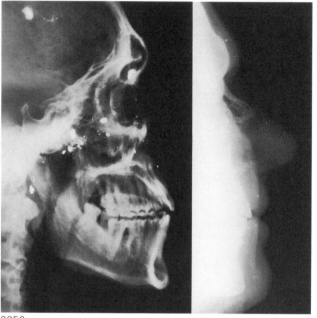

2356

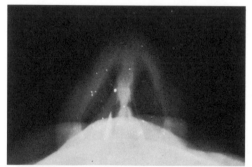

NOSE

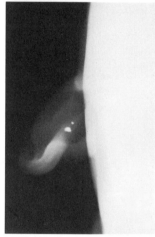

2357   EAR

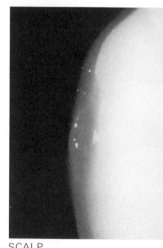

SCALP

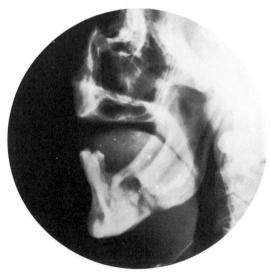

   2358   TONGUE

When an opaque foreign body is in the orbit and on lateral views its position varies with the eyes looking up and down then it is in or attached to the eyeball, but if unchanged in position it is in the surrounding orbital tissues. In (2359) a lateral and 30° occipito-mental film show a left sided glass eye and multiple extra-ocular and extra-orbital opaque foreign bodies. The small metal ring marks the orifice on the skin of a suppurating sinus.

In (2361) the large metallic foreign body lies antero-lateral to the odontoid peg, particular well localized on the submento-vertical view. In addition, there is another small opacity in the left supra-orbital ridge. A tangential view would be needed to show whether it was in the frontal sinus, embedded in bone or in the overlying soft tissues.

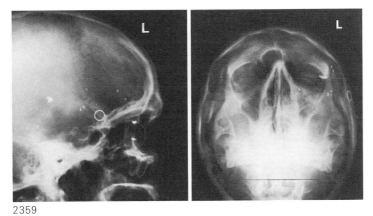

2359

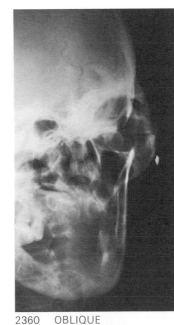 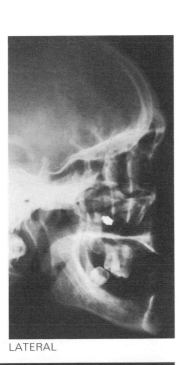

2360   OBLIQUE   LATERAL

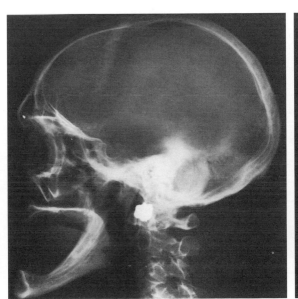 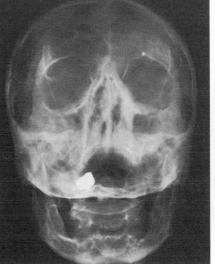 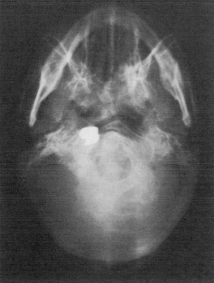

2361

Trunk

It may be difficult to localize foreign bodies in the region of the *shoulder* which may be in surrounding soft tissue, in bone, in the joint, on the pleura or even in the lung. A steep oblique view (2362) will usually displace the opacities away from the lung field to exclude an intrathoracic location. On occasion unusual views such as the supero-inferior view of the scapula (2364) will be needed to show the position of an opacity which in the example given, is a bullet in the spine of the scapula. Careful fluoroscopy is invaluable for showing foreign bodies in profile in this region.

For the clavicle there are several additional projections with the patient prone, supine or lateral. In the prone position, angling the tube 45° towards the feet may show a foreign body separate from other structures (2363) and these projections also produce clear views of the apices of the lungs.

Additional oblique projections (2365) and stereoscopy are usually necessary to localize foreign bodies near or in the *vertebral column*. Initially true antero-posterior and lateral views are essential (2366) but careful fluoroscopy may be decisive in difficult cases.

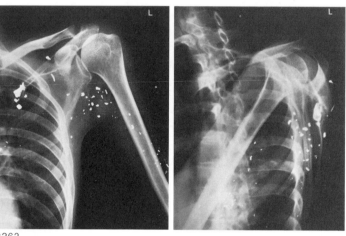

2362

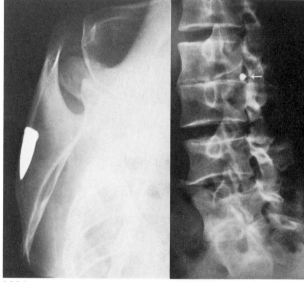

2364   OBLIQUE   2365   OBLIQUE

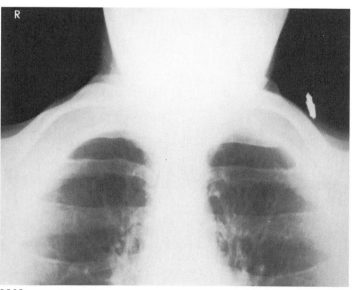

2363

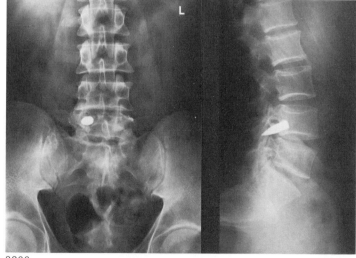

2366

For the *pelvis* a variety of oblique projections are possible, including the axial view over the pelvic brim for the pubis (2367), and posteriorly over the sacrum (2368). The bullet in (2368) is shown to be lodged in the sacrum. The projections for the hip joints are usually the general antero-posterior, lateral, lateral for the neck of the femur, general lateral and oblique views of the pelvis and stereoscopy. In one of a pair of stereoscopy films (2369) equal sized metal rings indicate the position of the surface wounds, the smaller ring being nearer the film.

Foreign bodies in the *thorax* may be in the overlying soft tissues, in the intercostal muscles, adjacent to or in ribs, or scapulae, attached to pleura or in the lungs. Only by very careful fluoroscopy can the position of some opacities be accurately established and in the example (2370) the metallic foreign bodies lie external, but very close to the pleura.

Due to the curved contours and movement during respiration *the diaphragm* presents a special problem. Projections tangential to the thoracic wall or to the diaphragm may be required to show whether the foreign body is above or below the diaphragm. Computed tomography producing axial sections is particularly useful in this respect, and will show not only whether the opaque foreign body is above or below the diaphragm but can localize it to a specific organ, such as the liver, heart, spleen or kidneys.

32

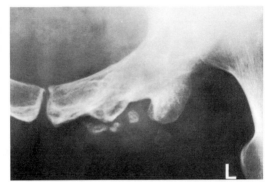

2367　PELVIS INLET POSITION

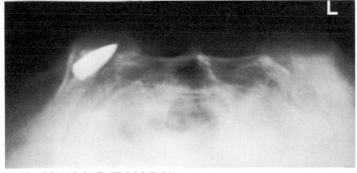

2368　PELVIS OUTLET POSITION

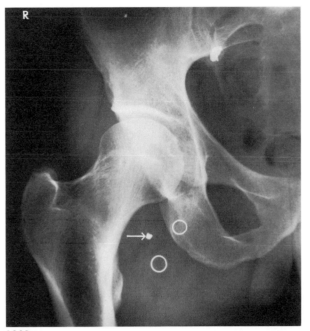

2369

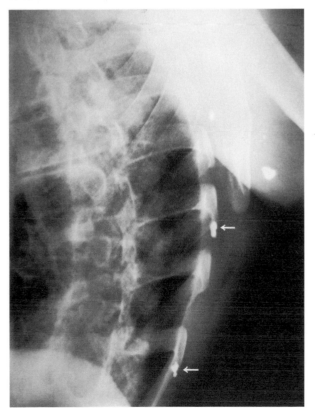

2370　OBLIQUE

Respiratory System

Foreign bodies may be inhaled and lodge in the larynx, trachea or bronchi. The commonly inhaled foreign bodies are non-opaque and manifest radiographically either as an area of collapse, ball valve obstructive emphysema or pneumonic consolidation. Inhalation of a peanut is not uncommon in children.

Penetrating injuries due to gunshot wounds and explosions are associated not only with foreign bodies, but also with injury to overlying soft tissue, pleura, ribs and lung. Haemo-pneumothorax, surgical emphysema, rib fractures and pulmonary contusion can be visualized on the chest radiograph.

Other inhaled and extraneous foreign bodies include, teeth, buttons, pins and glass beads. Pins and needles in the thoracic wall are best localized on fluoroscopy and by tangential views (2372, 2373, 2374). On fluoroscopy opaque foreign bodies can be seen to move with the thoracic wall on respiration. However, the initial films must include a straight postero-anterior and lateral film and must be sufficiently penetrated to show the mediastinum.

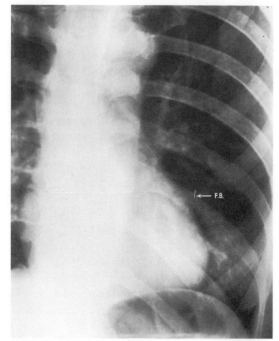

POSTERO-ANTERIOR (2372)

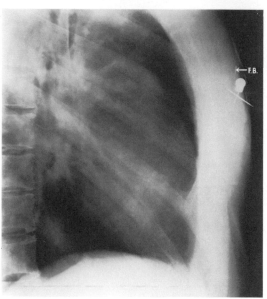

SLIGHTLY OBLIQUE (2373)

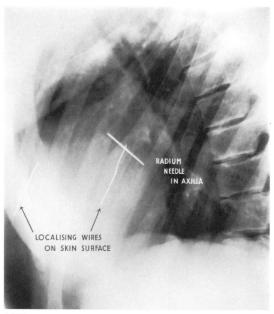

2371

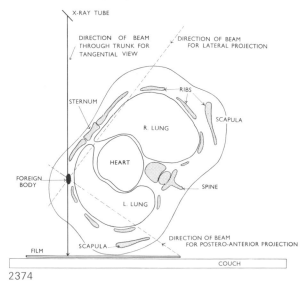

2374

When an opacity is over-shadowed by the diaphragm, it may lie above, below or in the diaphragm. Projections tangential to the diaphragm (2375, 2376) or computed tomography will then be required for its localization. Computed tomography is also of particular value in localizing foreign bodies in the mediastinum, adjacent to the heart, aorta and pulmonary artery.

For non-opaque foreign bodies or foreign bodies which are only slightly opaque, conventional tomography can be most informative. The foreign body may be seen in a bronchus or the obstructed bronchus may be visualized. Occasionally the related bronchus must be shown by bronchography (2377), but in most cases when a foreign body is strongly suspected, and not seen on radiographs, bronchoscopy will be done. Not only may the foreign body be seen by bronchoscopy, but can then also be removed.

Undetected foreign bodies cause a number of complications including pulmonary collapse, repeated attacks of pneumonia, bronchiectasis and pulmonary abscess. These complications may be avoided by careful and accurate radiography uncovering an otherwise undetected foreign body.

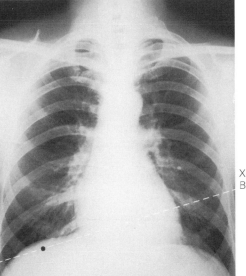

2375

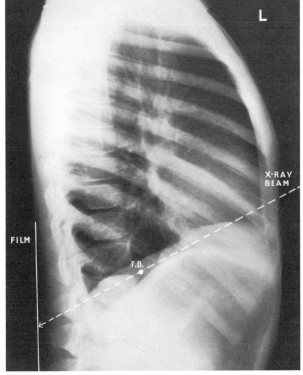

2376

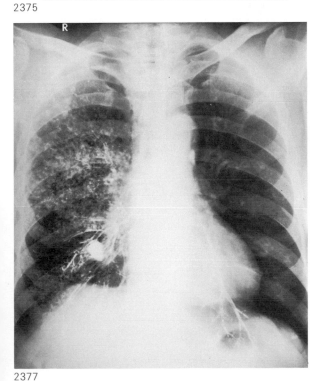

2377

Alimentary tract

Most smooth, small round foreign bodies, such as coins which are swallowed, pass through the alimentary tract without requiring radiography. However, sharp or jagged objects or if large may become impacted and cause obstruction or produce mucosal erosion, ulceration or haemorrhage. Such foreign bodies must be localized and removed.

Pharynx and upper oesophagus

Small bones are not infrequently swallowed and tend to stick in a vallecula above the epiglottis, in a pyriform fossa or just above the cricopharyngeus, and are most readily visualized on a soft tissue lateral view of the neck. The neck should be slightly extended, the shoulders depressed and the tube centred high up at the level of the third cervical vertebra to show the maximum amount of soft tissues above the dense overlying shoulders.

Previously a swallow of barium paste was recommended (2378) but in fact this seldom, if ever, uncovers a foreign body not already shown on the plain film. Foreign bodies come in all shapes and sizes including meat bones (2379), coins (2380), needles (2381) and dentures (2362).

Frequently the mucous membrane is abraded by the foreign body causing persistent pain for sometime after the foreign body has passed.

Oesophagus

Although an inhaled foreign body causes coughing and a swallowed foreign body dysphagia, the clinical distinction is not always clear-cut. A chest film will exclude an opaque foreign body in the trachea and bronchi, and a right anterior oblique view (2382) is used for the oesophagus. A non-opaque foreign body, such as a fruit stone or meat bolus can be shown as a filling defect on a barium swallow, the films being taken at fluoroscopy.

Gastrointestinal tract

A wide variety of opaque foreign bodies may be found in the stomach, small intestine or colon; coins, nails, and safety pins being quite common and seldom, if ever, produce complications. There is little to be gained by taking radiographs of smaller coins or other smooth objects which invariably pass.

Chewing or swallowing hair or persimmon fruit can produce a large "hair ball" or trichobezoar in the stomach which is shown on a barium meal.

Lead shot used especially in hunting wild fowl, not infrequently lodges in colonic diverticula and may be retained for many years.

Abdominal cavity

Foreign bodies outside the gastrointestinal tract are most commonly iatrogenic in origin. Aterial clips and opaque sutures are frequently shown in post-operative cases and intra-uterine contraceptive devices have characteristic appearances.

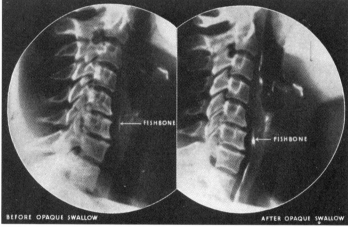

2378

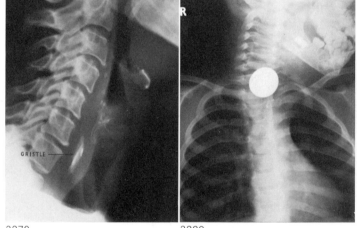

2379   2380

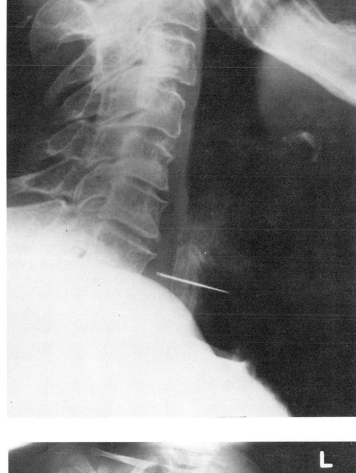

2381

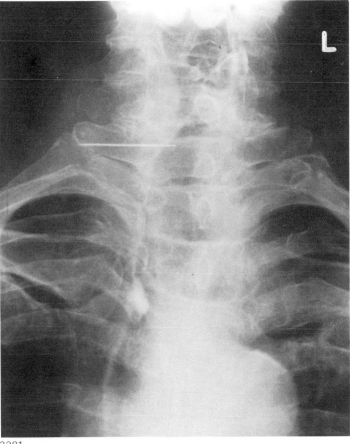

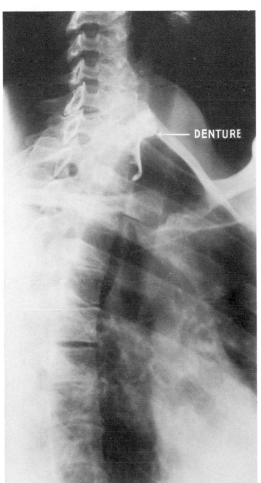

2382

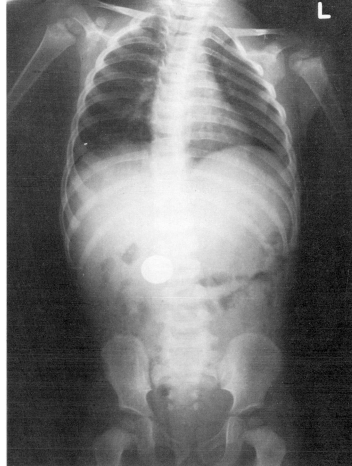

DENTURE

SWALLOWED COIN (2383)

Some of the numerous opaque foreign bodies which can be found in soft tissues have been illustrated. Many of these may remain in the body for many years without apparently producing any ill effects. However, occasionally an opaque foreign body may provoke abscess formation or cause arterial erosion. Intracranial, bronchial and cardiovascular foreign bodies are most likely to produce complications, but intramuscular metallic foreign bodies are usually quite harmless.

The image intensifier with television monitoring is invaluable for the localization of a foreign body giving a clear view with a relatively low radiation dose.

Marking the skin surface

During the fluoroscopy using a very small diaphragmatic aperture, a metal marker is positioned to coincide with the opaque foreign body and the skin labelled accordingly. Fluoroscopy is then done in a plane at right angles to that previously, again with a small aperture and the skin overlying the foreign body marked again (2384). However, in the vast majority of cases the foreign body can be left in situ unless it is close to a large artery or vein.

Tube centring

To accurately relate the position of an opaque foreign body to a mark on the skin the X-ray beam must be perfectly vertical or horizontal over the foreign body (2384), so that the X-ray tube, skin mark and foreign body are in a straight line. Accurate collimation and alignment of the X-ray beam are therefore essential.

Foreign bodies can now be very accurately localized by computed tomography or ultrasonography which provide highly reliable measurements of their position within the body.

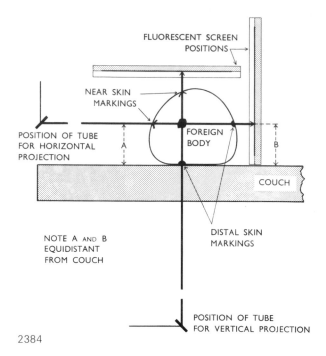

FLUORESCENT SCREEN POSITIONS

NEAR SKIN MARKINGS

POSITION OF TUBE FOR HORIZONTAL PROJECTION

FOREIGN BODY

A

B

COUCH

NOTE A AND B EQUIDISTANT FROM COUCH

DISTAL SKIN MARKINGS

POSITION OF TUBE FOR VERTICAL PROJECTION

2384

Tube shift

However, if neither ultrasonography nor computed tomography is available the depth of a foreign body can be calculated by the tube shift method.

The tube movement can be equidistant about the centring point for the foreign body when employing a localizer (2391, 2392) or in spectacle eye localization (page 772). Alternatively the tube shift may be only to one side of the centring point (2389). All automatic steroscopic tube shift measurements should be checked before being accepted as correct.

The tube shift should be at right angles to the long axis of the opaque foreign body (2385a, 2385b), and all shift measurements should be between the same points on the foreign body shadows. Only half the exposure is given for each tube position to obtain the correct density where the images are superimposed (2386).

Theatre processing and fluoroscopy

Small automatic 90 second processors are now available for the operating theatre and localizing films can rapidly be available to the surgeon. Moreover, C-arm mobile image intensifier units are ideally suited for localizing foreign bodies in the operating theatre. The region can be viewed in two planes at right angles to each other and the skin marked accordingly without moving the patient.

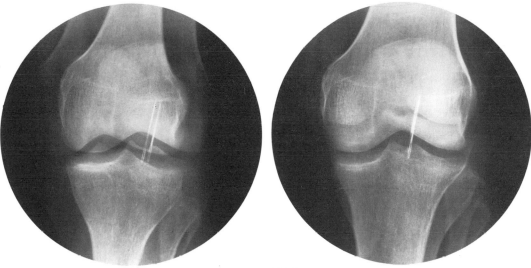

2385a TUBE SHIFT DIRECTION-CORRECT   2385b -INCORRECT

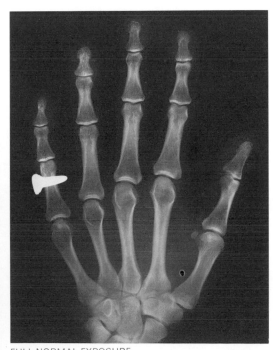

FULL NORMAL EXPOSURE

2386

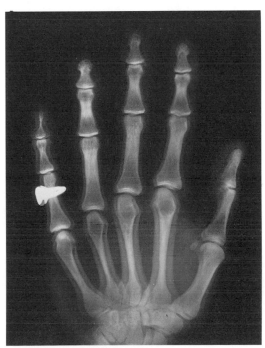

HALF NORMAL EXPOSURE FOR
EACH TUBE POSITION

Focus-to-table-top distance of an undercouch tube can be determined with a flat metal object such as a small coin on the top of the couch. A film is supported a known distance above the coin and exposed and the tube is then moved a known distance, say 10 cm (4 ins), and a second exposure made (2387). The displacement of the two shadows of the metal object is measured and the following formula applied.

$$D = \frac{T \times d}{S}$$

where D = focus to table top distance
$\quad T$ = tube shift
$\quad d$ = table top to film distance
$\quad S$ = shadow shift distance on film

In the example given in (2387)

$$D = \frac{10 \times 20}{4 \cdot 4} \text{ cm} = 45 \cdot 45 \text{ cm} \left(\frac{4 \times 8}{1 \cdot 8} \text{ ins} = 17 \cdot 7 \text{ ins} \right)$$

The exposure used is 50 kVp and 15 mAs for each tube position on non-screen film.

Practice localization

The method of depth localization can easily be demonstrated with two wooden blocks, 15 cm (6 ins) high. A small piece of metal is fixed to one of the opposing surfaces and exposures made to determine the depth of the piece of metal.

The exposure technique is 50 kVp, 30 mAs at a FFD of 60 cm using non-screen film. The total exposure is one second using 0·5 seconds for each tube position.

Depth localization can also be practiced on a variety of objects, such as a bread loaf, marrow or turnip using the tip of a knitting needle as the "foreign body".

To represent the eyeball a 2·5 cm (1 in) sphere can be cut out of a potato or moulded from paraffin wax and wedged with cotton wool into the orbit of a dried skull. The pupil can be marked on the model eye.

Lead shot or a small piece of metal in or behind the model eyeball acts as the "foreign body" for localization.

A suitable exposure would be 50 kVp, 40 mAs, FFD—50 cm using standard dental film. The total exposure is 1·5 seconds, 0·75 seconds for each position of the tube.

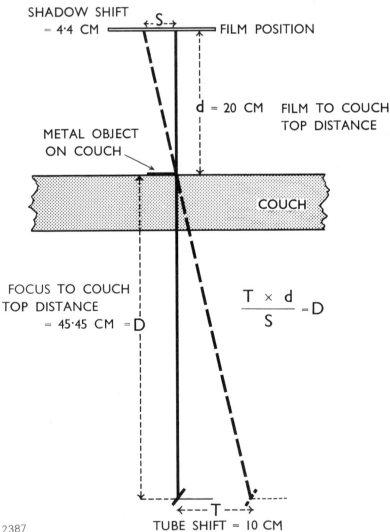

SHADOW SHIFT = 4·4 CM ←-S-→ FILM POSITION

d = 20 CM FILM TO COUCH TOP DISTANCE

METAL OBJECT ON COUCH

COUCH

FOCUS TO COUCH TOP DISTANCE = 45·45 CM = D

$$\frac{T \times d}{S} = D$$

TUBE SHIFT = 10 CM ←--- T ---→

Geometric projection

For depth localization measurements must be derived from flat radiographs, which are essentially two dimensional views; stereoscopic 3-dimensional views being more suitable for localization in depth. Most radiographic localization methods therefore, use the displacement of shadows after displacement of the tube between two exposures and is the basis for "triangulation" on which most methods depend (The Mackenzie-Davidson Method). The localizing chart serves as an accurate reference for applying the formula.

$$D = \frac{A \times S}{T + S}$$

where D = depth of foreign body
A = focal-film distance
T = tube shift
S = shadow shift

Margin of error

While radiographic localization is in theory extremely precise, in practice the slight body movements between the tube-shift detracts from the final result. In general work an error of not more than 5 mm is permissible, but in the eye it should not exceed 1 mm.

In each method the surface position over the foreign body is marked and the depth of the foreign body below the skin surface is calculated.

Other methods depend on parallax, namely the apparent displacement of an object caused by displacing the point of observation. On fluoroscopy, when the tube is moved parallel to the screen any object between the X-ray tube and screen moves in the opposite direction and the amount of movement increases as the distance of the object increases from the screen.

If a metal pointer is then positioned between the screen and couch top by a process of trial and error, till the movement on the screen is the same, the pointer and the foreign body must be at the same level. Thus the pointer can be used to indicate the depth of the foreign body below the skin surface.

Localization Chart for a Tube Shift (T) of 60mm, FFD (A) of 500–800 mm, and Shadow Shift (S) of 0·5 – 20 mm Resulting in Depths of Foreign Bodies (D)

SHADOW SHIFT (S) 0·5	1	2	3	4	5	6	7	8	9	10	11	12	13	14	15	16	17	18	19	20
FFD (A) — Depths of Foreign Bodies (D)																				
500 — 4·1	8·2	16·1	23·8	31·2	38·5	45·4	52·2	58·8	65·2	71·4	77·4	83·3	89	94·6	100	105·3	110·4	115·4	120·2	125
510 — 4·2	8·4	16·5	24·3	32	39·2	46·4	53·3	60	66·5	72·8	79	85	90·8	96·7	102	107·4	112·6	117·7	122·7	127·5
520 — 4·3	8·5	16·6	24·8	32·5	40	47·3	54·3	61·2	67·8	74·3	80·6	86·6	92·8	98·4	104	109·5	114·8	120	125·1	130
530 — 4·4	8·7	17	25·2	33·1	40·8	48·2	55·4	62·3	69·1	75·7	82·1	88·3	94·4	100	106	111·6	117	122·3	127·5	132·5
540 — 4·5	8·9	17·4	25·7	33·8	41·5	49	56·5	63·5	70·4	77·1	83·7	90	96·2	102·2	108	113·7	119·2	124·6	129·9	135
550 — 4·5	9	17·7	26·1	34·4	42·3	50	57·5	64·7	71·7	78·5	85·2	91·7	98	104	110	115·8	121·4	126·9	132·3	137·5
560 — 4·6	9·2	18	26·7	35	43·1	50·9	58·5	66	73	80	86·8	93·3	99·8	105·8	112	117·9	123·6	129·2	134·7	140
570 — 4·7	9·3	18·4	27·1	35·6	43·8	51·8	59·6	67	74·4	81·4	88·3	95	101·5	107·8	114	120	125·8	131·5	137·1	142·5
580 — 4·8	9·5	18·7	27·6	36·2	44·6	52·7	60·6	68·2	75·7	82·8	89·9	96·6	103·3	109·7	116	122·1	128	133·8	139·5	145
590 — 4·9	9·7	19	28·1	36·9	45·4	53·6	61·6	69·4	77	84·3	91·4	98·3	105·1	111·6	118	124·2	130·2	136·1	141·9	147·5
600 — 5	9·8	19·3	28·6	37·5	46·3	54·5	62·7	70·6	78·3	85·7	93	100	106·9	113·5	120	126·3	132·4	138·4	144·3	150
610 — 5	10	19·7	29·1	38·1	46·9	55·5	63·7	71·7	79·6	87·1	94·5	101·8	108·6	115·4	122	128·4	134·6	140·8	146·7	152·5
620 — 5·1	10·2	20	29·5	38·7	47·7	56·3	64·8	72·9	80·9	88·5	96·1	103·3	110·4	117·3	124	130·5	136·8	143·2	149·1	155
630 — 5·2	10·3	20·3	30	39·4	48·5	57	65·8	74·1	82·2	90	97·6	105	112·2	119·2	126	132·6	139	145·4	151·5	157·5
640 — 5·3	10·5	20·6	30·5	40	49·2	58·2	66·9	75·3	83·5	91·4	98·2	106·6	114	121·1	128	134·7	141·3	147·7	153·9	160
650 — 5·4	10·7	20·9	31	40·6	50	59	67·9	76·5	84·8	92·8	100·7	108·3	115·7	122·8	130	136·8	143·5	150	156·3	162·5
660 — 5·5	10·8	21·3	31·4	41·2	50·8	60	69	77·6	86·1	94·3	102·3	110	117·5	124·8	132	138·9	145·7	152·3	158·7	165
670 — 5·5	11	21·6	31·9	41·9	51·6	61	70	78·8	87·4	95·7	103·8	111·7	119·3	126·7	134	141	147·9	154·6	161·1	167·5
680 — 5·6	11·1	21·9	32·4	42·5	52·4	61·8	71	80	88·7	97·1	105·4	113·3	121·1	128·7	136	143·1	150·1	157	163·5	170
690 — 5·7	11·3	22·2	32·9	43·1	53·2	62·7	72·1	81·2	90	98·5	106·9	115	122·9	130·5	138	145·3	152·3	159·2	165·9	172·5
700 — 5·8	11·5	22·6	33·3	43·7	53·9	63·6	73·1	82·3	91·3	100	108·5	116·6	124·7	132·4	140	147·4	154·5	161·5	168·3	175
710 — 5·9	11·6	22·9	33·8	44·4	54·7	64·5	74·2	83·5	92·6	101·4	110	118·3	126·4	134·3	142	149·5	156·7	163·8	170·8	177·5
720 — 6	11·8	23·2	34·3	45	55·4	65·5	75·2	84·7	93·9	102·8	111·6	120	128·2	136·2	144	151·6	158·9	166·2	173·2	180
730 — 6	11·9	23·5	34·8	45·6	56·2	66·4	76·3	86	95·2	104·3	113·1	121·7	130	138·1	146	153·7	161·2	168·5	175·6	182·5
740 — 6·1	12·1	23·9	35·2	46·2	57	67·2	77·3	87	96·5	105·7	114·7	123·3	131·8	140	148	155·8	163·4	170·8	178	185
750 — 6·2	12·3	24·2	35·7	46·8	57·7	68·2	78·2	88·2	97·8	107·1	116·2	125	133·6	141·9	150	157·9	165·6	173·1	180·4	187·5
760 — 6·3	12·5	24·5	36·2	47·5	58·5	69·1	79·4	89·4	99·1	108·5	117·8	126·6	135·3	143·8	152	160	167·8	175·4	182·8	190
770 — 6·4	12·6	24·8	36·7	48·1	59·2	70	80·4	90·6	100·4	110	119·3	128·3	137·1	145·8	154	162·1	170	177·7	185·2	192·5
780 — 6·4	12·8	25	37·1	48·7	60	70·9	81·5	91·8	101·7	111·4	120·9	130	138·9	147·5	156	164·2	172·2	180	187·6	195
790 — 6·5	13	25·5	37·6	49·4	60·8	71·8	82·5	92·9	103	112·9	122·4	131·7	140·7	149·4	158	166·3	174·4	182·3	190	197·5
800 — 6·6	13·1	25·8	38·1	50	61·7	72·7	83·6	94·1	104·3	114·3	124	133·3	142·5	151·3	160	168·4	176·6	184·6	192·4	200

Screen and film triangulation is a precise method of depth localization not requiring special apparatus.

On fluoroscopy, the diaphragm is reduced to a small aperture and centred directly over the foreign body, the position is then marked on the skin surface, the diaphragm opened and the first exposure made at half the normal exposure time. The tube is moved a known distance, in this example 6 cm (2½ ins) and a second exposure made on the same film again at half the normal exposure time, to complete the double image (2388–2390). The focal-film distance is noted.

On the processed film the distance between the same point on the foreign body shadows is measured and the depth calculated by:

$$D = \frac{A \times S}{T + S}$$

where D = depth of foreign body
A = focal-film distance
T = tube shift
S = Shadow shift

In the example (2388, 2389),

$$D = \frac{600 \times 11}{60 + 11} \text{ mm} = 93 \text{ mm}$$

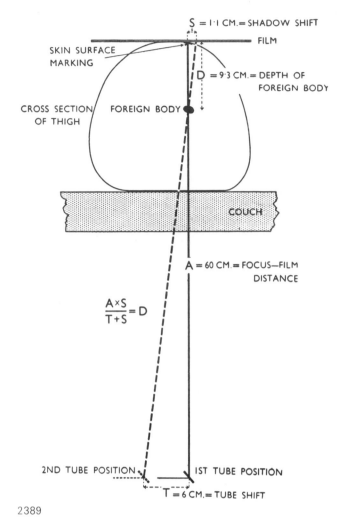

2389

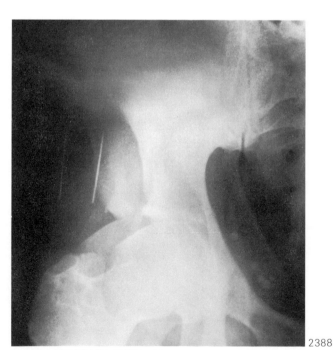

2388

NEEDLE IN BUTTOCK. DEPTH AT MIDDLE 12·2 CM
TUBE SHIFT 6 CM

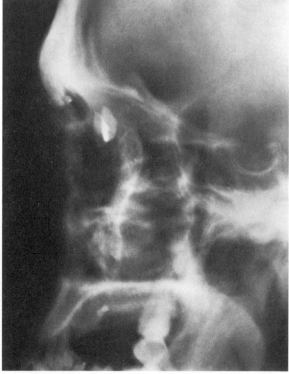

2390

TUBE SHIFT 6 CM

Screen and film parallax

There are various apparatuses for applying parallax to the localization of foreign bodies and an example is chosen for its simplicity and precision.

The localizer is a light metal right angled triangle with holes in the hypotonuse at intervals corresponding to the depth in centimetres from the film level, and is attached to the horizontal film or cassette by a spring clip (2392).

Application

At fluoroscopy the position of the foreign body is marked on the skin surface with the diaphragm closely collimated.

The diaphragm is then opened to include the whole localizer which is in line with the skin marking (2392). A convenient focus-film distance is used and although this does not need to be exact, the tube shift should be approximately one-tenth of the focus-film distance. Six centimetres ($2\frac{1}{2}$ ins) at a focal film distance of 60 cm (25 ins) is convenient. The two exposures are made from points equidistant from and on each side of the centring point. The tube movement must be at right angles to the long axis of the localizer (2392).

The shadows shift of the foreign body on the film is measured and matched with an equal shadow shift of a hole on the localizer (2392). The foreign body shadow is at the same depth as the hole causing the equal shadow shift; in the elevation view (2392) it is shown to be at 6 cm ($2\frac{1}{2}$ ins). The holes can be numbered to indicate the depth in centimetres and any intermediate values easily identified. In the localization radiograph (2391) the foreign body is at a depth of 7 cm.

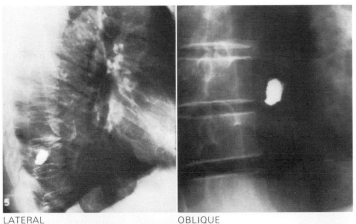

LATERAL   OBLIQUE

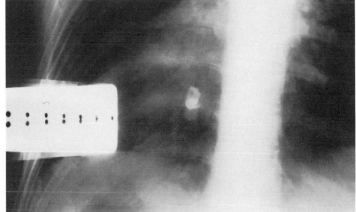

LOCALISATION
2391

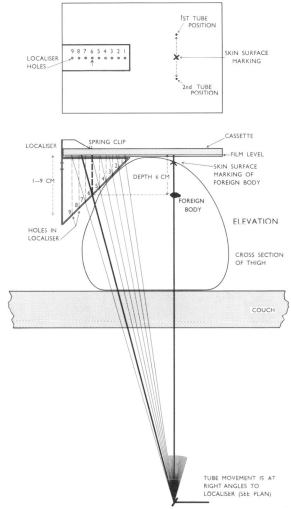

2392

General observations

Successful localization of a foreign body in the orbit with conventional radiography requires considerable experience and meticulous attention to detail. It is by and large a technique confined to specialist centres and the opacity must be quite radio-dense before being visible. However, with computed tomography foreign body localization in the orbit has been greatly simplified.

Radiographic localization falls into two parts, firstly in identifying the foreign body and secondly in determining its position. All exposures are made with the head immobilized by head clamps whether in the true lateral or occipito-mental position as required.

Soft tissue films showing good detail are essential and the intensifying screens must be pristine and free of any blemishes producing artefacts that could be confused with foreign bodies.

A special cassette holder to which fine cross wires are attached is adjusted to bring their point of intersection opposite the centre of the pupil when looking directly forwards. The holder can be made for a film large enough for two exposures, each half of the cassette being protected in turn and the cassette being moved into position for the second exposure (2395).

A focal-film distance of 100 cm (40 ins) is used which is sufficient to give negligible distortion for near film shadows. For foreign body localization the eyeball is regarded as being a somewhat flattened sphere with a maximum diameter of 2·5 cm.

Confirmation of a radio-opaque foreign body

Two lateral exposures are made on each half of a cassette, one with the eyes raised and the other with the eyes lowered. If a foreign body is attached to the eyeball a typical film (2395) will show the foreign body in two different positions in relation to the cross-wires.

To identify a foreign body in the anterior portion of the eyeball, the patient holds a small dental film during the exposure on the nasal side of the eye firmly and parallel to the median plane of the head. The eyelids are opened as widely as possible for the exposure.

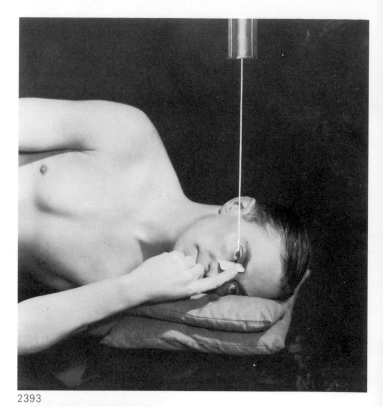

2393

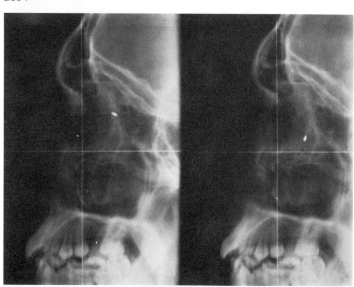

2394

kVp	mAS	FFD	Film ILFORD	Screens ILFORD	Grid
40	42	75 cm (30″)	Fast dental	—	—

EYES LOWERED
2395

EYES RAISED

Localization of foreign body

There are two main methods, firstly to determine the position of the foreign body relative to the centre of the eye for which no special apparatus is required (pp. 769–771), and secondly determining the depth of the foreign body from a plane tangential to the centre of the cornea and charting its position in three dimensions. The second method requires specialized equipment and two variations are described, namely; with localization spectacles and with a limbal ring, as well as, the charting of the 3-dimensional localization within a sphere which is similar to the charting of other methods such as that of Bromley and Sweet.

Localization of a foreign body with a specialized instrument depends on precise tube alignment and alignment of the corneal axis with a definite point on the film. The corneal axis must also be perpendicular to the film in the postero-anterior projection and parallel in the lateral projection.

The calculated position of the foreign body as related to the corneal axis is extremely accurate, but the relationship to the sclera depends on the assumption that the diameter of the globe is 2·5 cm (1 ins). These methods can also be done with a magnification technique using a fine-focus tube.

Ocular fixation

The patient must be able to keep both eyes fixed on a given mark, such as a small black disc placed directly in front of the eyes. Unless the patient has this ocular fixation the procedure cannot be carried out. Any impairment of eye movements will also effect the result.

Position of foreign body relative to centre of eye

If a foreign body lies anteriorly it will move upwards when looking up, but a foreign body lying posteriorly will move downwards, while the position of a foreign body in the centre will remain unchanged (2396). Also the shadow of an irregular foreign body will change its shape.

Similar an anterior foreign body will move inwards on adduction of the eye while a posterior foreign body moves outwards (2397).

Five films are therefore exposed to show the displacement of the shadow of the foreign body within the orbit.

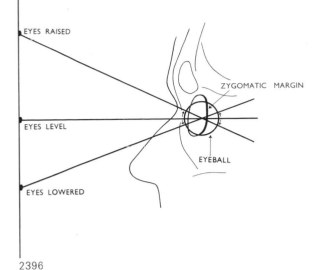

EYES RAISED

ZYGOMATIC MARGIN

EYES LEVEL

EYEBALL

EYES LOWERED

2396

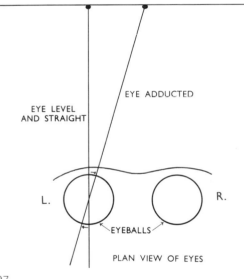

EYE ADDUCTED

EYE LEVEL AND STRAIGHT

L.   R.

EYEBALLS

PLAN VIEW OF EYES

2397

For postero-anterior exposures the intersection of the fine cross-wires in the supporting frame is in line with the centre of the pupil, while for lateral exposures the horizontal wire is at the level of the centre of the pupil.

The head is well immobilized before the following two postero-anterior and three lateral exposures are made.

(a) Modified occipito-mental (25°) with eyes level and looking straight at the disc (2398).
(b) Modified occipito-mental (25°) with the affected eye adducted (turned to nose (2399)).
(c) Lateral with patient looking at disc (2401).
(d) Lateral with eyes raised (2402).
(e) Lateral with eyes lowered (2403).

With these five films the opaque foreign body can be localized whether in the eyeball or in the adjacent muscle (2400).

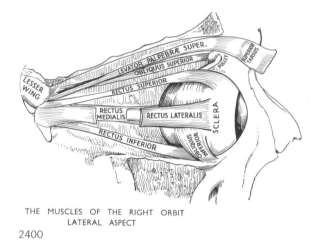

THE MUSCLES OF THE RIGHT ORBIT
LATERAL ASPECT

2400

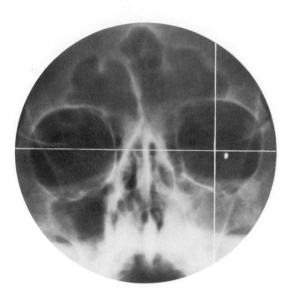

EYES LEVEL AND STRAIGHT

2398

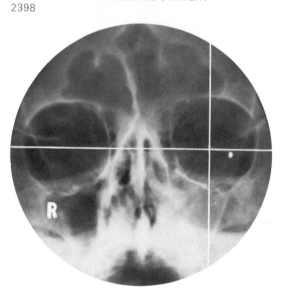

LEFT EYE ADDUCTED

2399

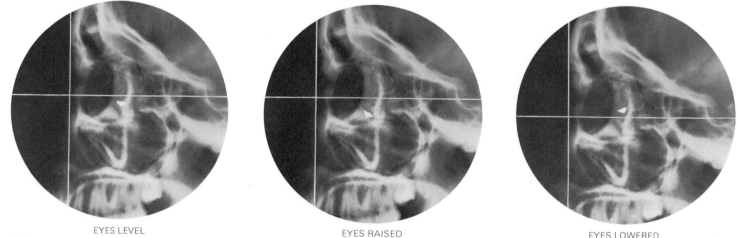

EYES LEVEL

2401

EYES RAISED

2402

EYES LOWERED

2403

On tracing of the three lateral projections showing the shadow of the foreign body in three different positions, straight lines are drawn between corresponding positions of the adjacent shadows (2404). If the opacity is attached to the eyeball the centre of the arc described by the shadows during movement should correspond to the centre of the eyeball. Therefore, lines are drawn to bisect the previous lines at right angles, and indicates the position of the centre of the eyeball if their point of intersection lies slightly anterior to the zygomatic border of the orbit. If the point of intersection is remote from the zygomatic border the opacity lies outside the eyeball.

A second tracing of the two postero-anterior films will show the lateral movement of the foreign body relative to the centre of the pupil, which corresponds to the intersection of the cross-wires (2405).

The five films, therefore, define the position of the foreign body in the orbit.

If the foreign body is outside the eyeball but changes its position with eye movements, it is in one of the eye muscles (2400) and can be localized by reference to the known anatomical positions of the eye muscles. In the example shown diagrammatically a pellet from an air gun is in the superior rectus muscle (2406, 2407). The centre of the arc of the foreign body shadows lies well outside the eyeball (2407).

Compared to computed tomography this method is slow and cumbersome, but relatively simple if compared with other conventional radiographic techniques.

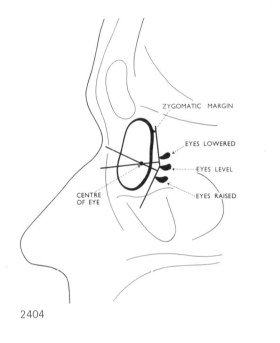

2404

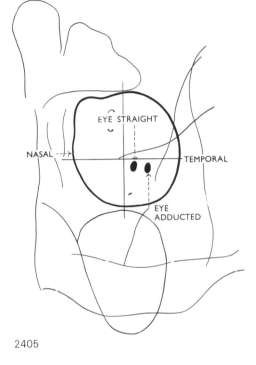

2405

2406

2407

Spectacles method

The spectacles method is performed only after a foreign body has been clearly demonstrated in the orbit and if ocular fixation is possible using the following stages:

(a) Exposing the shadow-shift film
(b) Estimating the position of the foreign body
(c) Calculating the depth measurement
(d) Charting the position of the foreign body

(a) Exposing the shadow-shift film

The spectacles are specially designed with a frame having an adjustable nose-piece and cross-wire eyepieces which can be lowered to the level of the eye by a controlling screw in a side piece also serving as a rest for the film.

When correctly positioned the eyepiece is parallel to the couch and to the direction of the tube movement, with the indicator raised vertically over the intersection of the cross-wires (2408, 2409).

The patient's head is immobilized with the neck resting on a sandbag and the eyes fixed on the overhead mark. The eyepiece over the eye being examined is adjusted to bring the point of intersection of the cross-wires immediately over the pupil. The eyes are then closed, the eyepiece lowered until there is gentle compression on the eyelid and by fluoroscopy the tube is centred to the point of intersection of the cross-wires with the raised indicator immediately above. The diaphragm is then opened and a dental film is placed on the eyepiece with the sound eye looking at the overhead mark. Two tube shift exposures are made on the one film, the tube positions being 3 cm on either side of the point of intersection of the cross-wires. A small weight, such as a penny, on the film maintains good contact (2409).

The position of the film is recorded by a small metal projection on the eyepiece indicating the upper or lower temporal quadrant of the eye. The focus-film distance and tube-shift must be noted and the procedure must be standardized. The film will show the foreign body in a particular quadrant.

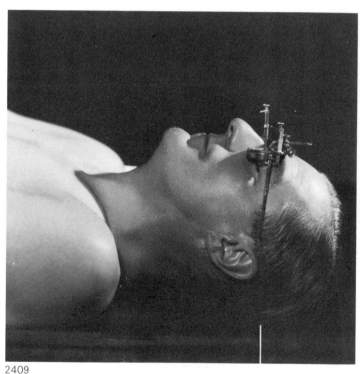

2409

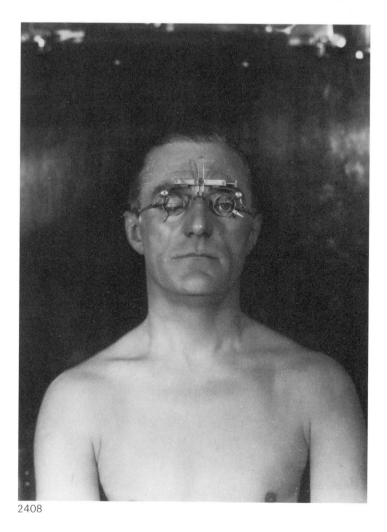

2408

(b) Estimating the position of the foreign body

The distance on the film between the shadows of the foreign body is measured and then marked on chart E (2410) lined in units of 1 mm.

Each tube centre position (T_1 and T_2) is joined to the respective shadow positions (S_1 and S_2), and their point of intersection indicates the actual position of the foreign body as seen from the front of the eye (2411).

(c) Calculation of depth

The film shadow-shift of the foreign body is measured and the formula applied.

$$D = \frac{A \times S}{T + S}$$

which in the example in (2411) is

$$D = \frac{550 \times 2 \cdot 5}{60 + 2 \cdot 5} = 22 \text{ mm}$$

or the depth can be obtained by referring to the table.

In both cases the depth is taken from a plane tangential to the cornea.

(d) Charting the position of the foreign body

Chart D (2411) has two diagrams representing elevation and plane views of the eyeball respectively with the position of the foreign body on the exposed film shown on the line running through X-4. The position of the shadow of the foreign body F on Chart C (2410) is transferred to the elevation diagram (2411) as P. A horizontal line $A–C$ is drawn through P and the part above, within the circumference of the circle, represents the diameter of the part of the orbit within which the foreign body lies. From the point at which the line $A–C$ cuts the circumference, perpendicular lines are dropped to the major axis of the lower diagram at $d–e$ completing the plan view (shaded).

From the point P on the elevation a perpendicular is dropped to the film line X-4 on the plan view which it meets at P and the calculated depth of the foreign body is set against this line, which in the example given was 22 mm, at P, the position of the foreign body on the plan view.

A foreign body lying within the heavy black line is in the eyeball but if outside the heavy black line is outside the eyeball, but within the orbit.

ELEVATION

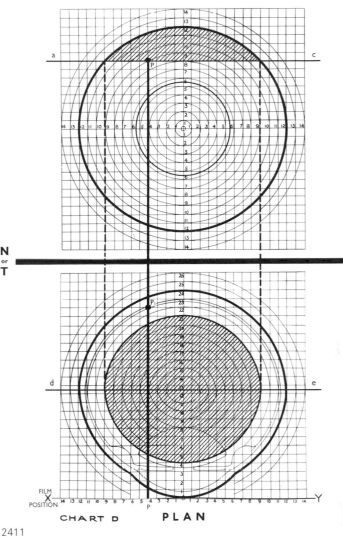

CHART D   PLAN

2411

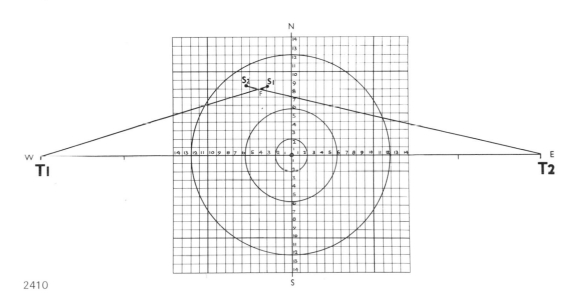

The position of the opaque foreign body in the right orbit in the example given is therefore,

8 mm above the central corneal axis
4 mm to the temporal side of the central corneal axis and
22 cm deep to the plane tangential to centre of the anterior surface of the cornea.

The full technique can be practised on a dry skull with a phantom eye, a curtain ring fitted with a fine cross-wire and an improvized quadrant indicator.

A typical localization chart (2412a) is usually somewhat larger, includes the patient's name, age and hospital number, and is suitable for charting eye localization by other methods as well.

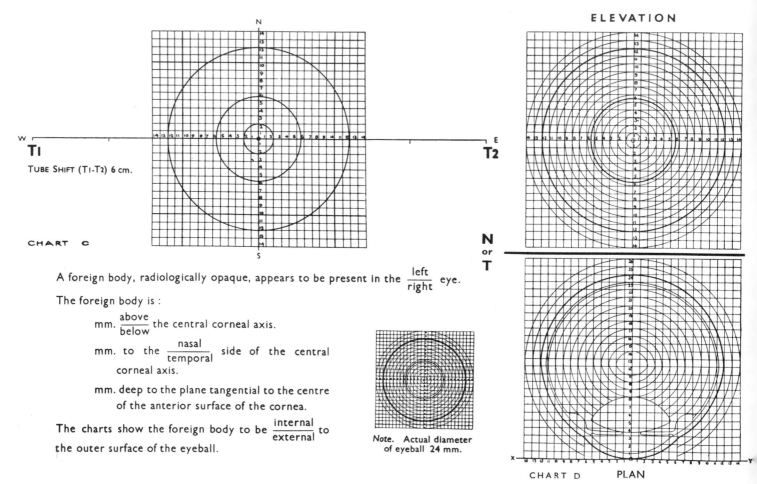

CHART C

TUBE SHIFT (T1-T2) 6 cm.

ELEVATION

CHART D   PLAN

A foreign body, radiologically opaque, appears to be present in the $\frac{left}{right}$ eye.

The foreign body is :

mm. $\frac{above}{below}$ the central corneal axis.

mm. to the $\frac{nasal}{temporal}$ side of the central corneal axis.

mm. deep to the plane tangential to the centre of the anterior surface of the cornea.

The charts show the foreign body to be $\frac{internal}{external}$ to the outer surface of the eyeball.

Note. Actual diameter of eyeball 24 mm.

2412a

774

The Limbal Ring method

The position of a foreign body in the orbit can be defined with the Limbal Ring method whether it is within or outside the eyeball. A metal wire ring 12 mm in diameter is first sutured to the junction of the cornea and conjunctiva. Alternatively a metal ring or 4 small metal balls or short lengths of wires at N, S, E, and W are embedded in a contact lens. The fixing of the limbal marker, therefore, requires local anaesthesia and or surgery, but is independent of the film-focus distance.

Radiographs are taken in antero-posterior and lateral projections with the tube centred to the centre of the wire ring or circle of markers (2413b).

A chart in square mm is subsequently prepared from a template of the limbal ring (2412b) to show the position of the foreign body.

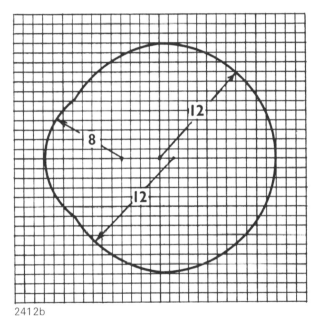

2412b

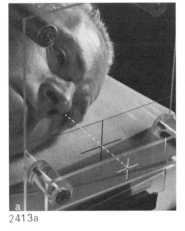

2413a

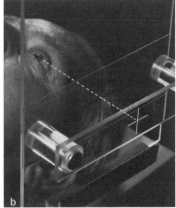

2413b

The radiographs are labelled as indicated (2414, 2416a) and the position of the foreign body in relation to the centring point is then transferred to the chart (2412b). Frontal and plan projection diagrams are also prepared (2415, 2416b) using the radii shown in (2412b), page 775.

Points S_1 and S_2 are then joined to their respective centring points T_1 and T_2. The position of the foreign body is along these lines and is located by

$$T_1B_1 = \frac{\text{Diameter of ring} \times T_1S_1}{\text{Diameter of ring image}}$$

and this distance is then marked along the line from T_1. A line parallel to the corneal axis through this point intersects the line T_2S_2 and so localizes the position of the foreign body in the frontal aspect.

The localization is completed by transferring the measurements onto the chart as in the spectacles method (2412a).

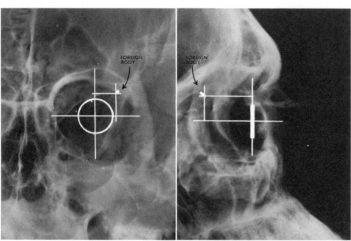

2414

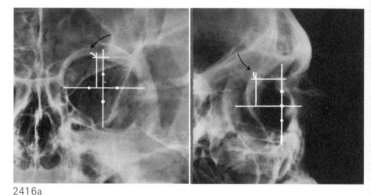

2416a

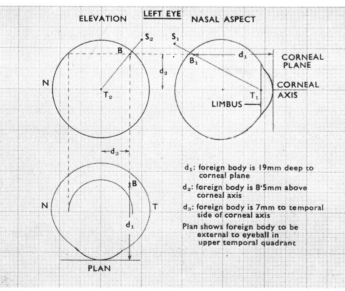

ELEVATION   LEFT EYE   NASAL ASPECT

d_1: foreign body is 19mm deep to corneal plane

d_2: foreign body is 8·5mm above corneal axis

d_3: foreign body is 7mm to temporal side of corneal axis

Plan shows foreign body to be external to eyeball in upper temporal quadrant

2415

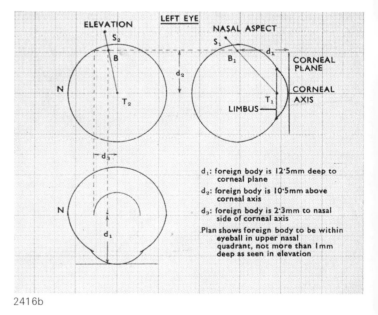

ELEVATION   LEFT EYE   NASAL ASPECT

d_1: foreign body is 12·5mm deep to corneal plane

d_2: foreign body is 10·5mm above corneal axis

d_3: foreign body is 2·3mm to nasal side of corneal axis

Plan shows foreign body to be within eyeball in upper nasal quadrant, not more than 1mm deep as seen in elevation

2416b

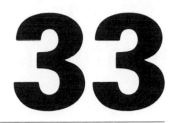

MINIATURE RADIOGRAPHY

MINIATURE RADIOGRAPHY

The X-ray fluorescent screen image can be used in two ways,

(a) Miniature radiography. A single exposure is recorded.

(b) Cineradiography. A rapid series of exposures are recorded, which on projection, forms a "moving" picture (Section 34).

Miniature radiography

Also known as photo-fluorography or radio-photography is similar to indirect cineradiography, but is concerned only with taking individual exposures of the fluorescent screen image, either singly or as a series and is used mainly for chest examinations and for angiography.

A uniformly high standard is required, but even the best results do not compare with direct chest radiography. Nevertheless, as a screening method especially for the detection of tuberculosis, miniature radiography is incomparable because the examinations are done quickly and cheaply.

Mass miniature radiography is used mainly for population surveys, especially for factory workers, and the armed forces. If there is any doubt as to the appearances on the "mini" film a full examination with a large film and often with more than one view will be required.

The use of the larger "mini" films of 70 to 100 mm in chest hospitals and for preliminary films in general hospitals is no longer recommended because of the somewhat higher radiation dose.

General procedure

The image produced on a fluorescent screen is photographed on small film either as 35 mm or 70 mm wide, roll film or as 100 mm cut film. Some cameras allow maximum sized images by eliminating perforations at the edge of the film (2424, 2426, 2427).

The examinations are performed erect. The whole apparatus is designed for rapid positioning and exposure for radiography of a large number of persons in quick succession. The "mini" apparatus uses a shorter focal-film distance than standard film apparatus (2417) and produces a miniature (indirect) radiograph.

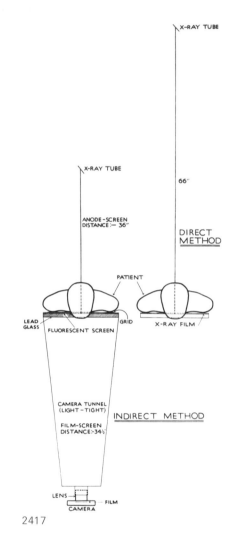

X-RAY TUBE

X-RAY TUBE

66"

DIRECT METHOD

ANODE-SCREEN DISTANCE :— 36"

PATIENT

LEAD GLASS

FLUORESCENT SCREEN

GRID

X-RAY FILM

CAMERA TUNNEL (LIGHT – TIGHT)

INDIRECT METHOD

FILM-SCREEN DISTANCE :-34½"

LENS

FILM

CAMERA

2417

X-ray equipment

The three major parts of miniature radiography apparatus are the power unit, camera unit and control panel.

The power unit is usually a transportable four valve transformer with an output of at least 200 milliamperes at 90 kilovoltage peak with a standard rotating anode tube. The tube aperture can be varied for "mini" or large films if there is an adjustable diaphragm on the unit to suit the different focus-screen or focus-film distances.

If the faster optical system is used with 70 or 100 mm film, but eliminating large films, a low powered, self rectified unit can be used with 85 kilovoltage peak and 30–50 milliamperes. The mass miniature radiography units have efficient protection for the operator in view of the large number of exposures per day.

The camera unit is, of course, light proof and is pyramidal-shaped with the protective lead glass of the fluorescent screen and grid at one end and the film unit at the smaller end. The tunnel also carries the identification windows and accom-

modates 25 metres of 35 mm film (2418). The movement of the film in the camera occurs automatically after each exposure and there is a cutting device to remove the exposed film in the take-up cassette for development.

For the conventional lens system the camera has a fluoride coated two inch F/1·5 lens.

The coating on the lens surfaces eliminates internal reflections ensuring maximum definition, contrast and speed, and the focusing of the lens must be adjusted very precisely.

However, the lens system has now been replaced by a mirror optical system which has improved definition and increased speed and for some mobile units of low output, the mirror optical system can be used with a limited mains electrical supply. The system also has the advantage of being compact as it uses a right angled reflecting system allowing a vertically placed camera tunnel (2420) instead of projecting horizontally (2419).

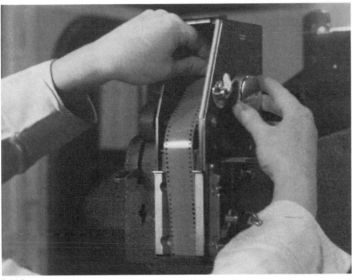

2418

2419

2420

The original Schmidt mirror optical system in astronomy was modified as the Schmidt-Helm system for miniature radiography, more generally known as the Odelca camera and shown diagrammatically (2421), with the mirror system inside the camera tunnel, but the curved cylindrical screen is not shown.

The 70 mm Odelca camera has a roll film magazine for 50 exposures and a "Rapidex" cassette for rapid serial exposures for angiography. There is also a 100 mm camera using cut film with 200 films packed in the separator cassette (2421). A blue sensitive film is used to match the blue fluorescing screen, but with a yellow green emitting screen, orthochromatic or panchromatic film is used.

The fluorescent screen is 40×40 cm (16×16 ins) to accommodate large chests, especially as there is some enlargement due to the short focus-screen distance of 90 cm (36 ins), and further reduced to 68 cm (27 ins) for the 70 mm film small output mobile unit. The tube aperture is adjusted to limit the X-ray beam to the fluorescent screen for better definition and for radiation protection.

The absorption of about 10 % of the fluorescence by the lead glass on the camera side of the screen is far outweighed by its protective value.

The patient's identification is photographed onto the lower margin of the radiograph from the record card (2421), placed in the slot provided on the apparatus and exposed automatically. The apparatus will, in fact, not expose unless the record card is in position.

A stationary grid is used to reduce scattered radiation and is placed in contact with the front of the fluorescent screen and adjacent to the patient. The grid lines are not visible on 35 mm film even when enlarged, but can be seen with the later mirror optical systems when viewed with significant enlargement.

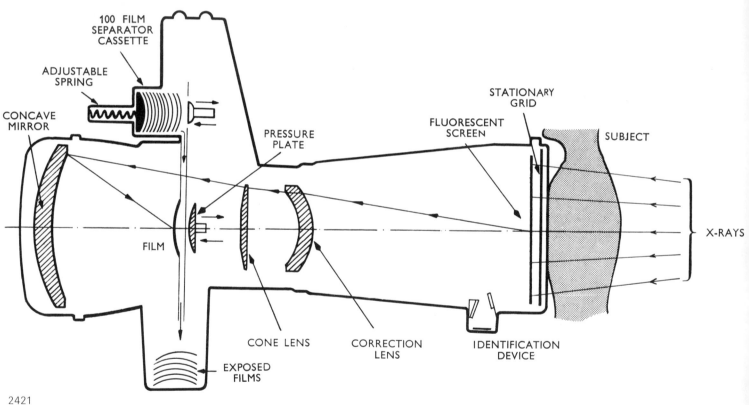

2421

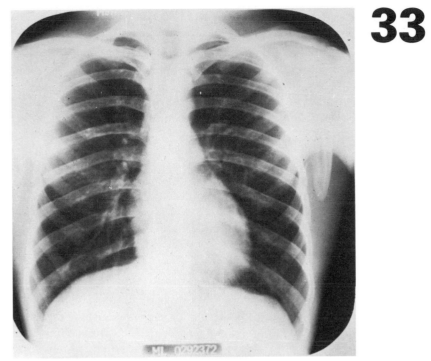

2424

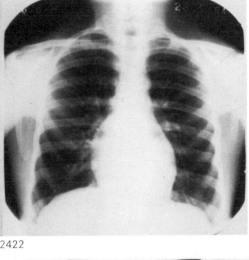

2422

2425

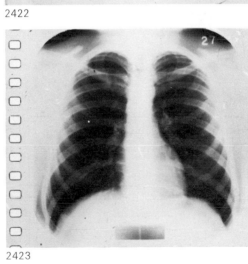

2423

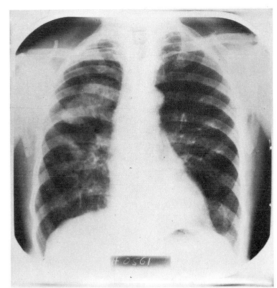

2426

Positioning in miniature radiography is critical because of the short focus-screen distance. The subject must be "moulded" to the screen (2427) by pressing the shoulders downwards and forwards, adjusting the arms to depress the clavicles and project the scapulae away from the lung fields. For patients with short arms the hands should be at waist level (2427); for elderly patients who are inclined to be stiff, the arms should be extended, rotated and brought forward (2428), and for patients with long arms the hands should be low down over the buttocks.

The position of the shoulders are of paramount importance and the position adopted by the arms and hands follows accordingly.

Correct alignment between the X-ray tube and the screen is essential and is checked by an optical centring device incorporated into the unit. Simultaneous adjustment of the X-ray tube and camera tunnel for different individuals is obtained in one unit by a flexible cable, and in another unit by a lift to move the examinee up to the screen.

The control table is designed to automatically rotate the tube, expose the record card, expose and then wind on the film, all in sequence, from a single control switch. There are metres and light indicators to detect failures in any part of the apparatus and there are limiting devices to prevent overloading of the X-ray tube.

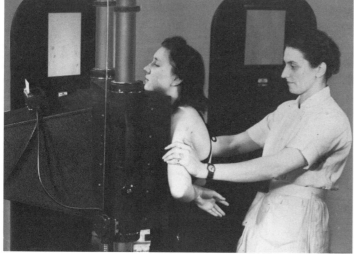

2427

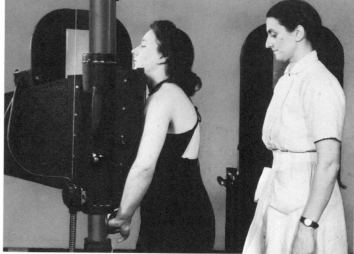

2428

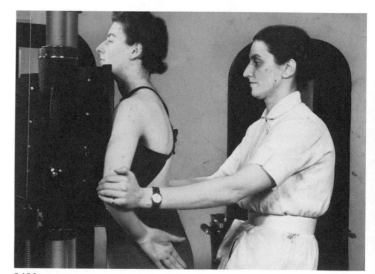

2429

Comparison of Large Film and Miniature Film Techniques

Large Film	Miniature
Direct radiation	Indirect radiation
Double coated	Single coated
Double intensifying screens	Single intensifying screens
Non-grid or grid	Grid
Film and screens in contact	Reduction in light intensity with inverse square law due to optical system

Light losses are greater in the miniature system with 35 mm film requiring $\times 9$ the normal large film X-ray exposure.

To maintain a suitable exposure time without introducing movement blurring, the focus-film distance is reduced to 90 cm (36 ins) from 180 cm (72 ins). Compared with the non-grid large film, an increase of 20 kVp is required to compensate for the grid in the miniature film system, but with the mirror optic system the disparity in exposure between the miniature and large film is reduced to $\times 3$.

Essentials of the miniature system

(a) A large aperture lens and short focal length lens system is required.
(b) The speed of the single screen must provide maximum emission with acceptable sharpness.
(c) Processing should be rapid with low grain and minimal fog.

Processing

Film is now available for automatic 90 second processing which allows rapid viewing and a decision as to whether a large film is required.

The colour sensitivity of the film used depends on the spectral emission of the fluorescent screen and is usually either monochromatic or orthochromatic film. The film must be handled carefully as any blemishes produced are magnified.

Viewing

Suitable projectors and viewing screens show the 35 mm film as 12×12 cm (5×5 ins) images or even larger. The projector must have a well corrected lens, easy transport mechanism which does not scratch the film and satisfactory illumination, usually a 100 watt lamp.

The projection screen has a white matt surface marked to the size of the image. Viewing the image no larger than 12×12 cm (5×5 ins) reduces eye strain and gives better definition.

Both 45 mm and 70 mm films are viewed by direct magnification to $\times 1.5$ their original size and the 100 mm film viewed directly on a marked illuminator.

Rolls of 35 mm film can be easily stored in shallow drawers and compared with large film the storage of even 70 mm and 100 mm film is very economical.

When large numbers of patients up to 500 per day are being examined, the organization must be extremely efficient, and then a photo-timer becomes essential. Usually all that is required to produce uniform exposures with a photo-timer is to adjust the kVp for small, medium or large individuals.

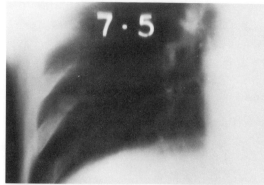

2434

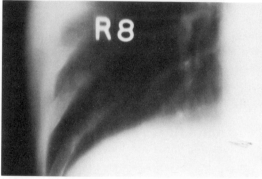

2435

Confirmation on large films

If any abnormality is seen on the miniature film, the person is recalled for a large film. The miniature films tend to accentuate pulmonary shadows and often the large films appear normal. However, even very small lesions can be detected on the miniature film (2430), and clearly shown on the large, such as the shadowing at the right upper lobe (2431). Similarly the nodular shadow was first detected on the "mini" (2432) shown on the large film (2433) and subsequently confirmed on tomography (2434, 2435).

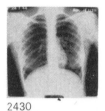

2430

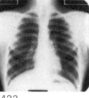

2432

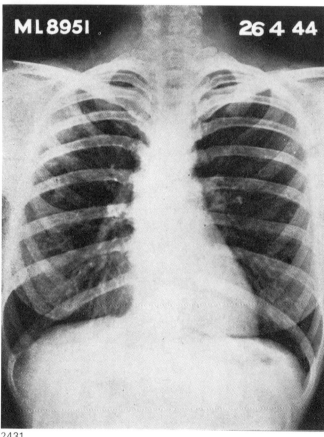

2431

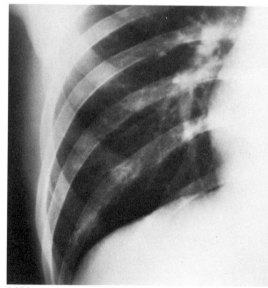

2433

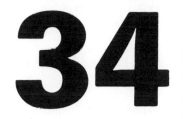

34

CINERADIOGRAPHY

CINERADIOGRAPHY

In cineradiography rapid sequential images of the fluorescent screen are photographed to produce a recording of the movements of internal organs, such as the cardiovascular and gastrointestinal systems after being visualized by contrast medium. Its main application is thus in cardioangiography, coronary arteriography and for the barium swallow. In the gastrointestinal system it has been largely replaced by video-tape recording.

To reduce the radiation dose cineradiography is used either with an image intensifier alone or amplified through a television camera system (2436). The image is photographed onto a 16 mm or 35 mm roll film.

The screen image is intensified by a combination of acceleration and linear reduction of the electrons as they pass between the two screens. The resulting intensification can be up to a factor of × 5000.

The image intensifier

An image intensifier is essentially a device which accelerates and concentrates photons, and is made up of a sealed bottle-necked container with an activated fluorescent screen or input phosphor at the broad end, and the cine photographic elements or output phosphor at the narrow end (2436).

The input fluorescent screen, on a thin curved aluminium support is at the broad end of the glass container with the convex surface towards the X-ray tube. The fluorescent coating on the screen is on the concave surface and is in turn covered by the photoelectric emitting layer and connected to the cathode end of the image intensifier tube by a 25 kilovolt direct-current supply.

A second fluorescent screen, the output screen, is at the neck of the tube with the small fine grain fluorescent surface facing the lens system of the cine camera.

An electron focusing device, just ahead of the smaller screen, directs the accelerated electrons from the larger to the smaller screen.

Thus the X-ray photons projecting the patient's image onto the larger fluorescent screen produce a similar pattern of photo-electrons which are freed from the negatively charged photo-electric layer and accelerated during their passage by the direct-current charge across the two ends of the tube. The electrons converge on the electron-focusing device and are projected onto the small viewing screen to reproduce the original image.

The input screens vary in size, the usual being 12·5 cm (5 ins), 23 cm (9 ins) and 30 cm (12 ins) and also producing an enlarged image of a smaller field size.

Image intensifiers can be used with a cine-camera, spot-film camera, television camera and television monitor or an optical viewing system, and up to three of these viewing-recording systems can be attached at any one time. There is an optical beam splitting mechanism or image distributor for rapid switching of the image from one part to another or to be shared between two to allow simultaneous recording and viewing. Thus recording can be by cine film, spot film or video tape and viewing can be through the optical viewer, but preferably on the television monitor.

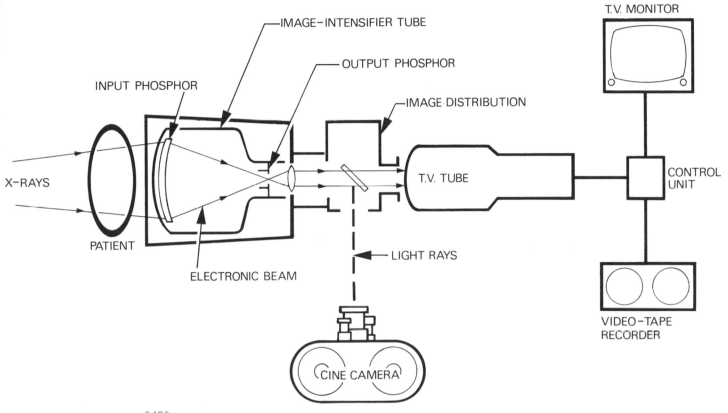

INPUT PHOSPHOR

IMAGE–INTENSIFIER TUBE

OUTPUT PHOSPHOR

IMAGE·DISTRIBUTION

T.V. MONITOR

X–RAYS

PATIENT

ELECTRONIC BEAM

T.V. TUBE

CONTROL UNIT

LIGHT RAYS

CINE CAMERA

VIDEO–TAPE RECORDER

2436

34 Cineradiography

There is a different method of image intensification using a mirror-lens system (2437) called the orthicon tube. The image formed on a 30 cm (12 ins) diameter fluorescent screen by a concentric mirror optical system is focused onto a tube of a television camera. The image is thereby transformed into an electronic signal, which is subsequently amplified to produce a sufficiently bright image to be recorded by cine, video tape or a spot film camera with a separate television monitor for viewing.

Television monitoring has many advantages. Following the introduction of television monitoring, fluoroscopy is no longer performed in the dark but in subdued light, relieving patients of much of their anxiety, abolishing dark adaptation with red goggles and allowing radiographers a view of the fluorescent image during the procedure. One or more television monitors can be anywhere in the room and it is now common practice to have a large television monitor near the X-ray couch and a smaller monitor at the radiographic control panel.

With television monitoring the image can be viewed simultaneously by many observers, can be transmitted for remote viewing or recorded by cine or video and used subsequently for reporting or teaching.

The line-focus tube: Because of the increased luminosity of the screen, currents of 0·2–2 mA can be used for fluoroscopy and television viewing. Using just the flourescent screen, flouroscopy for a wide range of examinations varies from 8–140 millirads with a 30 cm (12 ins) screen, but can be reduced to 20–30% with image intensification. With the lower milliamperage required fine tube foci of 0·3 cm and 0·6 cm can be used providing better definition for fluoroscopy, cine and spot films.

16 mm and 35 mm cameras: The detail on a 12·5 cm (5 ins) screen can be resolved by 16 mm cine film but the image quality is distinctly superior with a 35 mm unit and the difference is even more marked with progressive enlargement when viewing.

However, 16 mm film and systems for recording, viewing and storage are considerably cheaper. Furthermore, the faster lens systems are more readily available with 16 mm and for a similar output on a given fluorescent screen size, the 35 mm film is up to four times slower. The greater speed associated with the wider aperture lens on 16 mm cine allows shorter exposure times with lower radiation dose or a more extended examination. Alternatively a slower film can be used to produce greater definition and a more uniform image.

Recent developments in the efficiency of image intensifier systems have, however, tended to detract from the advantages of the 16 mm format.

Pulsed cine radiography: If the output of the X-ray tube is intermittent, coinciding with the stationary period of the film in the cine camera, there is a considerable saving in radiation to the patient, less scattered radiation and better definition on the film. Programming and electronic switching produces a pulsed output of the X-ray tube to coincide with the stationary phase of the cine giving extremely high quality 35 mm images.

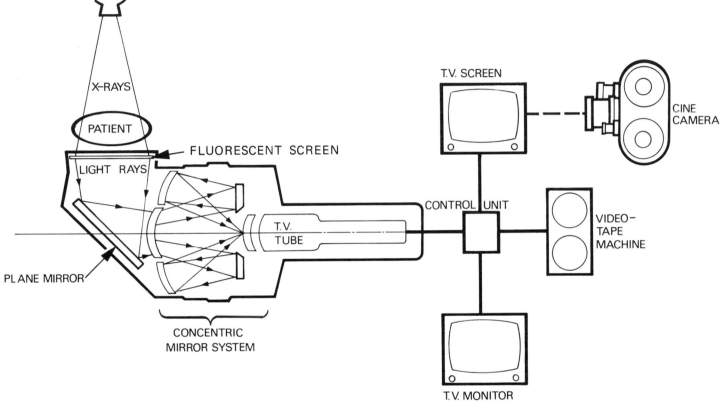

X-RAYS

PATIENT

FLUORESCENT SCREEN

LIGHT RAYS

PLANE MIRROR

T.V.
TUBE

CONCENTRIC
MIRROR SYSTEM

T.V. SCREEN

CINE
CAMERA

CONTROL UNIT

VIDEO-
TAPE
MACHINE

T.V. MONITOR

2437

34 Cineradiography

Cine frame speeds: Most cine cameras have a choice of speeds of 8, 48 and 64 frames per sec, and with modern 16 mm cameras 200 frames per sec, and modern 35 mm cameras 80 and 150 frames per sec are possible.

Cine radiography uses a considerable footage of film; with 16 mm there are 40 frames per foot and with 35 mm 16 frames per foot of film. Therefore, using 16 mm film at 200 frames per sec amounts to 5 feet of film per sec and for 35 mm at 64 frames per sec, 4 feet of film per sec. At these rates a typical run of 5 secs would use 25 feet of 16 mm film or 20 feet of 35 mm film.

Rapid speeds are used for cardioangiography in children and for coronary angiography, but for most of the examinations slower speeds are perfectly adequate.

Frame speeds higher than 50 frames per sec can only be achieved with constant high voltage and a camera independent of the television viewing screen.

The frame speed must be synchronized with the television system when the camera records directly from a monitor. Many systems have a triple scan of a thousand lines and with a pulsating high tension; 50 frames per sec requires careful synchronizing of the camera because lower frame speeds must be submultiples of 50 for a frequency of 50 cycles per sec.

Exposure control: The exposure is controlled by the frame speed for continuous tube discharge or alternatively by the pulsed exposure to each frame. Three systems are used:

(a) Continuous—the tube exposes throughout the cine run.
(b) Synchronized—the tube exposes to coincide with the open shutter, stationary film phase.
(c) Grid tube pulse control—pulsed millisecond exposure with shutter open, stationary film phase.

The radiation dose decreases progressively from a–c. With millesecond exposures there is no subject movement and each individual frame can be studied with sharp definition of the projected image and absence of movement blurring.

In the continuous and synchronized systems at a frame speed of 64 per sec the exposure time would be 1/128th second and with the grid tube pulse control system 2–5 millisec.

Selection of film: The film should be capable of recording the light intensity differences and detail on the screen image and be fast enough for the required exposures with sufficient contrast. Thus FP4 film attains the requirements with a reasonable compromise between all the factors. However, for maximum detail Pan F is more suitable and for faster speeds Mark V.

Processing: With the use of a leader most cine film can now be processed through automatic processors or when available through special automatic "mini" processors.

70 mm and 100 mm cameras: Most image intensifiers can now accommodate either a 70 mm or 100 mm camera. The 70 mm camera can take up to 6 frames per sec using roll film and the 100 mm camera up to 3 frames per sec and uses cut film. Using the image intensifier, exposure times can be down to $\frac{1}{10}$ of large films resulting in a considerable saving in cost with smaller film.

With magnification techniques in the image intensifiers the area of interest covers the whole film, and is very valuable for spot films in gastroenterology particularly for the duodenal cap and lesser curve of the stomach. In the 70 mm camera each magazine takes a film length of 150 feet or more. Rapid repetitive exposure times must be below 0·04 sec so that the film is stationary in the gate during the exposure.

Applications

Cine-radiography is extremely valuable in coronary angiography where the flow of contrast medium is so rapid, for the detailed study of the coronary vessels in different projections. It is also of considerable value in paediatric cardioangiography for selective contrast injections into different cardiac chambers to detect shunts. However, in gastroenterology cine-radiography has largely been replaced by video recording systems and in micturating cystoureterography by isotope studies.

Cineradiographs

The recordings have been enlarged and, therefore, there are no perforations in most of the examples shown.

(2438) is of a patent ductus arteriosus of an infant.

(2439) shows the aorta and left ventricle in cardioangiography.

(2440) shows a cerebral angiogram taken at 16 frames per sec.

(2441) is at the lower end of the oesophagus showing passage of barium into stomach, taken at 8 frames per sec.

(2442) is of a deformed duodenal cap with an ulcer, taken at 8 frames per sec.

(2443) is of calyces and pelvis of the kidney, taken at 8 frames per sec.

(2443) shows the bladder and urethra during a micturating cystogram.

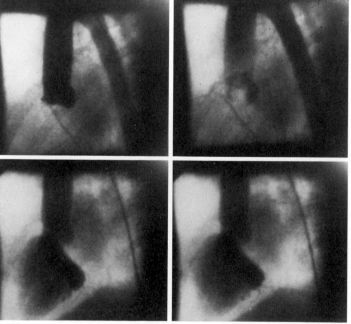

792   2439

2438

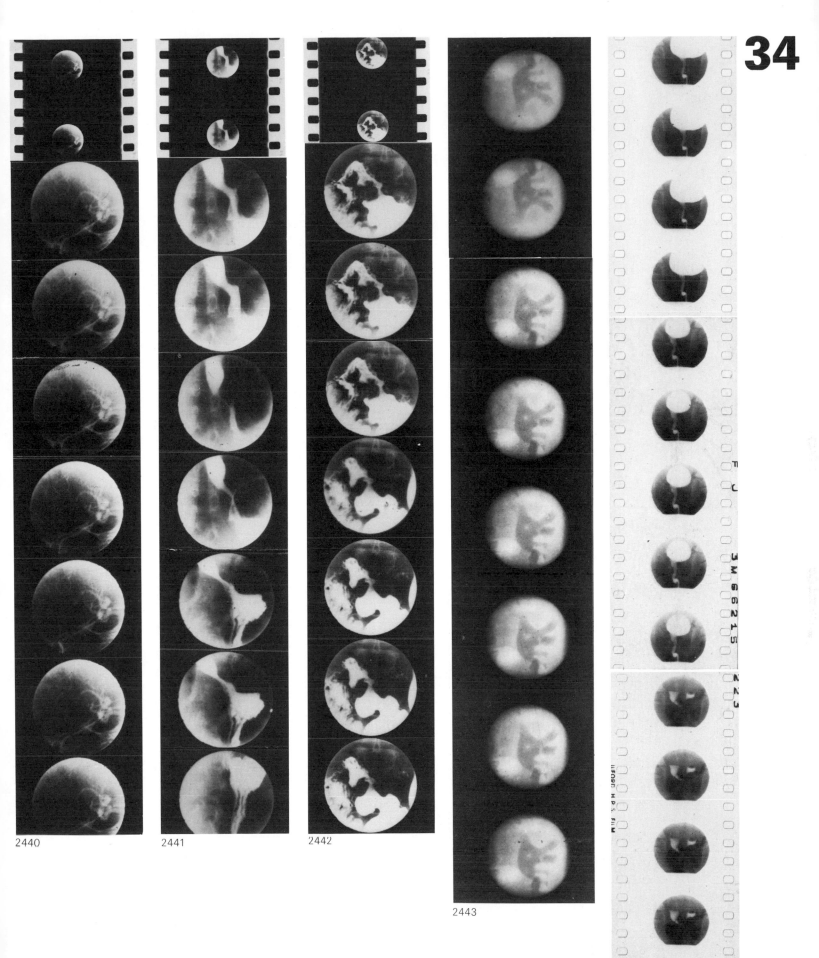

2440

2441

2442

2443

2444

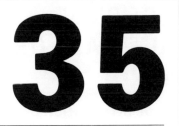

CONTRAST OR OPAQUE MEDIA

35

SECTION 35
CONTRAST OR OPAQUE MEDIA

Tissue attenuation or absorption

The radiographic differentiation of tissues is due to the varying absorption or attenuation of the X-ray beam as it passes through the body and depends on the atomic numbers in the tissues and its thickness. Substances with high atomic numbers including contrast agents and bone will cause marked attenuation of the X-ray beam producing maximum radiographic shadowing and appear white on radiographs. Air and fat have low atomic numbers, cause less X-ray attenuation and, therefore, appear black or grey on the radiograph. Thus the degree of blackening on the film or contrast depends on differential tissue attenuation of the X-ray beam.

Soft tissues are remarkably similar in attenuating the X-ray beam, apart from adipose tissue or fat, and therefore internal organs cannot be distinguished from each other unless there is an intervening fatty layer of adipose tissue. The reason the outline of the kidneys can be seen is precisely because it is surrounded by a fatty layer in the perirenal space. While the margins of internal organs can be defined by their surrounding fatty layer their internal structure can only be visualized by using contrast agents. The gastrointestinal system, gall bladder, kidneys, liver, bladder, aorta, and inferior vena cava cannot be examined radiographically without contrast medium.

There are two main types of contrast medium, low density and high density. The gases, air, oxygen and carbon dioxide can be used on their own to outline internal organs, but have been largely replaced by modern methods especially ultrasonography and computed tomography. Thus gynaecography, retroperitoneal pneumography, air encephalography, and diagnostic pneumoperitoneum are being performed less and less frequently, if at all while high density or positive contrast agents containing either barium or iodine are frequently used.

There are various barium sulphate preparations used largely, if not exclusively, for the gastrointestinal tract and iodine preparations for the kidneys, gall bladder, cardiovascular system pancreatic ducts, lymphatic system, and spinal cord. The iodine preparations are either water soluble or fat soluble compounds, only the water soluble compounds are used for intravenous or intra-arterial injections.

Liquid barium preparations are colloidal suspensions made up in 100% w/v concentrations for individual or in larger quantities for multiple examinations. There are also aerated liquid preparations for single examinations in disposable cans for barium meals and individually packed plastic bags for barium enemas. Proprietary names for barium preparations include Baritop, Barytgen, Micropaque and Unibaryt.

Barium preparations

Barium examinations are done either as single contrast or as double contrast examinations. The methods for obtaining double contrast examinations are different for the different parts of the gastrointestinal tract using swallowed air for the oesophagus, gas tablets for the stomach, methylcellulose water solution for the small bowel and air insufflation for the colon.

The technique of double contrast examinations of the oesophagus, stomach and colon have been developed in the last decade. The internal surfaces of these organs are shown by a thin layer of barium while being distended by gas thus producing a detailed view of their surface patterns.

Radiopharmaceuticals in isotope scanning and contrast agents in computed tomography must also be mentioned and will be dealt with in more detail in their respective sections.

The relative differences of X-ray beam attenuation between body tissues and contrast agents is shown by their approximate atomic weights.

Element		Atomic weight
Hydrogen	⎫	1
Carbon	⎬ soft tissues	12
Nitrogen		14
Oxygen	⎭	16
Calcium	bone	40
Iodine	⎫ contrast agents	127
Barium	⎭	137

Barium sulphate ($BaSO_4$) (Fig. A, B)

Barium sulphate is supplied either as a powder or in liquid form. The powder may come in large containers for multiple examinations or in a packet for each individual examination which is subsequently made up to 100–130% w/v suspensions or to 170% w/v for high density (HD) preparations.
(see pp. 801–802 for figures A to H).

Applications

Barium swallow

The barium suspension for a barium swallow is usually the same as for the barium meal and performed as part of the upper gastrointestinal examination. The double contrast view is usually obtained in the right anterior oblique projection when the patient rapidly swallows a small quantity of barium, and as the barium passes down there is a phase of oesophageal dilatation with air producing a double contrast study.

Barium meal

A 50–80 % w/v barium suspension is used for the single contrast barium meal either prepared from powder or as a proprietary liquid suspension and 200–300 ml is used per examination. For the double contrast examination either special liquid barium such as Baritop 100 % w/v is used or powder is mixed as 120–130 % w/v suspensions. Some high density bariums are given as 170 % w/v suspensions; lesser volumes of barium suspension suffice for double contrast examinations, usually 120–200 ml. Gas granules, powder or tablets are swallowed just before the barium to produce the double contrast effect. These preparations contain citric acid and sodium bicarbonate giving off carbon dioxide in the stomach as they absorb water.

Small intestine-follow through examinations or small bowel enema

For the follow through examination after a barium meal a further 300 ml of barium suspension is given which should be a non-flocculating preparation and preferably hydrophilic.

The small bowel enema is performed after passing a Bilboa-Dotter oesophago-gastro-duodenal tube. A colloidal barium suspension, 150–200 ml is injected down the tube and followed by a solution of methylcellulose in water to produce a double contrast examination.

Barium enema

Dilute barium of approximately 50 % w/v is used for the single contrast enema and 500–600 ml given to fill the colon to the caecum.

For the double contrast examination of the colon 100–120 % w/v barium is used and 200–300 ml given till the barium reaches the hepatic flexure. The barium from the rectum and descending colon is then drained off, followed by air insufflation to propel the residual barium into the caecum and distend the colon.

Organic iodine compounds

Organic iodine compounds are used for renal and cardiovascular examinations, for biliary examinations, for the lymphatic system and in gastroenterology. There are three main groups of iodine contrast agents, the water soluble compounds that can be given intravenously, those for oral cholecystography, and the oily contrast agents.

Iodine has a high atomic number and is, therefore, radiopaque, but as sodium iodide is both irritant and toxic. The iodine atom is, therefore, incorporated into an organic molecule of very low toxicity which can be used as a safe contrast agent.

Hypersensitivity to organic iodine

Pre-testing for hypersensitivity to organic iodine compounds has largely been abandoned except in patients who have a specific history of allergy or asthma. If the examination is essential for the outcome of the patient's illness, prophylactic antihistaminics or steroids should be given. It is worth emphasizing that severe reactions can be caused by even small intravenous injections of contrast medium.

Precautions for organic iodine compounds

The patient should always be questioned for previous allergic or hypersensitivity reactions and for asthma. All patients must be well hydrated particularly those with renal failure who must also be given a non-sodium containing contrast agent.

Any reactions must be reported to the radiologist immediately and a resuscitation kit containing emergency drugs and apparatus for artificial respiration must be available in all examination rooms using intravascular contrast agents.

Excretion of organic iodine compounds

The modern pyelographic and angiographic contrast agents are 2:4:6, tri-iodinated benzene ring derivatives which are water

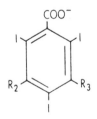

soluble and in usual concentrations are excreted by the kidneys, but, in renal failure and in high concentrations can be excreted by the liver into the gall bladder and gastrointestinal tract.

The oral cholecystographic agents are also tri-iodinated benzene ring derivatives, are polar lipids, have only two side chains.

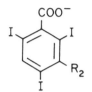

and are excreted by the liver and concentrated in the gallbladder after 12–14 hours. The intravenous cholangiographic agents are dibasic acid dimer derivatives of 2:4:6 tri-iodinated benzene rings,

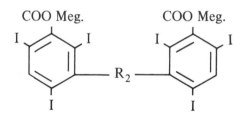

which are excreted by the liver, showing the bile ducts after $\frac{1}{2}$ to $1\frac{1}{2}$ hours and after 2–3 hours accumulate in the gall bladder. Following an injection of iodinated contrast medium some iodine is extracted by the thyroid and it may take up to 20 weeks for this iodine to be eliminated.

Water soluble compounds for urography and angiography (Figs. C, D, E)

The modern urographic and angiographic contrast agents are formed from 2:4:6, tri-iodinated benzene rings and also used for percutaneous cholangiography (Fig. F) and hysterogalpingography (Fig. G).

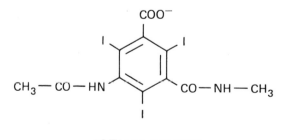

IOTHALAMATE

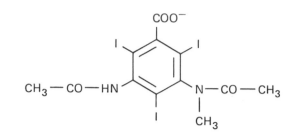

METRIZOATE

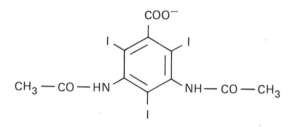

DIATRIZOATE

and the three commonly used anions are remarkably similar.

The usual cations used are Sodium and Methylglucamine (Meglumine).

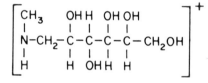

The sodium salts are much less viscous but more irritant during the intravenous injection and probably somewhat more toxic. In renal failure only the meglumine salt must be used and partial substitution of the sodium salt by calcium and magnesium appears to make these compounds less toxic. The toxicity is partly related to the hypertonicity and hyperosmolality.

Dimer compounds such as Ioxaglate (Hexabrix) have a much lower osmolality and cause less reactions both locally and systematically.

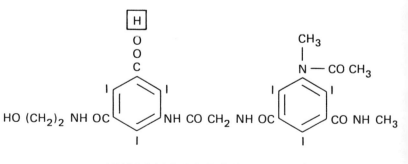

IOXAGLIC ACID (HEXABRIX)

An anionic water soluble contrast agent, metrizamide, has been developed which can be used intrathecally for myelography, cysternography and ventriculography, and has largely replaced myodil.

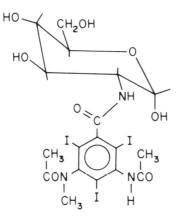

The important factor in deciding the dose of contrast to be given is the amount of iodine and the concentration of the compound; while there is some variation from one product to another the following table acts as a guide to the water soluble tri-iodinated compounds.

% solution	G iodine/100 ml
25	15
30	18
45	28
50	33
60	37
65	39
76	46

2. Cholecystography and cholangiography
(a) Oral cholecystography (Fig H)
The oral cholecystographic agents are also 2:4:6, tri-iodinated benzene ring derivatives, but have only two side chains.

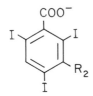

The best known is iopanoic acid (Telepaque).

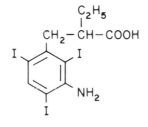

Biloptin comes in two forms, either as the sodium salt or as the soluble rapidly absorbed calcium salt Solu-Biloptin (Sodium or calcium ipodate).

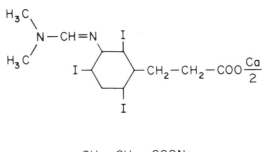

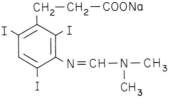

and other products include

Iocetamic Acid (Cholebrine)

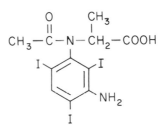

Sodium Tyrapanoate (Bilopaque)

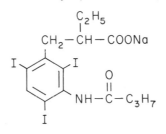

(b) Intravenous cholangiography
Intravenous cholangiographic contrast agents are megulamine dimer derivatives of 2:4:6 tri-iodinated benzene rings and are dibasic acid salts which are excreted by the liver showing the

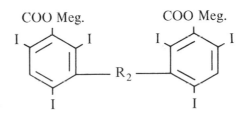

bile ducts in $\frac{1}{2}$–$1\frac{1}{2}$ hours and after 2–3 hours accumulates in the gall bladder. The best known is iodipamide (Biligrafin) which comes in two strengths.

% solution	G Iodine/100 ml
30 Biligrafin	14
50 Biligrafin "forte"	24

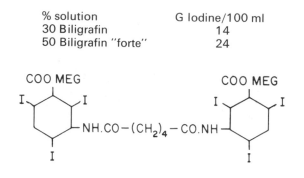

Other intravenous cholangiographic agents include:
  Iodoxamate (Choleone)
  Ioglycamide (Biligram)

3. Lymphographic contrast agents

There are two parts to the examination; the first is the injection of patent blue violet, which is a diamino derivative of triphenyl methane dye to stain the lymphatic vessels blue, prior to dissection.

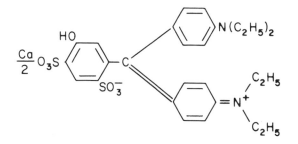

The radiographic contrast medium is lipiodol ultra-fluid or ethiodol which contains glyceryl esters of natural poppy seed oil, such as oleic, linoleic, palmitic and stearic acids.

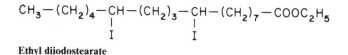

Ethyl diiodostearate

The lymphatic vessels are shown immediately after Ultra-fluid lipiodol is injected and the lymph nodes after 24 hours when the contrast has cleared from the vessels. The lymph nodes retain contrast for 6 months to a year after the original examination.

4. Bronchographic contrast agents

The commonly used compounds are now dionosil and hytrast.

  Dionosil aqueous is a 50% w/v opaque white suspension of propylidone crystals in water with carboxymethyl cellulose (CMC). Dionisil oily is a 60% w/v suspension of propylidone crystals in pure arachis oil. On standing a supernatant layer of oil separates out, half of which may be discarded before bronchography.

  Both preparations are warmed and shaken well before being used.

  Hytrast is a dispersion of a mixture of crystals of Iopydol and Iopydone which are diiodo-pyridone derivatives containing 1·5% w/v carboxymethyl cellulose.

5. Myelographic contrast agents

Myodil has largely been displaced by metrizamide (Amipaque) for myelography, cisternography and ventriculography, and has been discussed previously (p. 588). Because of its anionic properties it can be used wherever normo-osmolar compounds are indicated as for arthrography, endoscopic pancreatico-cholangiography, hysterosalpingography and sialography.

  Ethyl iodophenyl undecylate (Myodil) is a non-soluble oily contrast agent which was previously used for myelography,

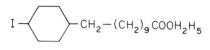

Ethyl iodophenyl undecylate

and contains 30% w/v iodine.

6. Water soluble contrast agents for gastrointestinal examinations

The main indications are in patients suspected of having a perforation or fistula within the abdomen, and for meconium ileus in infants. Gastrografin is sodium diatrizoate (Hypaque) with a flavouring agent and is used for stomach, small intestine and colonic studies. For sinuses and fistulae any of the tri-iodinated water soluble contrast agents can be used. Because of the hyperosmolality of these solutions they are *not* advised in infants for gastrointestinal studies apart from meconium ileus when a triiodinated water soluble contrast such as Hypaque or Conray is used.

A summary of contrast agents appears on pages 905–908.

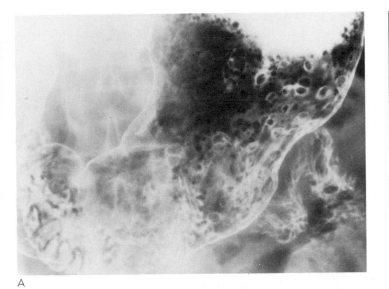

A

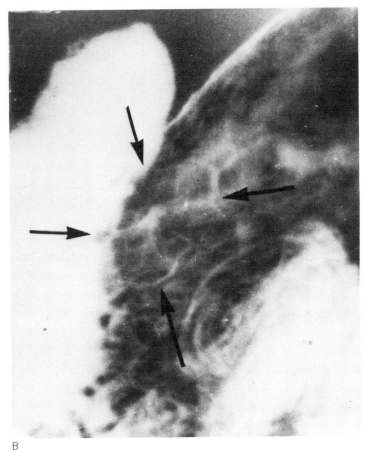

B

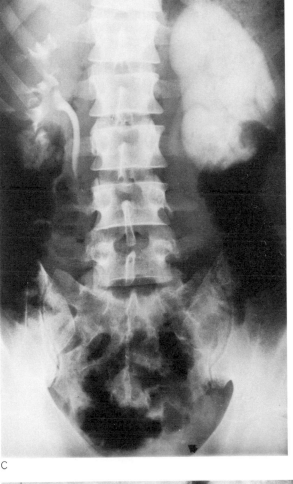

C

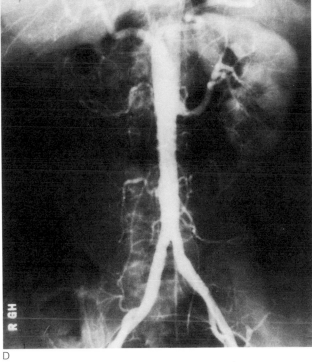

D

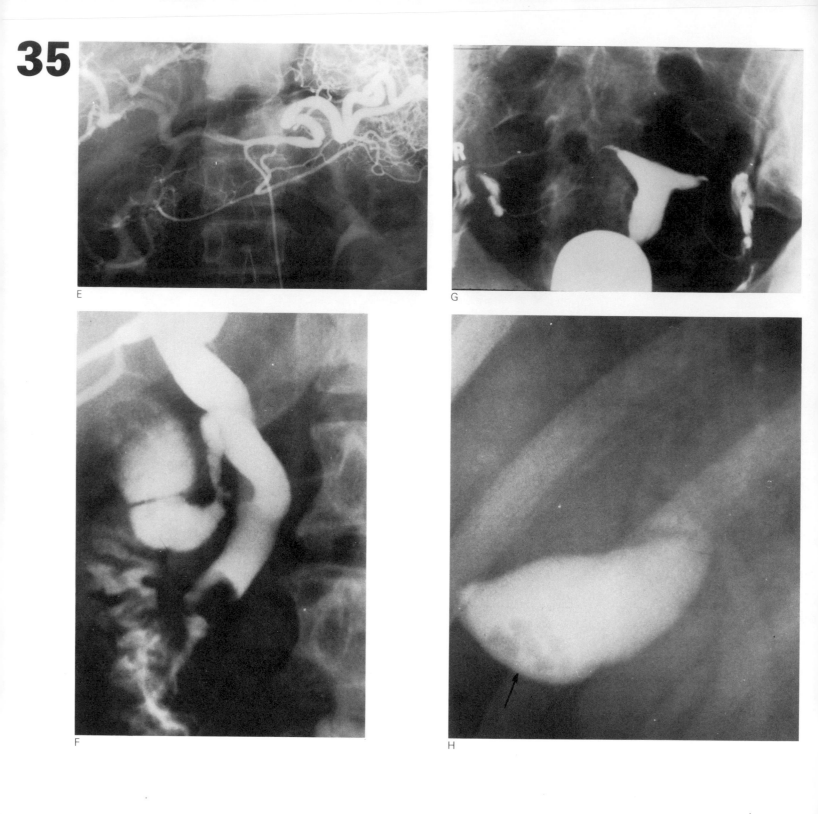

E

G

F

H

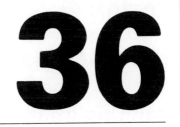

MEDICAL IMAGING

MEDICAL IMAGING

Scanning images

In the last decade diagnostic procedures in radiology departments have expanded and been transformed to such a degree that even the name of the department becomes inappropriate because not only X-rays are used. Examinations are now undertaken with ultrasound, thermography, isotopes and in the not too distant future, nuclear magnetic resonance. The pictures produced can hardly be called radiographs; images or scans (2445, 2446, 2447, 2448) would be more correct and the department could well be called a Department of Diagnostic or Medical Imaging.

The scanning procedures fulfil a basic need in morphological diagnosis due to the limitations of radiography. Radiographic contrast is insufficient to show soft tissue masses without contrast agents. In modern terms this is perfectly acceptable provided the contrast is given orally, rectally or intravenously, but when the procedure requires intra-arterial injections or is associated with significant adverse effects, a non-invasive method, if available, will be substituted. In obstetrics even ionising radiation should be avoided if at all possible.

Thus scanning or non-invasive imaging methods have been introduced because they delineate soft tissue planes to show mass effects or space occupying lesions. Computed tomography and ultrasonography have a high spatial and contrast resolution and isotope scanning relies on specific radionuclides being taken up by particular organs.

Departments of Radiology are thus being transformed into Medical Imaging Departments using a wide range of modalities including isotope imaging, ultrasonography, computed tomography, thermography, and possibly in the future zeugmatography (nuclear magnetic resonance scanning). These systems are based on cathode ray tube (CRT) display and use minicomputers, system discs, magnetic tape, floppy discs, video tape and various hard copy methods.

The modern radiographer will sooner or later be exposed to these new imaging technologies, will be required to perform the examinations, manage the equipment and have a working knowledge of the system as a whole.

In summary, therefore, conventional radiography has a limited role in demonstrating mass lesions unless invasive procedures are used and even with contrast agents functional studies are very limited. This has led to the development of non-invasive scanning methods for visualizing soft tissues by demonstrating mass lesions or by tissues taking up specific radioactive metabolites to overcome the deficiences of conventional radiography.

Scanning Modalities

1. Isotope scanning (IS) or nuclear medicine (NM).
2. Ultrasonography (U/S).
3. Computed tomography.
   (a) Transmission computed tomography (CT or X-ray CT).
   (b) Emission computed tomography.
      (1) Positron scanning
      (2) Twin detector rotation system
   (c) Nuclear magnetic resonance scanning (Zeugmatography) (NMR – CT)
4. Thermography

All scanning systems require
1. Source of energy
2. Detector system

The source of energy and the detector system are interlinked in x-ray computed tomography as the scanner gantry.

3. Processing or registering the data
4. Storage of data
5. Display and hard copy

The source of energy may be internal and spontaneous as for thermography which uses the infrared rays from the heat of the body, or internal but following an injection as for an isotope scan with γ-rays. For ultrasonography the energy source is both produced and received by the same transducer outside the body. In X-ray computed tomography (CT), an external photon beam passes through the body onto scintillation detectors while in nuclear magnetic resonance scanning the source of energy is from the protons of the hydrogen molecule and is therefore more like emission tomography.

(2445) Isotope image of the head and mandible in Paget's Disease showing areas of increased uptake.

(2446) Computed Tomography scan through the lateral ventricles, third ventricle, pineal and choroid plexuses.

(2447) Ultrasound scan of a fetal head showing midline structures.

(2448) Nuclear Magnetic Resonance Scan through the posterior, middle and anterior fossae showing frontal and temporal lobes and cerebellum.

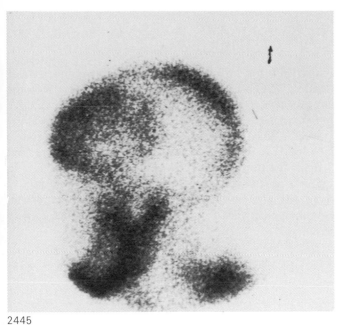

2445

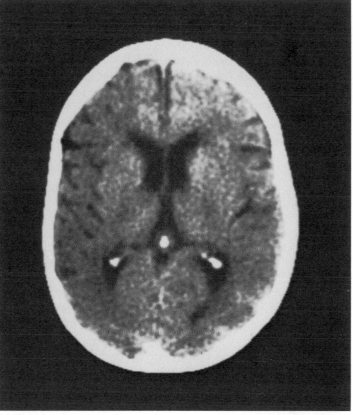

2446

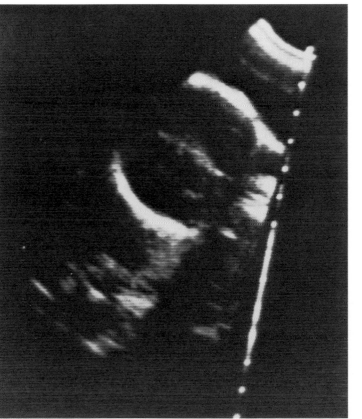

2447

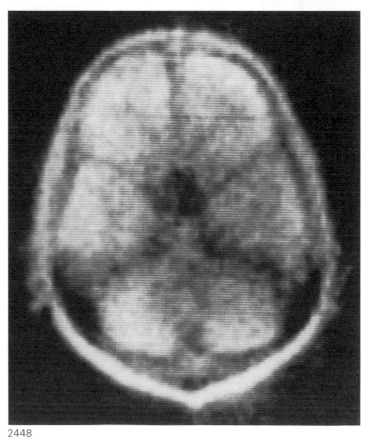

2448

All systems which use computers to process and record these energies, transform the readings into digital data which is subsequently displayed as anatomical information. (Table 1.)

All scanning or medical imaging systems, therefore, use the detection and subsequent recording of differences in energy levels in adjacent areas in the body and ultimately produce a picture display on a cathode ray tube (CRT), which is recorded on film or bromide paper as hard copy. The intermediate digital data can be stored on magnetic tape or on floppy discs for all systems using computers or can be stored as pictures in analogue form on video tape which is especially valuable in ultrasonography.

In some ways the various imaging methods produce similar information. The choice of the imaging method depends on the clinical problem, but also on local expertise and available equipment. In general terms the method of choice that gives the most specific information, is least expensive, is of course available, and can be scheduled as an outpatient is preferred but at all times the non-invasive procedures take precedence. In passing, it is noteworthy that the role of arteriography is also changing with increasing emphasis on its therapeutic possibilities for angioplasty or for perfusion of malignant disease with chemotherapy.

Table 1

Scanning system	Source of energy	Energy spectrum	Detector system	Area examined	Processing of data
Isotope Scanning (IS)	Injected Radioactive Isotopes	γ-rays (60–500 KeV)	Sodium Iodide	Individual organ	Electronic, bright spot CRT storage
Ultrasonography (U/S)	Piezo-electric transducers	Ultrasound 2–5 MHz	Piezo-electric tranducers	2–3 mm thick sections – multidirectional	Electronic, bright spot CRT storage – modified log compression for 'grey scale'
X-ray Computed Tomography	X-ray tube	X-rays 110–140 KvP	Scintillation detectors Sodium iodide (solid) or xenon (gas)	2–13 mm thick axial sections	Computer algorithm
Emission Computed Tomography (E-CT)	Injected isotope	γ-rays 20–500 KeV	Scintillation detectors	1–2 cm thick axial sections	Computer algorithm
Nuclear Magnetic Resonance Scanning (NMR –/CT) (Zeugmatography)	Radio frequency in magnetic field	Proton (nuclei) of hydrogen molecules ($\pm4\cdot5$ MHz)	Low noise, wide band radio-receiver	2–10 mm multidirectional sections	Computer algorithm (Fourier transform)
Thermography	Body heat	Infrared	Display on infrared sensitive materials	Body surface	

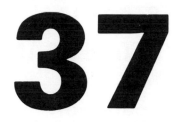

ISOTOPE SCANNING

ISOTOPE SCANNING (IS)
(Nuclear Medicine (NM))

Introduction

Nuclear medicine includes both organ imaging as well as functional studies such as the T_3 and T_4 tests for the thyroid or studies of differential renal blood flow and excretion. But by and large imaging or radiology departments are concerned only with imaging or scanning techniques. Any particular isotope examination shows only a specific organ such as the lungs, liver or brain or a specific system such as the osseous system without imaging the rest of the body.

The scan is carried out after a suitable interval following an injection of a minute amount of a radioactive labelled chemical which is taken up by the organ being examined. The radiopharmaceutical gives off γ-rays (gamma-rays) in the range of 20–500 KeV. Because the amount of chemical given is minute, toxicity and hypersensitivity is not a problem. (Table 2).

Previously scanning was done with a rectilinear scanner using a raster action, but has now been replaced by the gamma camera. The dispensing of radio-pharmaceuticals has also been simplified and most examinations can be carried out with commercially available products without the need of an on-site laboratory.

The Apparatus

There are three types of isotope scanners, the recti-linear scanner, the gamma camera and the hybrid scanner.

(a) The rectilinear scanner has a $7 \cdot 5 \times 5$ cm (3×2 ins) or $12 \cdot 5 \times 5$ cm (5×2 ins) scintillation detector and a focused collimator which moves to and fro across the patient with a raster action. Later models are dual headed, quadruple headed or even have up to ten crystals which greatly shortens the time of the examination.

The gamma ray interacts with the thallium activated sodium iodide crystal to produce a light photon which is converted by a photo multiplier tube to an electrical pulse with a voltage proportional to the light produced. The electronic impulse at the anode end of the photo multiplier tube stimulates a cathode ray tube and exposes x-ray film to produce a photo scan. (2449)

The older models have a long scanning time which can take up to 2 hours for the liver, but if a full examination can be achieved the accuracy is as good as for a gamma camera, Recti-linear scanners have now largely been replaced by the gamma camera except for thyroid scans.

(b) *The Gamma camera* (2450)

(1) Anger Camera

A 27–30 cm (11–12 ins) thallium enriched sodium iodide crystal is viewed by an array of 19–40 photo multiplier tubes associated with a computing circuit. The computing circuit detects the positions of the scintillations in the crystal and transmits signals to an oscilloscope where they are shown as bright dots. Pulse height analysis and summation of signals from the photo tubes are an essential part of a gamma camera.

The image produced on the oscilloscope is recorded on film or photographic plate (2451) or can be stored on magnetic tape preferably in digital form which can be further manipulated by computers. Mobile, bedside gamma cameras are now also available (2452).

(11) *The Autoflouroscope* (Bender-Blau Camera)

Sodium iodide crystals each 5 cm (2 ins) thick and 1 cm ($\frac{3}{8}$ ins) square are arranged in a 14×21 rectangle. The 22–15 cm (9×6 ins) rectangle contains an array of 294 Thallium enriched sodium iodide crystals from which the light impulses are transferred by light pipes to a photo multiplier tube. Thus a photon from each crystal produces a simultaneous pulse in a photo tube specific for that crystal. Multiple channel collimators are used with this type of camera.

The data is stored on a magnetic card and can be transferred to an oscilloscope or magnetic tape. Because this system can record a high count ratio, it is particularly valuable in cardiovascular imaging.

(c) *The Hybrid Scanner*

The hybrid scanner has two interlinked rows of 10 thallium activated sodium iodide crystals one in front of the patient and another behind. Each bank of crystals is 24 ins long and each crystal is connected to a photo tube.

The interlinked banks of scintillation detectors move longitudinally at right angles to the long axis of the body covering the region from the toes to the groin (2453) usually at a speed of 10 cm per min and the groin to the head at 5 cm per min.

The examination with the hybrid scanner is often used as a screening procedure, any pathological areas being rescanned with the gamma camera.

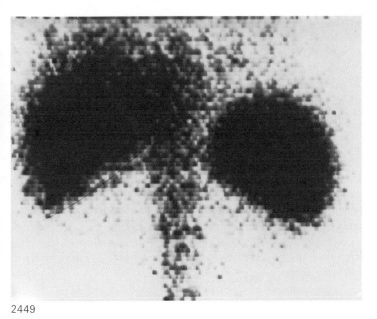

2449

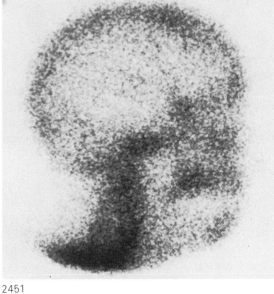

2451

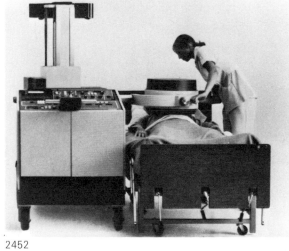

2450

2452

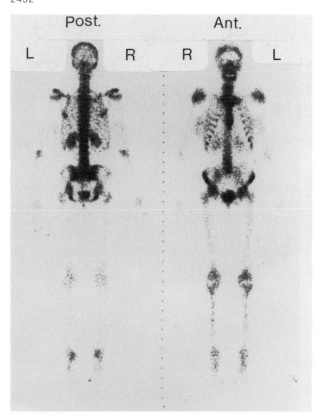

(2449) Isotope image of the liver and spleen taken on a rectilinear scanner.

(2450) Lateral view of the skull and spine showing 'hot spots' in a patient with metastases from a breast carcinoma.

(2451) Gamma camera positioned over the abdomen for a frontal view.

(2452) Mobile gamma camera for cardiac scanning taken to the bedside.

(2453) Posterior and anterior whole skeleton imaging with a hybrid scanner.

2453

37 Isotope Scanning

Radiopharmaceuticals

Radiopharmaceuticals or radioactive drugs used for diagnostic purposes, produce no effects due to chemical toxicity and the radiation produced is well below any somatic effect. (Table 1). For an external imaging system the radioactive nuclide must have a gamma emission between 20 and 500 KeV and a physical half life of between 1 hour and 1 year.

The ideal agent should be easily produced, readily available, inexpensive, and should have a high specific activity with no possible physiological or toxic effects. Its physical half life should be only a few hours and not much longer than the time required for completing the imaging examination. It should have a gamma emission of about 150 KeV, allowing efficient collimation and demonstration of lesions at some depth in the body. The radionuclide which at present most closely approaches the ideal is 99 mTc (99m Technetium).

The commonly used radionuclides are shown in the table.

Table 1

Radionuclide	Dose	Weight (grammes)	Half Life
99m Tc (Technetium)	20 mCi	3.4×10^{-9}	6 hrs
67-Ga (Gallium)	4 mCi	6.7×10^{-9}	3.25 days
201-Tl (Thallium)	2 mCi	6.5×10^{-9}	3.04 days
111-In (Indium)	1 mCi	2.4×10^{-9}	2.81 days
81-Kr (Krypton)	15 mCi (inhalation)	1.5×10^{-12}	10.8 years

Production of Radionuclides

There are three methods available for producing radionuclides, (i) the nuclear reactor, (ii) the cyclotron and linear accelerators, (iii) chromatographic columns containing parent/daughter nuclides—the parent nuclide being made in a reactor or linear accelerator. In hospital practice, in the vast majority of cases, radiopharmaceuticals are made from a chromatographic column (a 'cow' or 'super-cow').

A radioisotope generator is made up of a glass cylinder at the bottom of which is a porous disc containing a column of chromatographic ion-exchange medium on which the parent nuclide is absorbed. The daughter activity grows as the parent activity diminishes by decay. The daughter activity is removed by elution with a suitable solvent, which must be sterile and free of radiochemical contaminents. The column can be flushed again after a suitable interval has been allowed for regrowth of the daughter activity amounting to four half lives of daughter nuclide. The eluted radiopharmaceutical from a 'cow' or radioisotope generator is carrier-free, unlike most reactor produced materials. 99 mTc (99m Technetium) is produced in a generator containing 99 mo (99 molybdenum) with a half life of 2.7 days. The porous column is made of alumina and the radiopharmaceutical is eluted from the 'cow' into physiological saline.

The radionuclides produced are tagged onto a carrier or vehicle which varies for the organ being imaged.

Radiopharmaceutical Properties for Imaging

There are two different mechanisms whereby isotope imaging becomes possible. The radiopharmaceutical can concentrate selectively in a normal organ leaving a 'bare' area at the site of the lesion, whether it is due to a tumour, cyst, haemorrhage or compression/displacement, or the radiopharmaceutical can concentrate within the lesion itself as in brain scanning or scanning with 67-gallium or 111-Indium which show abscesses and tumours. 99m-Technetium phosphate compounds are concentrated in bone but reach higher concentrations in bone tumours, infections or fractures showing as 'hot spots' or areas of increased activity.

Interpretation of Isotope Images

Whereas the isotope is highly specific for a particular organ it has a low specificity for pathological processes. Thus 99m Tc-sulphur colloid localizes to the reticulo-endothelial system of the liver and spleen, but 'filling defects' or cold spots can be due to tumours whether benign or malignant, cysts, abscesses, or pressure effects from enlarged adjacent organs such as the kidney or suprarenal. Furthermore in bone Paget's disease, fractures, degenerative spondylosis and osteophyte formation as well as tumours and infections can all produce regions of increased isotope uptake. It is thus imperative to compare the isotope images with bone radiographs in interpreting bone pathology. Even 67-gallium scans may be positive with both tumours and abscesses and therefore tends to be used more in localizing a disease process than in diagnosing the nature of the pathology. Due to this lack of specificity isotope imaging is more a screening procedure than the other scanning modalities which have greater powers of tissue characterization.

Table 2

Agent	Vehicle	Time after injection to start of scan	Organ
99m Technetium	Pertechnetate (Tc$_4$)	20–30 minutes 30–60 minutes	Thyroid Brain
	Phosphates e.g. Methylene Diphosphonate	2–3 hours	Bone
	Microspheres (perfusion)	1–3 minutes	Lung
	Sulphur colloid	5–10 minutes	Liver Spleen
	Diethyl-IDA (Amino-diacetic acid)	At 5 minute intervals from 0–45 minutes and then AFM every 10 to 90 minutes	Gall-bladder Bile ducts (acute cholecystitis)
	Iron-ascorbate	Immediate for blood flow $1\frac{1}{2}$–2 hours for static scans	Kidneys
^{201}Thallium	Thallium Chloride	7–10 minutes Delayed at 4 hours	Myocardium
^{123}Iodine	Sodium iodide	4–6 hours Delayed at 24 hours	Thyroid-retrosternal
^{111}Indium	Leucocytes	13 minutes Delayed at 24 hours	Abscesses
^{67}Gallium	Gallium citrate	1–3 minutes Delayed at 24 and 48 hours	Tumours

The Lungs

Most pulmonary imaging is done for the detection of pulmonary embolic disease but defects also occur with bullous formation, pneumonia and lung carcinoma. Therefore, the chest radiograph must be compared with the isotope scan in all cases.

There are two, quite distinct lung imaging methods, the perfusion scan and the inhalation scan. For *perfusion* scans a radioactive particle 10–50μ in size is injected into a peripheral vein, 99mTc microspheres are now commonly used, which are trapped in their first pass through the pulmonary capillary bed. After some hours the particles are broken down, pass through the capillary bed and are cleared from the bloodstream by the reticulo-endothelial system. 133-Xenon is used for *ventilation* scans which is re-breathed through a disposable mouth piece with a closed-circuit spirometer for multiple views. Patients with pulmonary tuberculosis must not have ventilation scans as they can contaminate the apparatus. The radiopharmaceutical for perfusion scans is usually injected very slowly with the patient supine, but both ventilation and perfusion scans are performed upright whenever possible.

Positioning in isotope scanning resembles that in fluoroscopy rather than conventional radiography which uses an overcouch tube. In Isotope scanning the patient is initially in approximately the correct position. The final position is judged by the view obtained on the persistence oscilloscope which allows accurate centring to the gamma camera face, but whichever view is chosen the patient must be as close as possible to the gamma camera, in fact touching the camera face.

Projections

1. Anterior (2454)
The patient sits facing the gamma camera with a point midway between the xisphisternum and manubrium sternum centred to and in contact with the camera face, breathing normally during the exposure.

2. Posterior Erect (2455)
The patient sits erect with the spine towards the camera, D6 centred to the camera face, the scapulae rotated forwards and breathing normally during the exposure.

3. Right and Left Lateral: (2456, 2457)
The patient sits upright with the median sagittal plane parallel to the camera face, the arm towards the camera raised above the head and a point in the midaxillary line at the level of D6 centred to and touching the camera face.

The four views of the chest in quiet breathing for both inhalation and perfusion scans are required for a pulmonary isotope scan.

Additional views (2458, 2459) may be required especially for functional studies such as the single breath technique or washout studies and to show pulmonary defects.

For a combined ventilation perfusion study the ventilation scan is done followed by perfusion scan.

(2454–9) Six views of lung scan taken on a gamma camera

2454 Anterior	2457 Right lateral
2455 Posterior	2458 Right posterior oblique
2456 Left lateral	2459 Left posterior oblique

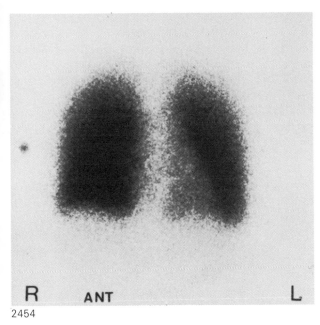

R   ANT   L

2454

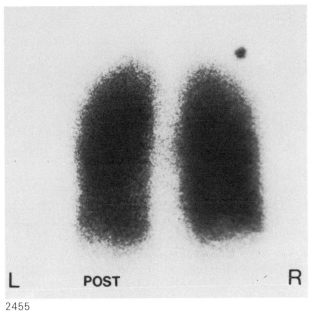

L   POST   R

2455

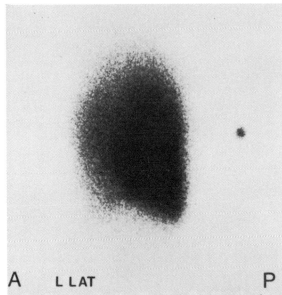

A   L LAT   P

2456

P   R LAT   A

2457

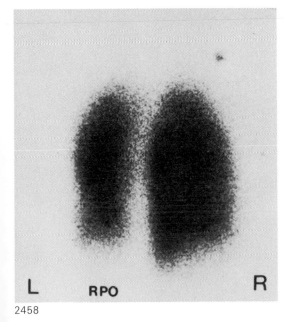

L   RPO   R

2458

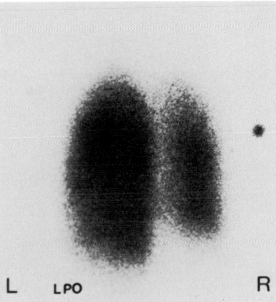

L   LPO   R

2459

813

PERFUSION

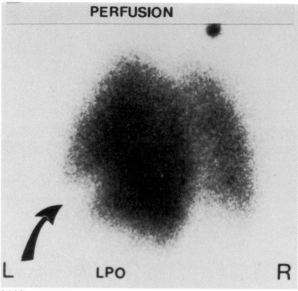

L   LPO   R

2460

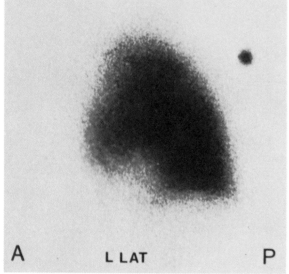

A   L LAT   P

2462

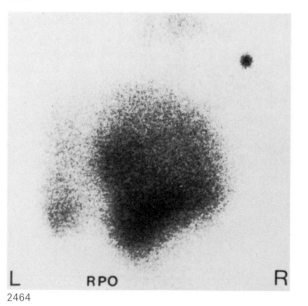

L   RPO   R

2464

VENTILATION

L   LPO   R

2461

L LAT

2463

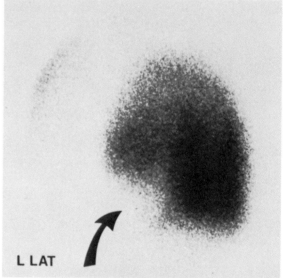

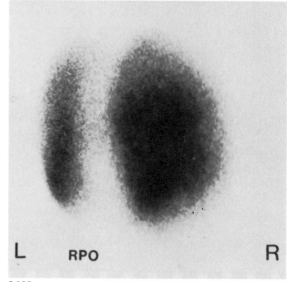

L   RPO   R

2465

The Thyroid

The most common indication for thyroid imaging is a nodular goitre to show the size and number of nodules and can also be used for the detection of a retrosternal goitre. Thyroid imaging is contraindicated in pregnancy and lactation and is performed with either 123-Iodine or 99 m Technetium. The rectilinear scanner produces high quality images of the thyroid. If a gamma camera is used an anatomical marker accessory is essential to obtain accurate localization of a nodule. 123-I is administered orally 6–8 hours before the examination in a dose of 100 mCi but 99 mTc is given intravenously in a dose of 3–5 mCi, 20–30 minutes before scanning. 123-I is used for the detection of a retrosternal thyroid.

Projections

1. The preferred view is with the patient supine and the head extended to clear the salivary glands out of the field. If a retrosternal gland is suspected scanning continues caudally to cover the anterior aspect of the chest.
2. For the gamma camera the patient is seated facing the camera with neck extended and the median sagittal plane at right angles to the camera face.

The lateral extent of the field should cover the lateral skin margin, and the position of the sternal notch must be indicated on the scan as well as any palpable nodules.

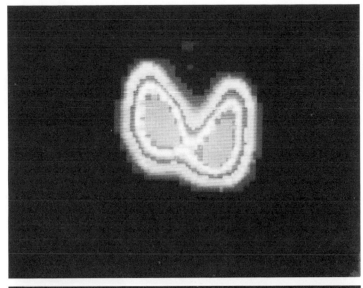

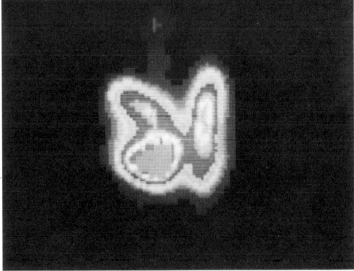

2465a

(2460–5) Lateral and oblique views of Perfusion and Ventilation scans showing that the defect remains unchanged indicating it is *not* due to an infarct but probably bullous emphysema or a blocked bronchus. In a pulmonary infarct the perfusion scan is abnormal, but the defect disappears on the ventilation scan.

(2465a) Digital processed thyroid scans showing normal thyroid (above) and 'hot' nodule (below).

(2465b) Isotope angiography showing poor flow in common iliac artery associated with a stenosis.

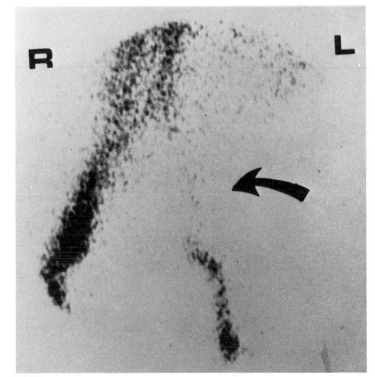

2465b

The Cardiovascular System

There are three methods for imaging in the cardiovascular system, namely blood pool imaging, direct myocardial imaging, and imaging of thrombus.

Blood pool imaging is now most easily achieved with 99m Technetium pertechnetate by correct timing of sequential images and by gating techniques. Isotope angiography and angiocardiography is performed for superior and inferior cavography, pericardial effusions, cardiac output, myocardial dyskinesia and the aorta and major branches.

99 m Tc-pyrophosphate localizes the regions of acute myocardial infarction and Rubidium-81 studies could well show areas of diminished cardiac perfusion.

Radioactive fibrinogen localizes to freshly forming clots and can be detected by a point counting method.

For cardiovascular isotope studies multiple sequential images are required necessitating the use of a gamma camera and data processing especially for determining cardiac output.

Projections

1. Anterior

For the superior vena cava, inferior vena cava, and aorta the patient lies supine with the camera over the chest or abdomen.

2. Anterior Dynamic Study

The patient is seated or lying supine with the camera centred to and touching the anterior aspect of the chest.

The radiopharmaceutical is injected as a compact bolus and the appearance of the image is watched on a persistance oscilloscope. Exposures are taken to show superior vena cava, right atrium and right ventricle, pulmonary artery, left atrium and ventricle, and aorta.

3. Left Anterior Oblique Dynamic Study

The patient sits facing the camera in the left anterior oblique position with the left chest towards and touching the camera and the right chest away forming an angle of 50° to the camera face.

4. Myocardial studies

Myocardial imaging studies are usually done in three projections: right anterior oblique, anterior and left anterior oblique. The left ventral view may also be required. (2466,a,b).

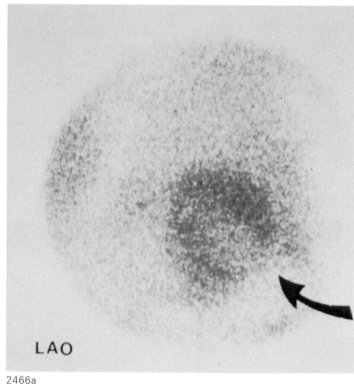

LAO

2466a

L LAT

2466b

(2466a, b,) Two views of a myocardial scan showing a defect due to a myocardial infarct.

The Liver and Spleen

Approximately 85 % of the cells of the liver are hepatocytes and the remainder are mainly Kupfer cells forming part of the reticulo-endothelial system which can clear nearly 95 % of the blood passing through the liver of particles in one passage. Thus the liver can be shown by labelling the Kupfer cells with a radiocolloid such as 99 m Tc sulphur colloid, some of which also localizes in the spleen. In liver cirrhosis there is an increase in the uptake of radiocolloid in the spleen. (2467b)

Bile formation on the other hand is a function of the hepatocytes and rose bengal is extracted from the blood stream by the hepatocytes. Methionine is also extracted from the blood stream by hepatocytes because of their protein synthesis function. Thus 131-Iodine and 75 Se—selenomethionine are used for 'hepatocyte' liver scanning. However, the IDA (amino diacetic acid) compounds have now replaced Rose Bengal, 131-Iodine and 75-Se products for 'hepatocyte' scans.

Isotope imaging of the liver is used mainly as a non-specific screening procedure to detect space occupying lesions whether hepatomas, metastases, cysts, or abscesses appearing as areas of non-uptake or 'cold' areas. (2467a) Cirrhosis produces patchy uptake with the isotope showing an enlarged spleen. (2467b)

Combined liver and blood pool imaging show pericardial effusions and combined liver and pulmonary imaging is used for the detection of subphrenic abscesses.

75 Se—selenomethionine may show hepatomas as 'hot areas' and 67-gallium-citrate can demonstrate hepatomas, abscesses or lymphoma in a similar way.

The rectilinear scanner and the gamma camera produce adquate visualization of the liver and spleen, but the gamma camera is much quicker.

In isotope imaging of the liver, surface markings on the xiphisternum and costal margin are important and multiple views essential.

Currently 99 mTc sulphur colloid is the agent of choice in liver imaging with a dose of 1–3 mCi intravenously and scanning starts after 5–10 minutes.

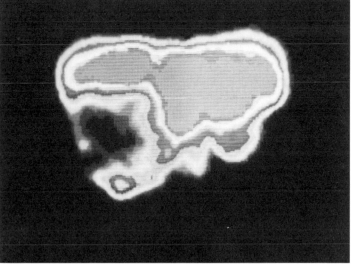

2467a

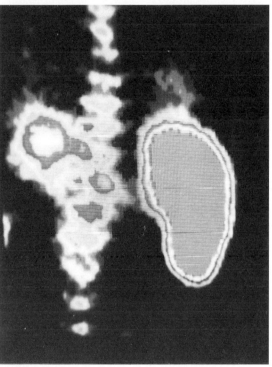

2467b

(**2467a**) Digital processed liver scan showing a large filling defect in the right lobe of the liver due to a tumour.

(**2467b**) Poor uptake of isotope in the liver due to cirrhosis. The large spleen is well shown.

(Figs. 2465a, 2467a, b by kind permission of Dr P. J. Robinson, St. James University Hospital, Leeds.)

Projections

(2468–73) The liver and spleen are usually examined with the patient horizontal.

1. Anterior
With the patient supine the camera is centred over the costal margin slightly towards the right to include the whole of the lower right thoracic cage with the camera face touching the skin surface. The first anterior image is produced with one million counts, and each subsequent projection is then done for a similar length of time. The anterior scan is then repeated with a costal margin marker. (2468, 2469).

2. Anterior Oblique—Right
With the patient supine the camera face is at 45° to the horizontal over the lower thoracic cage at the anterior axillary line for the right anterior oblique. (2470).

3. Anterior Oblique—left
The left anterior oblique projection is centred over the left anterior axillary line with the camera face at 45° to the horizontal to include the whole of the spleen.

4. Lateral, Right and Left
With the patient horizontal and moved towards the right edge of the couch the camera face is vertical against the right lower costal margin to show the lateral view of the liver. The lateral projection is also done on the left side for the spleen with the patient moved to the left edge of the couch and the camera face vertical. (2471, 2472).

5. Posterior (Liver)
With the patient prone and the camera face horizontal, the camera is centred to the ninth intercostal space to include the whole of the right costal margin. (2473).

6. Erect anterior view
This view of the liver is a routine projection in some centres. Often the change in position of the liver when the patient is erect can uncover a lesion not visible in the other projections.

(2468–73) Isotope imaging of the liver and spleen.

(2468) Anterior view showing patchy uptake in the liver with a markedly enlarged spleen.

(2469) Anterior view with costal margin 'marker'.

(2470) Anterior oblique view taken over the spleen (R. indicates right side).

(2471) Right lateral view of the liver.

(2472) Left lateral view of the spleen.

(2473) Posterior view again showing enlarged spleen.

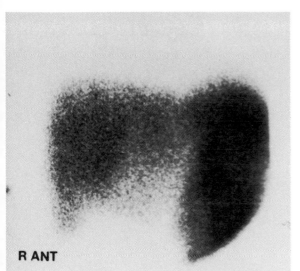

R ANT

2468

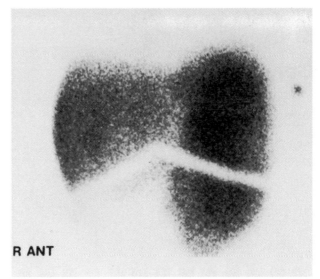

R ANT

2469

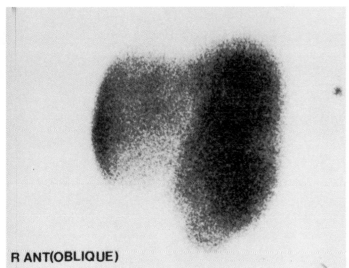

R ANT(OBLIQUE)

2470

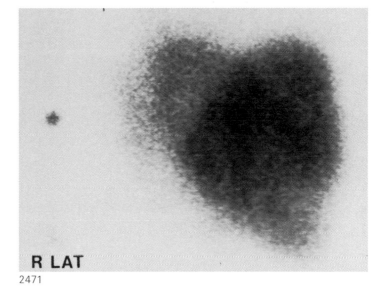

R LAT

2471

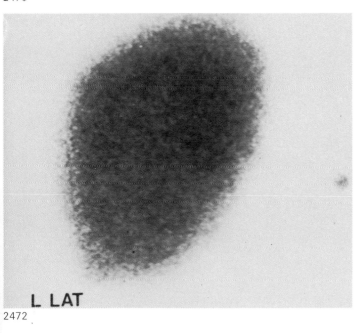

L LAT

2472

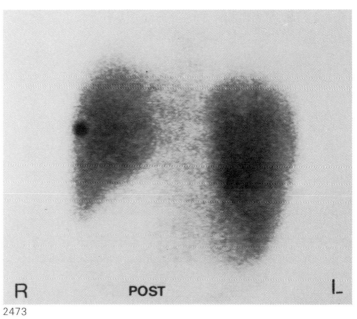

R   **POST**   **L**

2473

The Gall Bladder

The hepatocyte agents labelled with 99 mTc such as HIDA (diethyl-acetanilido-iminodiacetate) are excreted by the liver into the bile. (2474–85). The gall bladder and biliary system can thus be imagined. Failure to show the gall bladder in a non-choleystectomised patient indicates obstruction to the cystic duct and is present in acute cholescystitis. An obstructed dilated bile duct may be demonstrated with no radioactivity reaching small bowel but normally the radiopharmaceutical appears in the small bowel 15–30 minutes after the injection.

Positioning

With the patient supine or erect, frontal views of the gall bladder region to include the common bile duct and duodenum at 0–35 mins and after injection of a 'fatty meal' are taken. However, in cystic or biliary duct obstruction imaging is repeated at 4 and 24 hours.

(2474–85) Isotope imaging of the gall bladder.

(2474–82) Sequential scans showing first the liver and then concentration of the radioactive agent in the gall bladder up to 35 minutes.

(2483–5) Contraction of the gall bladder with isotope showing in the duodenum and proximal small bowel.

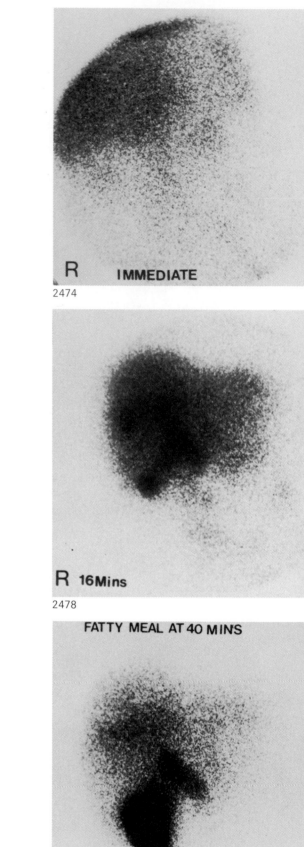

R   IMMEDIATE
2474

R   16 Mins
2478

FATTY MEAL AT 40 MINS

R   35 Mins
2482

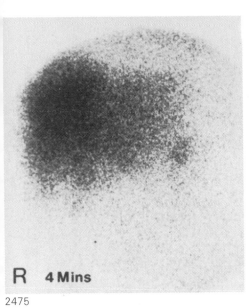

R   4 Mins

2475

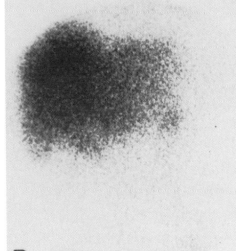

R   8 Mins

2476

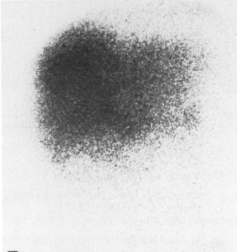

R   12 Mins

2477

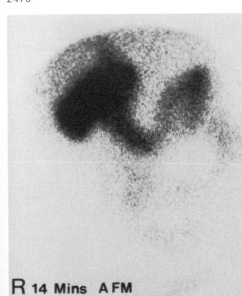

R   20 Mins

2479

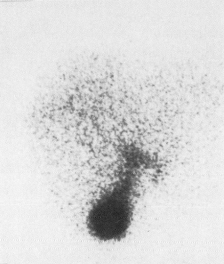

R   25 Mins

2480

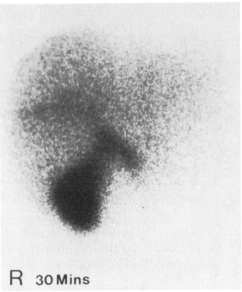

R   30 Mins

2481

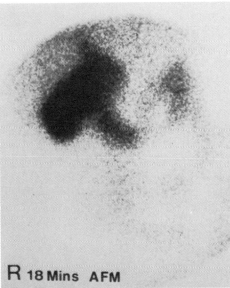

R   14 Mins   AFM

2483

R   18 Mins   AFM

2484

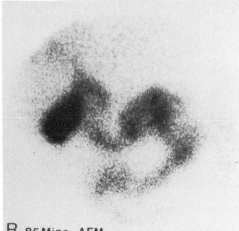

R   85 Mins   AFM

2485

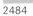

The Pancreas

Isotope scanning of the pancreas with 75 Se-selonomethiomine has been almost completely abandoned in favour of computed tomography and ultrasonography.

The Kidneys

There are three types of isotope renal images: static morphological images, (2486, 2487) perfusion or blood flow studies and excretion studies.

1. Static morphological images

Previously 197-Hg -Chlormerodrin was used in a dose of 100–200 μCi but has been replaced by 99 mTc-iron ascorbate which gives an immediate blood flow study with 10 mCi and a static image at 2 hours.

2. Blood flow radionuclide angiography

99 mTc-Pertechnetate is given as a rapid bolus injection of 10–15 mCi and the first exposure is taken 10 seconds later with repeat exposures every 4 seconds. With a data processor 0·5–1 sec exposures can be obtained.

3. Excretion studies

For excretion studies the kidneys are imaged with ^{131}I-ortho-iodohippurate using 200–300 μCi intravenously. In patients with a raised blood urea the dose is 400 μCi. Lugol's solution is given before the examination to block the thyroid and serial 5–10 minute scintigrams are taken with an exposure at 24 hours if delayed function is to be detected.

For the 'triple' study the static images for localisation are first performed then the blood flow images and lastly excretion studies.

Positioning

With the patient supine the gamma camera is positioned posteriorly under the table. The legs should be slightly flexed at the knees to flatten the lumbar lordosis, bringing the kidneys as close as possible to the table top and gamma camera face. The gamma camera must be parallel to and touching the under surface of the table.

The kidneys can also be examined in the erect sitting position with the back of the patient against the camera face. However in the erect position the kidneys tend to move caudally and anteriorly with slight forward rotation of the lower poles.

Transplant kidneys lying in the iliac fossae are examined with the patient supine and the gamma camera anteriorly; the camera face being parallel to the table top and as close as possible to the anterior abdominal wall.

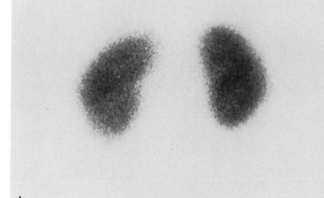

2486

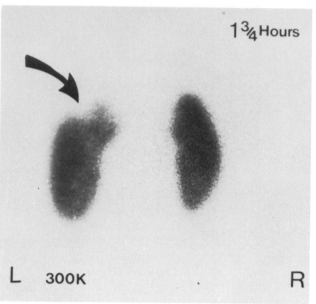

2487a

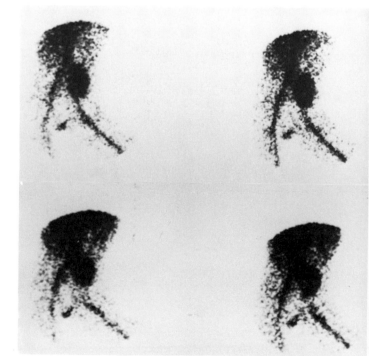

2487b

(2486) Normal isotope image of the kidneys.
(2487a) Filling defect in the upper pole of the left kidney.
(2487b) Isotope angiography after renal transplant to iliac fossa.

The Skeletal system

Isotope imaging of bone for the detection of disseminated lesions from metastases, Paget's disease or sarcoidosis has been greatly simplified with the hybrid scanner or gamma camera and 99 m Tc labelled phosphate compounds. The rectilinear scanner was far too slow to cover the whole body and strontium-85 and fluorine-18 had too many disadvantages as radionuclides.

The commonly used bone seeking isotope is 99 mTc methylene diphosphonate which produces a uniform pattern of uptake in the ribs, spine and other flat bones but in adolescents areas of active growth such as the ends of long bones, also show increased activity.

Imaging starts 2–3 hours after an intravenous injection of 10 mCi of 99^mTc methylene diphosphonate, recording 300,000 counts for the pelvis and 100,000–200,000 counts for other regions. The radionuclide is cleared by the kidneys into the bladder. Although no preparation is necessary for a bone scan the bladder must be emptied prior to the scan or the activity in the urine may hide abnormal areas in the pubis or sacrum.

Bone abnormalities whether due to osteomyelitis, tumour, (2488–93) fracture or Paget's disease (2494–9), show as areas of increased uptake. The isotope scan must always therefore be compared with radiographs of the relevant region to assess the nature of the pathology.

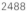
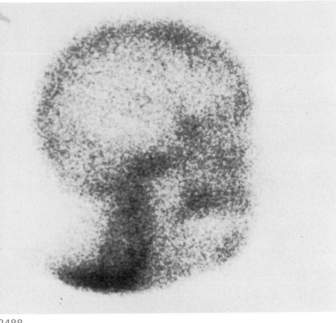

2488

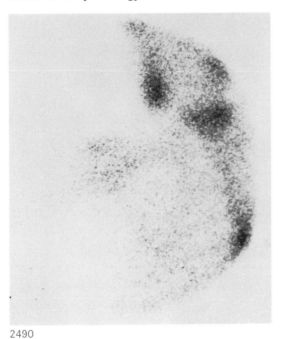

2490

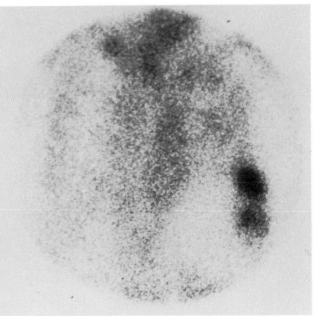

2489

2491

(2488–93) Isotope imaging of the osseous system to show metastases from breast carcinoma which appear as 'hot' spots.

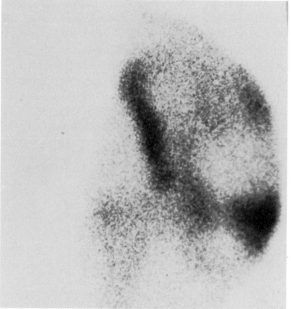

2492

2493

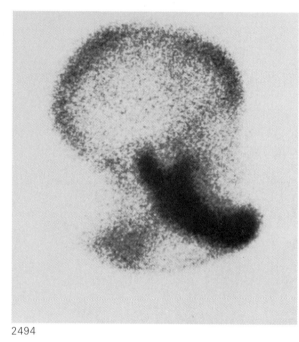

2494

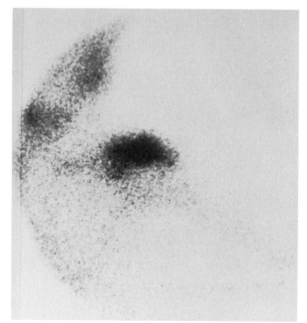

2495

(2494–9) Paget's Disease on isotope imaging showing as large areas of increased uptake.

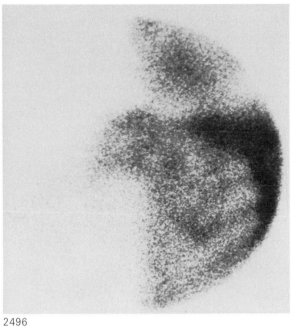

2496

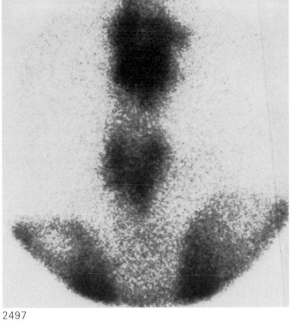

2497

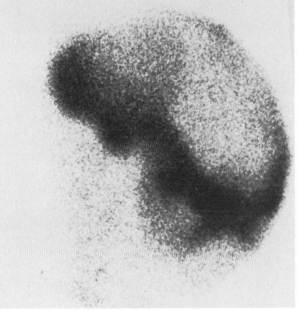

2498

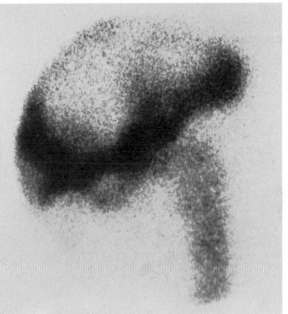

2499

Positioning

The patient lies supine or prone with the central median plane of the body in the centre of the table. Using the hybrid scanner the head is in the antero-posterior position but with the gamma camera the head is turned to each lateral position in turn. (2500b).

With the hybrid scanner the scintillation detectors and photo tubes move more rapidly over the legs than over the trunk at approximately 10 cm per minute from toes to groin and 5 cm per minute from groin to head (2453).

To cover the whole skeleton 16 views must be taken with the gamma camera, 11–13 being needed if the forearms and legs are excluded from the examination. (2500b) With the patient prone the following images are required.

1. Skull—left lateral
2. Skull—right lateral
3. Dorsal spine and posterior ribs
4. Shoulder, arm and scapula—left
5. Shoulder, arm and scapula—right
6. Dorso-lumbar spine
7. Lumbar spine and sacrum
8. Lateral sacrum and hip—left
9. Lateral sacrum and hip—right
10. Femur—left
11. Femur—right

The patient is then turned supine and two additional images are made

12. Thorax—anterior view
13. Both knees—anterior view

The examination can also be performed with the patient supine, on a mobile couch, the gamma camera under the couch and the mobile couch re-positioned for each area in turn.

Isotope bone imaging has become the screening test for detection of metastases but occasionally during the course of a skeletal examination with 99 mTc-methylene diphosphonate soft tissue metastases particularly in the liver from colon, bronchial and breast carcinoma, will also be detected. Local views of the particular region should then be taken.

As indicated previously, if the hybrid scanner is used for skeletal imaging, any abnormal areas shown can subsequently be more clearly defined by localised views of the involved skeleton using the gamma camera.

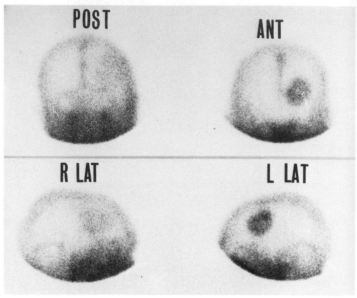

2500c

(2500a) High resolution bone scan showing multiple small metastases. (By kind permission, Dr M. Merrick.)

(2500b) Normal osseous system on isotope bone scan.

(2500c) Brain scan showing area of increased uptake in the left frontal region due to a cerebral tumour.

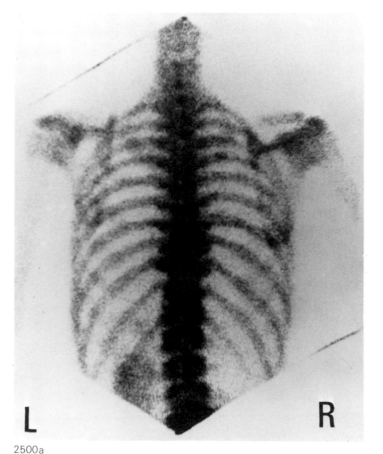

2500a

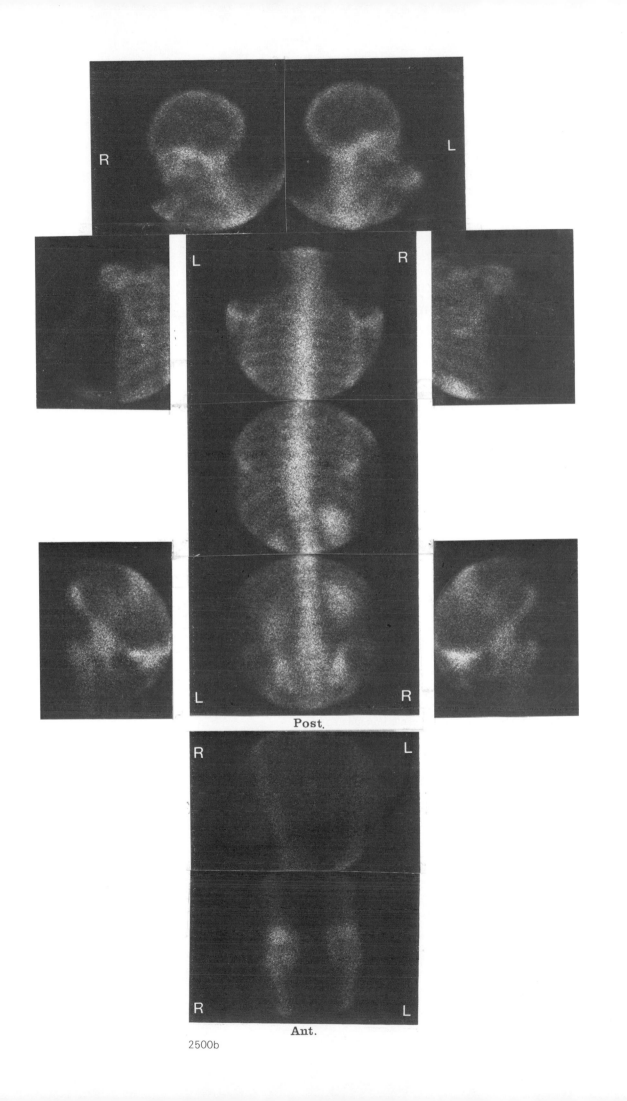

L   R

R   L

Post.

Ant.

2500b

Abscesses and tumours

A tumour or abscess seeking isotope with a high degree of specificity would be a great boon for diagnostic imaging. At present 67-Gallium, [111]Indium and Bleomycin are used but have only a limited success in showing such lesions and furthermore cannot distinguish between an abscess or a tumour; both conditions may show as hot areas or areas of increased uptake. It is certainly possible however that in the future a more specific and sensitive agent may be produced.

Gastro-intestinal haemorrhage

99 m Tc-Sulphur colloid is normally cleared from the circulating blood by the liver but if there is active gastro-intestinal bleeding, the injected isotope accumulates at the bleeding site. The accumulation of isotope at the bleeding site then shows as an area of increasing activity. (2501–6).

Positioning

With the patient supine and lying under the gamma camera, 12 mCi of 99 m Tc-Sulphur colloid is injected intravenously. The gamma camera is positioned over the abdomen to cover the area from the lower edge of the liver to the pelvis. Serial images are taken after each time 500,000 counts have accumulated on the persistance oscilloscope. Any area of increasing isotope activity outside of the liver is positioned in the centre of the gamma camera field.

In cases indicating the presence of active intestinal haemorrhage, the procedure is completed by immediately thereafter collecting the stool in a plastic container for a scintogram. The specimen of stool should have a similar degree of radioactivity to that seen in the abdomen.

(2501–6) Isotope scan to show active bleeding from the gastro-intestinal tract with accumulation of isotope in the bowel to produce a localised 'hot' area in the abdomen.

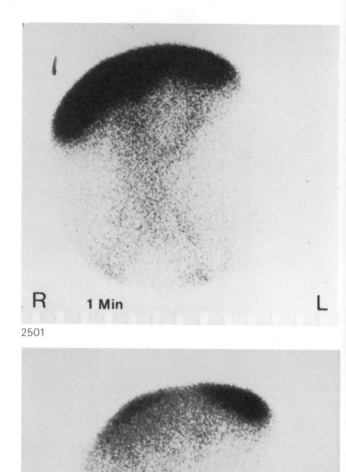

2501

2504

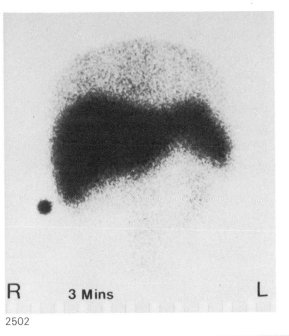

R 3 Mins L

2502

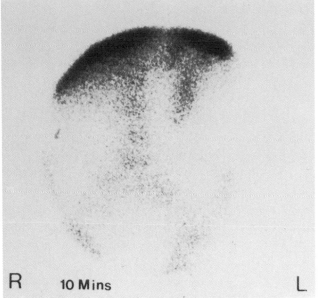

R 10 Mins L

2503

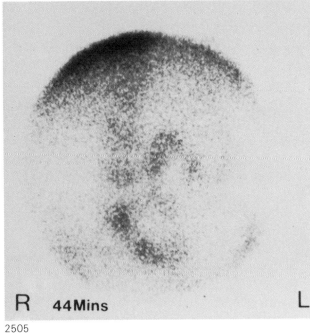

R 44 Mins L

2505

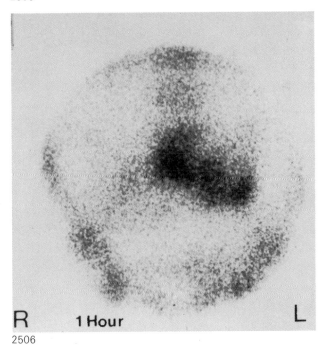

R 1 Hour L

2506

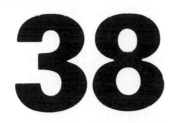

ULTRASONOGRAPHY

ULTRASONOGRAPHY

History

Roentgen discovered X-rays in 1895 and immediately produced the first radiograph, which was of his wife's hand. Paradoxically ultrasonography was produced in 1880 by the Curie brothers, who demonstrated the piezo-electric effect, but was only successfully applied medically in 1949 when Ludwig and Struthers proved the possibility of showing gallstones and soft tissue foreign bodies. Only then were the first cross sectional 'ultrasonographs' produced by Howry from Denver, Colorado in 1950 with subjects immersed in a water bath.

Direct contact ultrasonography was pioneered by Ian Donald of Glasgow who, together with MacVicar and Brown, developed the first two-dimensional contact scanner in 1958 followed by its immediate application to obstetrics and gynaecology. The modern high resolution pictures taken with ultrasound use the grey-scale technique first described by Kossoff of Australia in 1972, imaging both the small echoes from tissues as well as the large echoes from organ boundaries.

Theory of ultrasonography

Diagnostic images created from ultrasound are formed from mechanical vibrations similar to sound but with much higher frequencies. Audible sound has a range of 20–20,000 oscillations per second whereas for ultrasonography 1–15 million oscillations per second (1–15 MHz) are needed and produced by a transducer using the piezo-electric effect.

The piezo-electric effect is the conversion of electricity into mechanical vibrations and, vice-versa, the conversion of mechanical vibrations into electrical impulses, a property of many naturally occurring crystals such as quartz. For ultrasonography transducers are made of synthetic crystals such as barium titanate and lead zirconate titanate to produce the piezo-electric effect. When electrical pulses of very short duration excite the crystal, ultrasonic pulses are produced; about 1 % of these are reflected back from tissue interfaces and detected by the transducer to produce the pulse echo system which is the basis of ultrasonography.

The physics of ultrasound

Diagnostic ultrasound has a frequency about 150 times greater than the sound waves we can hear and is also due to small pressure changes in the air caused by mechanical vibrations, having similar physical properties related to speed, frequency and wave length.

Speed

Ultrasound travels in the form of a wave, and the particles of the medium through which it is passing vibrate backwards and forwards with the frequency of the wave. The speed of the ultrasound wave is constant for the medium through which it is travelling, is measured in metres per second and varies with different tissues in the body.

Tissue	Speed of u/s in m/s
Bowel gas	330
Fat	1450
(Water	1510)
Liver	1550
Blood	1570
Muscle	1580
Bone	4000

Wavelength

The wave length (λ) is the distance between two adjacent crests of the wave which is approximately 0·77 mm for 2 MHz wave in average tissue, 0·1 mm for 1 MHz and 1·5 mm for 15 MHz.

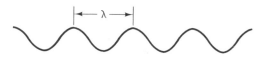

The frequency

The frequency is the number of times in one second the pressure wave reaches its maximum and the unit of frequency is the hertz (Hz) which is one pressure cycle per second. Ultrasound frequency is in the megahertz (MHz) range of a million cycles per second.

The speed of ultrasound is the product of its wavelength and frequency.

$$c = \lambda \times f$$

c = speed; λ = Wave length; f = frequency.

Because the speed of ultrasound is constant in a tissue, increasing the frequency must shorten the wave length and when the speed increases by passing from one tissue to another, because the frequency is constant, the wavelength must increase.

To produce a well defined beam of ultrasound the size of the transducer must be at least ten times that of the wavelength. For a 2 MHz probe, its diameter must be at least 1 cm. Significantly smaller sized probes will produce divergent beams.

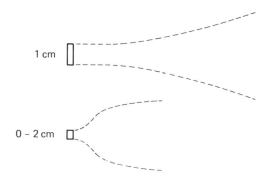

Smaller wavelengths produce better spatial resolution as they more effectively discriminate between adjacent objects.

Attenuation

The intensity of ultrasound is reduced as it passes through tissues, especially at echo-producing interfaces (the reflective component as well as the absorption of energy) by a more complex mechanism called the 'relaxation processes'.

The attenuation of ultrasound increases directly with frequency and therefore if the frequency is doubled the attenuation of the ultrasound will also be doubled. Higher frequency pulse—echoes which penetrate tissues less readily than low frequency pulses—are therefore used for more superficial tissues.

Attenuation also increases with depth and is dissipated exponentially but this varies with different tissues. Thus if one unit of tissue will reduce the intensity by a half, two units will reduce it by a quarter, but fluids, especially cyst-fluid, urine and liquor amnii, attenuate ultrasound much less than muscle or fat. Bone greatly attenuates ultrasound.

Reflectivity

Some of the energy of an ultrasound wave, often only 1–2%, will be reflected from the interface of tissues with different densities much in the same way as light is reflected from a mirror. This is known as reflective or specular energy. When ultrasound strikes much smaller objects the reflected energy is much weaker spreading out in all directions—scattering energy. Specular echoes are a hundred times stronger than scattered echoes.

The interface between gas and tissue forms an almost complete reflector of ultrasound and therefore bowel gas forms an inpenetrable barrier. Gas must also be excluded between the transducer and the patient by using a 'coupling agent' on the skin such as oil or a gel.

The decibel scale

The intensity of ultrasound is measured in decibels but because the strongest echoes are tens of thousands of times greater than the weakest echoes it is more convenient to use a logarithmic scale.

Ultrasound Images
(Registration of pulse-echo)

A-scope

The A-scope defines and measures the positions of acoustic interfaces and is used particularly for fetal cephalometry to show the size of the fetal head and position of the midline echoes. Basically the A-scope depends upon the time-delay between the production of the ultrasound pulse and the return of the echoes and is related to the velocity of the propagated wave and its path length.

As a pulse of ultrasound is emitted, it produces an upward deflection on the scope and the bright spot is then driven horizontally across the face of the oscilloscope by a time base.

When the ultrasonic pulse is reflected from an acoustic interface and returns to the transducer it produces an electrical signal which shows as a vertical deflection on the oscilloscope.

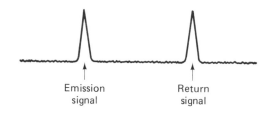

Emission
signal

Return
signal

The distance between the two signals is proportional to the distance between the probe and the reflecting boundary. Of course multiple reflecting boundaries will produce multiple return signals but because the further echoes from deeper structures are weaker it is necessary to include a *time-gain compensation* (TGC) which increases the gain in proportion to the depth from which the signals return. The A-mode provides information of an object in only one specific direction at a time.

B-scope or brightness modulated display

The B-scope shows the signals from the returning echoes as stationary bright spots on the oscilloscope and the brightness of each spot can be related to the value of the corresponding echo amplitude. There are two main display systems used in medical imaging based on the B-scope. In the first, *movement* is recorded by a time—position method and in the second, two-dimensional *tomographic sections* display anatomy.

(i) Time—position recording (M—mode)

The returning signals from one specific direction are represented as bright spots on the oscilloscope and a relatively slow speed time base is moved at right angles to the line of returning signals. By convention the signals from deeper tissues are towards the bottom of the record and the earlier signals towards the left. The 'M-scope' is used almost exclusively in cardiology and is particularly valuable for studying valve or ventricular wall motion.

(ii) Two-dimensional B-scanning
(Ultrasound tomography)

An ultrasonography scanner has the direction and position of the B-scope time base on the oscilloscope linked to the ultrasonic beam in the patient and the transducer can move only in the direction of the preselected plane. The signals are stored on the display while the transducer moves in contact with the skin through the coupling agent, scanning in all directions in the selected plane. The transducer may be moved manually, mechanically or electronically.

The signals may be stored directly onto photographic plate, or electronically, but electronic recording is either by a persistence oscilloscope or a scan converter with a television display. When only bistable black and white images were required a direct view storage tube was adequate while for grey-scale pictures a scan converter with a television monitor is required. (2507, 2508, 2509)

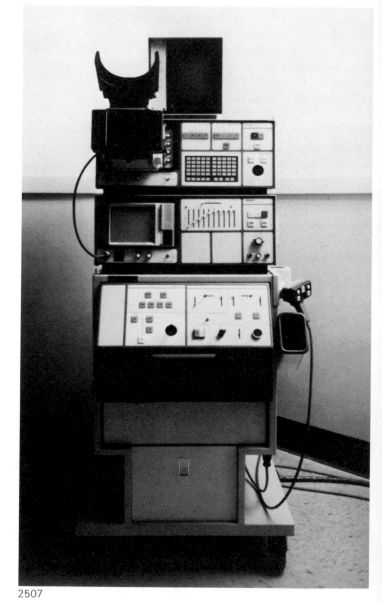

2507

(2507) B-scanner apparatus with a digital mini computer facility which also allows A-mode and cardiac scanning. The viewing monitor sits on top of the device adjacent to the polaroid camera with the alpha numeric keyboard. The patient's data and scanning planes can be printed out on the hard copy.

(2508) The scanner is being operated with the monitor displaying a B-scan.

(2509a, b) Smaller scanners with both static B-scan and real-time facility.

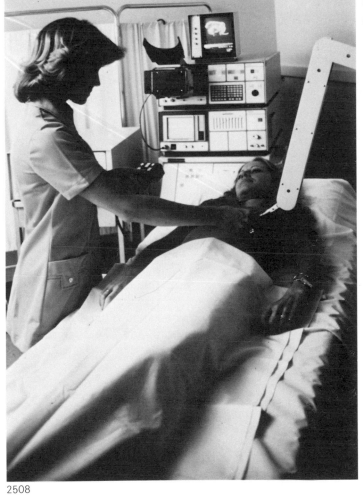

2508

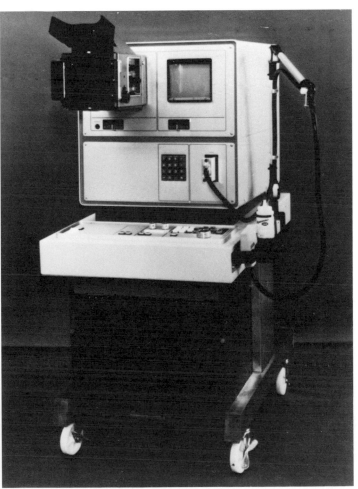

2509a

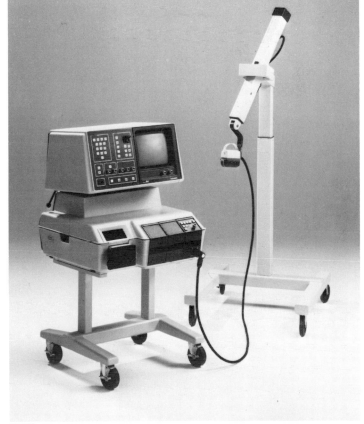

2509b

Real-time tomographic sections

An instantaneous two dimensional image can be produced by moving the ultrasound beam very rapidly through the section being examined. The resulting scan is shown on a non-storage oscilloscope or processed by a digital scan converter to be shown on a television monitor. The images are refreshed at frame rates of 15–200 per second, and visualise moving structures (in 'real time') virtually instantaneously.

The ultrasound beam may be moved either mechanically or electronically and the image is either a rectangular or a fan-shaped sector depending on the type of transducer.

The successful mechanical transducers are either of the rotating type or rotating with a parabolic mirror. In the rotating type two or more piezo-electric elements are rotated in a wheel and produce a sector scan. (Nuclear Enterprises, Bruel and Kjaer, RTS). The rotating type with parabolic mirror incorporates the rotating elements in a large water-filled applicator and the ultrasound beam and signals are reflected from a steel parabolic mirror resulting in a rectangular scan (Sieman's Vidison).

The electronic real-time transducers are multi-element either as linear array or phased array.

The multi-element linear array transducer has a row of small piezo-electric elements set in a block and excited singly or in small groups. When the echoes have returned, the next transducer or group is excited. These transducers produce a rectangular parallel line image. (Kretz ADR, Diagnostic Sonor System 85, Unirad Sonofluoroscope, Philips Sono-Diagnost).

The multi-element phased array transducers are electronic sector scanners and also use a block of identical piezo-electric elements, but their excitation pattern produces a wave front which is deflected away from the forward axial direction and can also be used to 'focus' the beam to a particular depth in the area of interest. These transducers can be much smaller than the linear array scanners, providing small acoustic windows and are especially useful in cardiology.

It is essential that real time scanners have a 'freeze frame' facility to record an image. The resolution of real time scanners is constantly improving and may well soon approach that of static B-mode scans. (2510, 2511)

Two dimensional Doppler scanners

The Doppler scanner issues a continuous beam of ultrasound with range gating to show the depth of the returning signals formed by moving structures, and is used for imaging blood vessels, especially the carotid arteries in the neck. The blood vessel is imaged by moving the transducer to and fro across the overlying skin.

Internal probe

The Radial Scanner was developed for examining the pelvis, using a rotating transducer and plan position indication (PPI), a display system based on radar with scan lines radiating from a central point. The transducer, with its outer stationary tube and inner assembly of a radial ultrasonic beam axis, can both rotate and move longitudinally up and down. The transducer is covered with a thin rubber condom which is filled with water to make contact with the rectal or vaginal wall.

For the prostate, transverse scans are made at 1 cm intervals beginning at the level of the seminal vesicles behind the bladder. The transducer emerges through a hole in the seat of a chair and the patient sits with the transducer in position in the rectum.

The 'Octoson'

The patient lies on a plastic membrane that is in contact with a water bath in which the scanning mechanism is mounted on a large semicircular frame. The frame both angulates and rotates and can be moved up and down on a set of rails.

Eight large transducers are fixed to the semicircular frame, each being able to rock through 30° to produce a scan.

(2510) A compact real-time scanner.

(2511) A compact real-time scanner showing the linear array transducer. It has a freeze frame facility and A and M mode displays.

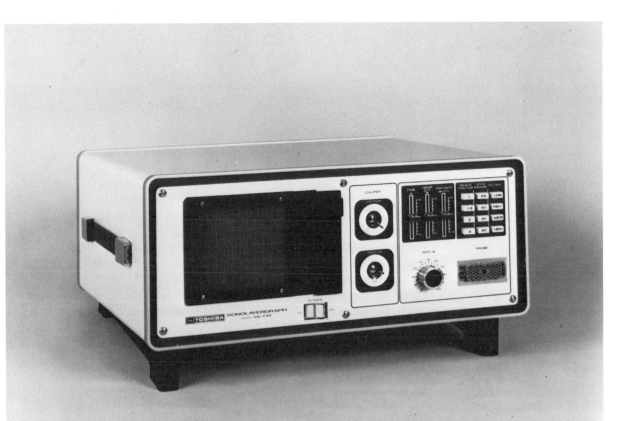

2510

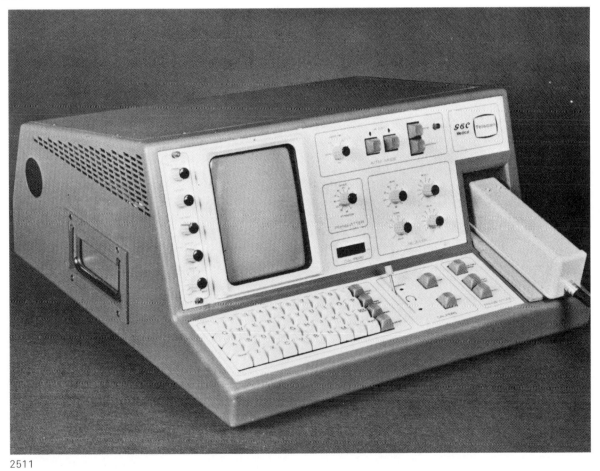

2511

The Electronic System

To obtain the best results in ultrasonography it is extremely helpful to have a working knowledge of the components of an ultrasound scanner. By its very nature the equipment must generate ultrasound pulses, then detect the returning echoes, and measure the time intervals between each pulse and the returning echo. It must also compute the position of the origin of each echo and then display the information obtained by these processes.

The basic components are represented diagramatically in figure (2512) and consist of a number of electronic modules. The control circuitry co-ordinates the entire system, the transmitter energises the piezo-electric transducer to produce short ultrasonic pulses, and the receiver detects the returning echoes. The signal processing circuitry prepares the echoes for display and the position-sensing circuitry determines the position of the transducer and its direction. The final information is then shown on the display system.

The control circuitry orders the stages of the scan cycle to ensure correct timing of the transmitted pulse and starts the time-base which must be repeated many hundreds of times per second. It includes a 'clock' or 'pulse repetition frequency' generator (PRF) to initiate each cycle.

The Transmitter generates the electrical impulse which produces a short ultrasound pulse from the transducer which is excited by a very brief voltage spike or step. The magnitude of the voltage spike or step largely determines the acoustic output of the transducer.

The Receiver includes an amplifier which boosts the very small returning echo to a level suitable for display and must obviously work at ultrasonic frequencies, being known as a 'radio-frequency amplifier'. The 'gain' is in fact the factor by which the amplitude of the signal is increased and is measured in decibels (dB). The amplifier usually also corrects for the attenuation of the echoes through the tissues, a function known as 'time-gain compensation' (TGC).

Echoes originating near the surface are proportionally far too large compared with deep echoes, and can be compensated for by making the receiver amplifier increase exponentially as the deeper echoes are recorded. The rate for increasing the gain is adjusted by the TGC slope control.

Signal Processing is required because the unprocessed amplified echo information is in the range of 100 dB while the display device only has a range of 30 dB. Additional functions such as edge enhancement can also be performed by the signal processor.

Position sensing circuitry ensures that the display spot should start at a point correctly representing the position of the transducer and then the spot should move in a direction in which the ultrasound pulse is propagated into the tissues. Therefore it must accurately locate the position of the probe in space, the direction in which it is pointing and the time delay of the pulse-echo assuming a value for the velocity of sound in tissues.

The Display System must be able to show a spot in its defined position on the screen and for B-scans the spot requires to be moved to any position and in any direction, at the correct speed. The main display units are oscilloscopes, storage oscilloscopes and grey-scale displays.

Oscilloscopes With the conventional cathode ray oscilloscope (CRO) the image fades rapidly and must therefore be recorded on photographic plate or repeatedly refreshed (real-time scanner).

Storage Oscilloscopes retain the image for some time after it is produced on the tube face, and come in two types. The bistable type retains its image until erased while with the variable persistence oscilloscope the rate at which the image fades can be controlled. However the spot sizes are larger in storage oscilloscopes which also have a limited dynamic range of display (5–10 dB).

Grey Scale requires a wide range of brightness levels and although this can be achieved with conventional oscilloscopes and also with photographic film there is no doubt that the best results are obtained with television monitors. Television monitors have a dynamic range of 30 dB and the spot size is more than adequate, but to show the B-scan requires a scan convertor to make the B-scan data compatible with the television system and may be either analogue or digital in type.

Machine Controls either control the picture or the signals. Picture controls adjust the image size, position on the screen, brightness, focus, and contrast whereas signal controls adjust the formation of the picture before it reaches the display. But before the examination even starts a frequency will be chosen, as will the type of scan—real-time, A, B, or M-scan. To ensure picture sharpness the calibre pips are placed on the time base and focused by being made as small as possible. With a scan convertor the contrast and brightness controls of the TV monitor must also be adjusted.

Centring the scan

The gantry must be centred on the patient lying on the couch. If a static scanner is used the picture is then centralised on the display but in modern equipment this happens automatically. If there is difficulty in finding the time base the picture must be made as small as possible and the time base brightness slightly increased. The X-direction shift control should be adjusted first. After locating the time base the probe should be placed centrally over the patient and the time base centred on the display. The picture can then be enlarged to the required size and the time base brightness reduced to its correct level.

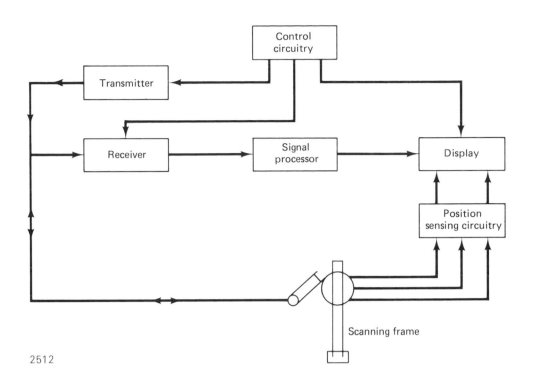

2512

Summary of preliminary adjustments

1. Switch on
2. Select transducer and amplifier
3. Adjust time base velocity
4. Choose display
5. Adjust focus
6. Set time base brightness.
7. Adjust dynamic grey scale range
8. Fix grey-scale contrast and brightness
9. Set suppression to minimum
10. Position patient,
11. Centre gantry
12. Select small display scale
13. Centre picture

Signal Controls

Varying the sensitivity in ultrasonography changes the number and distribution of the signals and is an essential part of producing a diagnostic image.

With high sensitivity there is a large number of echoes of all amplitudes but if too high the saturated signals hide details and there is an increase in artefacts due to noise and reverberations with the masking of the 'acoustic texture' of the tissue.

With low sensitivity only high amplitude echoes are visible and major organ boundaries well displayed. If too low a sensitivity is used then tissue texture is invisible and if small echoes are lost a false diagnosis of a cyst can be made because the tissue appears 'anechoic'.

Thus low sensitivity shows organ boundaries well, and high sensitivities are used for 'tissue texture'.

There are two main methods of changing sensitivity, firstly by varying the radio frequency amplifier ('far gain') and secondly by adjusting the intensity of ultrasound pulse from the transducer by an output attenuator.

Metreweli* has produced a practical guide to the signal controls. When there are *too many echoes overall* change to higher frequency transducer or increase attenuation or suppression. With *too few echoes overall or too few small amplitude echoes* ensure good skin coupling is present, have minimal suppression, reduce attenuation, use more sensitive transducer and lower frequency, or lower frequency transducer.

With *too many near echoes* increase slope delay or decrease slope or use a water bath. With *too many far echoes* decrease slope delay or increase attenuation and slope, use higher frequency or higher frequency transducer.

With *too few near echoes* reduce slope delay or increase slope and with *too few far echoes* decrease transducer attenuation and add slope delay, use lower frequency or lower frequency transducer.

With *too many echoes in a '? cyst'* increase suppression or transducer attenuation.

* *Practical Abdominal Ultrasound*, C. Metreweli. Heinemann Medical Books Ltd.

The major clinical indications for ultrasonography

Ultrasonography in medicine was developed for, and continues to be used mainly in, obstetrics, to show the placenta, estimate fetal maturity and demonstrate fetal abnormalities. However in recent years non-obstetric abdominal diagnosis has become increasingly important, particularly for the kidneys, liver, gall bladder, pancreas, enlarged lymph nodes and the aorta, in showing mass lesions and distinguishing between solid tumours and cysts.

A detailed knowledge of the anatomy of the abdominal soft tissues in axial and longitudinal sections is essential in ultrasonography, not only in interpretation but also in performing the scans. The high resolution of the new real-time grey-scale equipment is extremely valuable in familiarising the student with the basic appearances in abdominal ultrasonography and like conventional radiography there is now a recognised technique for examining each region and each organ. The ultrasonic examination is also like conventional radiography in being directed towards a particular organ, attention being focused on the particular clinical problem rather than producing a general survey.

The Kidneys

Indications for ultrasonography of the kidneys include mass lesions and a 'non-functioning' kidney seen on the intravenous urogram. Perinephric haemorrhage, especially from trauma, tumours, cysts and hydronephrosis can be visualised, and ultrasonography is now the major imaging method following renal transplantation.

Position

All scans of the normally situated kidneys are done in deep arrested inspiration to bring the upper poles into view below the rib margin.

Prone (standard)

The patient lies prone with the arms to the side and the head turned towards the side being examined. (2513a)

Supine

If the upper pole of the right kidney is not shown in the prone position it can be shown with the patient supine, especially on deep inspiration, and the supine position is also the position for showing the presacral kidney, transplant kidney and horse-shoe kidney.

Right lateral decubitus

When the left kidney is not well shown with the patient prone it can be examined from the left side with the patient lying on the right and scanning longitudinally in the mid axillary line. This is also the position for scanning the adrenal gland. The right adrenal is examined with the patient in the left decubitus position.

Scanning planes

The longitudinal scans are performed with the transducer initially pointing upwards towards the head with a single sweep or only one return pass. The transverse scans require compound arc and sector scans.

1. With the patient prone, longitudinal serial scans are made at 0·5 to 1 cm parallel to the spine in the sagittal plane, extending beyond the lateral margin of the kidney. Scans in the true sagittal plane are more easily related to the intravenous urogram than oblique scans.
2. Scans along the long axis of the kidneys are preferred by some workers. The upper poles are nearer the spine and the long axis tends to be at about a 20° angle to the spine.
3. With the patient prone, scans are made at 0·5–1 cm intervals at right angles to the vertebral column in deep inspiration, starting just below the twelfth rib. Transverse or axial scans do not usually show the upper poles of the kidneys.
4. Supine longitudinal scans in deep suspended inspiration are made over the liver for the right kidney.
5. Longitudinal scans over the left side parallel to the mid-axillary line with the patient lying on the right side, can be used for the left kidney. This is also the position used for the adrenal gland.
6. With the patient supine, longitudinal scans are made along the mid and anterior axillary lines, particularly to show the left kidney.
7. Supine longitudinal and transverse scans in the iliac fossae of renal transplant patients are made to show the kidney and bladder.

Normal appearances

On longitudinal scans the kidneys appear as sonolucent ovoid areas with a smooth margin due to renal parenchyma and a thick central band of intense echoes due to the renal sinus with its calyces and surrounding fatty tissue. The superior pole lies more posteriorly than the inferior pole. (2513a, b).

In transverse and oblique sections the kidneys appear as U-shaped sonolucent areas with the central renal sinus producing intense echoes and facing anteriorly and medially. (2514, 2515a, b)

The capsule of each kidney is seen as a smooth thin echogenic line surrounding the sonolucent parenchyma.

(2513) Real time scan. (a) Longitudinal prone section of a normal left kidney showing well defined margins, low level parenchymal echoes and high density echoes in the hilum of the kidney. (b) Longitudinal supine scan of right kidney through the liver with more obvious hilar echoes. (c) Horizontal supine scan of the right kidney through the hilus.

(2514) Oblique supine view of the right kidney with the renal pelvis lying behind the inferior vena cava giving off the renal vein.

(2515a, b) Transverse supine section through both kidneys with the vertebral body between and lying in front of it are inferior vena cava and aorta with the left renal artery. An enlarged portal vein lies anterior to the right kidney shown as both (a) negative and (b) positive prints.

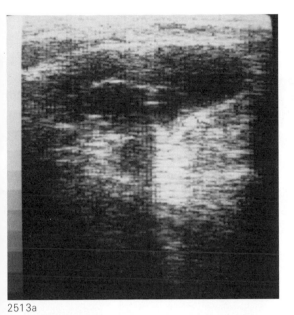

2513a

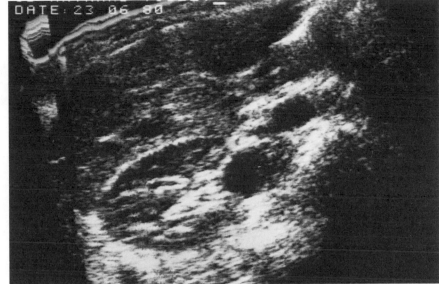

2514

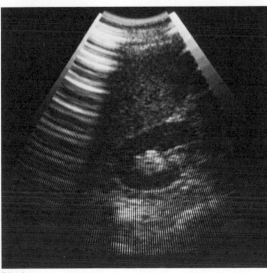

2513b

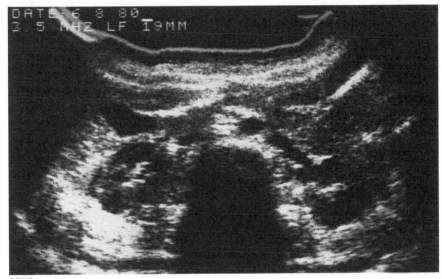

2515a

2513c

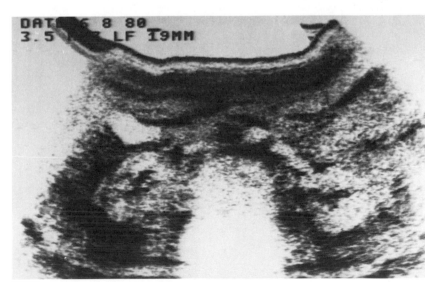

2515b

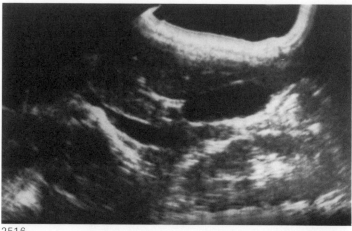

2516

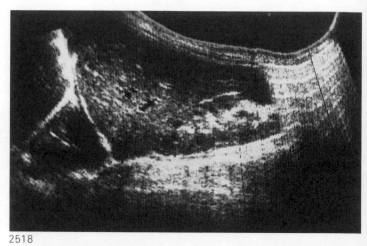

2518

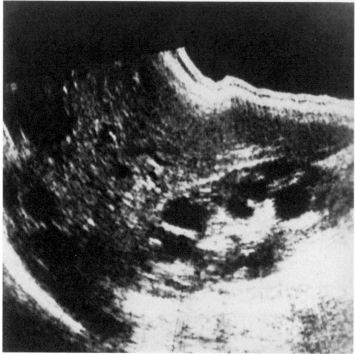

2517

2519

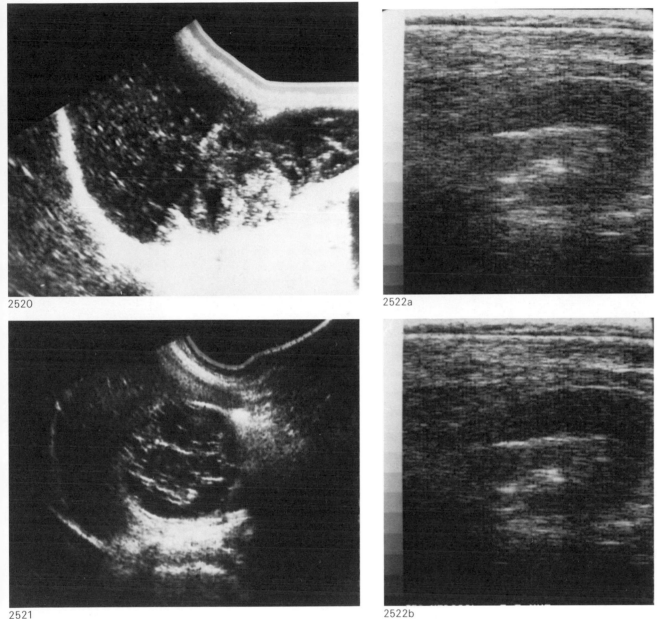

2520

2521

2522a

2522b

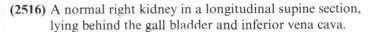

(2516) A normal right kidney in a longitudinal supine section, lying behind the gall bladder and inferior vena cava.

(2517) There is a renal cyst at the lower pole of the right kidney with increased ultrasound transmission behind.

(2518) The renal cyst is considerably smaller after aspiration.

(2519) Polycystic right kidney shown in the supine position through the liver.

(2520) Mass in the right kidney shown as dense echoes. This proved to be an adenoma of the kidney.

(2521) Complex kidney mass due to a renal tumour.

(2522) Oblique prone scan (right kidney) showing dilated renal pelvis in an early hydronephrosis due to a ureteric calculus. (Two different polaroid settings.)

The Liver

Clinical indications for ultrasonography

1. In obstructive jaundice.
2. To show dilated bile ducts and possibly the obstructing mass.
3. Metastases in the liver.
4. For space occupying lesions shown on isotope scanning, to distinguish tumours from cysts.
5. Subphrenic and intrahepatic abscess.
6. Upper abdominal mass lesions which may be intrahepatic.

Transducer

For the thick right lobe a 1·5 MHz transducer is required to visualise the postero-superior aspect. Minimal suppression must be used if the small liver echoes are to be shown. To start, select a TGC slope of 1·5–2 dB cm^{-1}.

Scanning planes

Longitudinal scans at 1–2 cm intervals start to the left of the midline and are done in deep arrested inspiration progressing to the right.

1. Longitudinal scans

With the patient supine or in the right anterior oblique position, the skin of the upper abdomen well oiled and the patient in deep arrested inspiration, angle the transducer steeply towards the head from the subcostal position. Perform a tight sector scan till the transducer is vertical and then complete with a longitudinal movement to the inferior edge of the liver.

2. Transverse scans

(i) With the transducer angled 10° towards the head and the skin of the upper abdomen well oiled start at the umbilicus and proceed caudally at 1 cm intervals in deep arrested inspiration allowing one inspiration per scan.

(ii) Transverse scans are usually compound scans with more than one pass.

(iii) Final scans at or near to the costal margins are done with a 30° caudal tilt on the transducer.

3. Oblique scans

With the patient supine and in deep arrested inspiration, angle the transducer 25–30° caudally along the line parallel to the lower costal margin.

Oblique scans on occasion show an abnormality more clearly than transverse axial scans.

Normal appearances   (2523, 2524, 2525)

The liver is triangular with the base towards the diaphragm and the right and the apex towards the feet and the left side anteriorly. The diaphragm is seen above the liver as a thick arc of intense echoes. The liver hilum and falciform ligaments produce intense echoes and the liver parenchyma a uniform pattern of small echoes broken up by portal and hepatic veins seen as rounded or linear branching sonolucencies. Portal veins have marked surrounding echoes whereas hepatic veins have no surrounding echoes. The normal intrahepatic bile ducts and hepatic arteries are not visualised on ultrasonography.

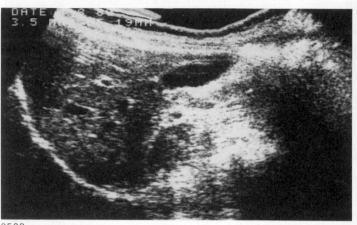

2523

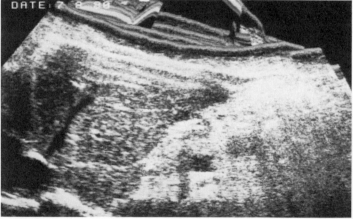

2524

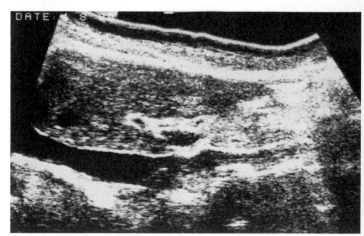

2525

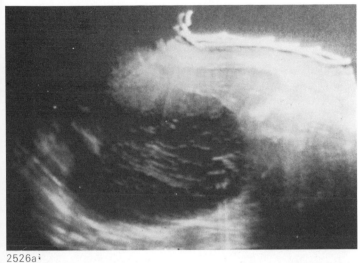

2526a

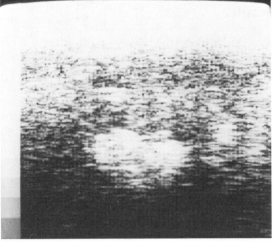

2527

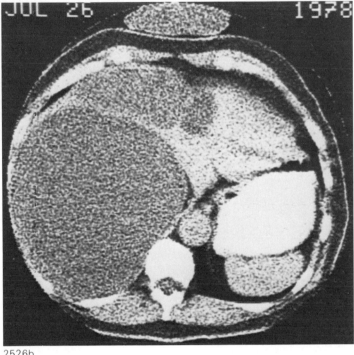

2526b

(2523) Normal liver parenchyma with portal veins which have echogenic walls and hepatic veins which show as small echolucent areas. The normal gall bladder is visible and the upper pole of the right kidney. The liver is bounded above and behind by the diaphragm showing as a thick echogenic line.

(2524) Normal liver with branching hepatic vein draining into the inferior vena cava.

(2525) Normal liver in longitudinal section showing the inferior vena cava with the portal vein in front and the common hepatic duct anterior to it.

(2526) Large hepatic cyst on (a) ultrasonography and on (b) computed tomography for comparison.

(2527) Two different settings to show multiple liver metastases with a real time scanner.

(2528) Complex mass lesion in liver shown to be abscess.

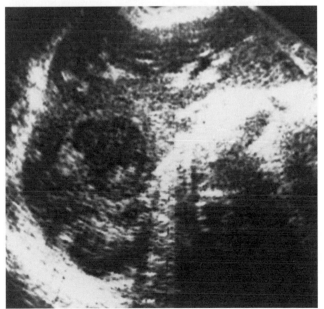

2528

The Gall Bladder

Ultrasonography is now commonly used in the diagnosis of gall-bladder disease and this is a major indication for its use in non-obstetric conditions of the abdomen. The patient must have a fat free diet for 24 hours prior to examination and no fluid or food for 4 hours before the examination.

Indications

1. Diagnosis of gall stones (upper abdominal pain, jaundice, dyspepsia).
2. 'Non-functioning' gall bladder on oral cholecystography.
3. Jaundice.

The transducer and ultrasound settings are similar to those for the liver which can then also be visualised, and similarly scans are done in deep arrested inspiration. Most scans will be done with the patient supine but decubitus scans can be helpful in showing layered small stones, bile sludge and 'limey' bile and in distinguishing a gall stone from a tumour.

Scanning planes

1. With the patient supine and in deep arrested inspiration perform longitudinal scans at 1 cm intervals starting 2 cm to the right of the midline and proceeding towards the right side. The transducer must be tilted 10° caudally under the rib cage at the start of the sector sweep.
2. Transverse scans at 1 cm intervals from just below the gall bladder, and proceeding cranially, are then performed, again in deep arrested inspiration.
3. Oblique transverse scans along the line of the costal margin in deep arrested inspiration may show the gall bladder to better advantage.
4. Oblique 10–15° longitudinal scans from lateral to medial at 0·5 cm intervals over the long axis of the common bile duct, completes the examination.

Normal appearances (2529, 2530)

The gall-bladder produces an ovoid or a pear shaped sonolucent area with increased echoes behind the posterior margin and lies under the triangular liver edge on longitudinal scans. It appears as a round sonolucency on the transverse scan.

(2529) Normal gall bladder with increased echoes posteriorly lying in front of the right kidney.

(2530) Longitudinal scan of a normal gall bladder with increased echoes behind. The inferior vena cava lies posteriorly.

(2531) Small stone in the gall bladder casting acoustic shadow.

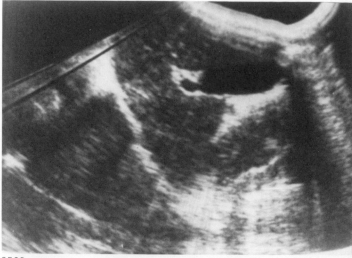

2529

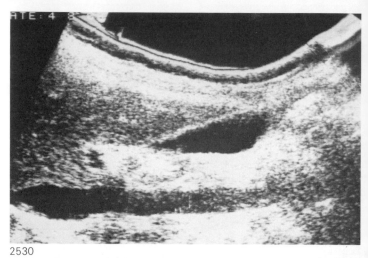

2530

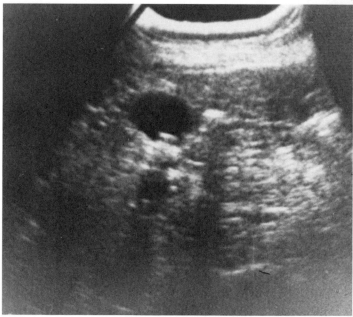

2531

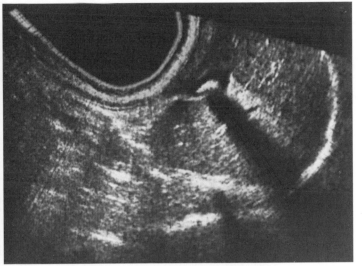

2532

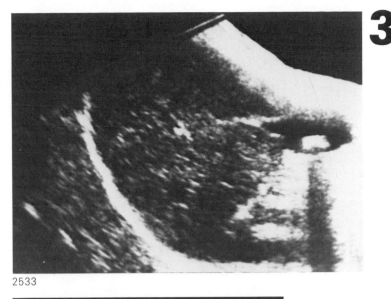

2533

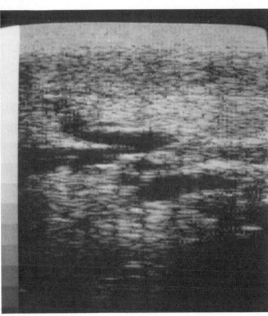

2534a

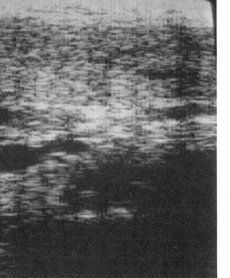

2534b

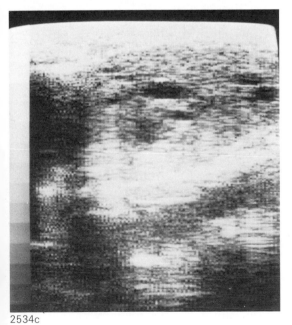

2534c

(2532) Moderate size gall stone with marked acoustic shadowing.

(2533) Gall stone showing acoustic shadowing.

(2534a, b, c) Dilated bile ducts in obstructive jaundice with a large mass in the hilum of the liver due to a cholangiocarcinoma.

The Spleen

It is often difficult to demonstrate the normal spleen with ultrasonography because it lies behind the stomach and splenic flexure of the colon. However the enlarged spleen can be examined from the left side with the patient either supine or in the right lateral decubitus position using longitudinal scans. Ultrasonography is used to distinguish focal disease, especially splenic cysts, from diffuse parenchymal disease or portal hypertension, and is also useful for the diagnosis of splenic rupture and perisplenic haematoma after trauma.

Scanning planes

1. Transverse scans are performed with the patient supine using a marked caudal tilt of the transducer with sections 1–2 cm apart and in deep arrested inspiration.
2. Longitudinal scans with the patient supine are done starting with a 70–80° tilt of the transducer under the costal margin, in the mid axillary line and directed far posteriorly.
3. Right lateral decubitus scans may be necessary to show a small spleen and are done as transverse and longitudinal scans.
4. Oblique supine scans done parallel to the costal margin may also be useful.

The Pancreas

In about 15–25 % of cases the pancreas cannot be visualised due to overlying bowel shadows, the tail of the pancreas being an especially difficult region. In such circumstances scanning with the patient sitting erect and the stomach filled with water to provide an acoustic window has been advocated. However most patients are scanned supine but occasionally prone scans will show the tail of the pancreas.

Clinical indications

1. For pancreatic tumours, especially carcinoma of pancreas.
2. For pancreatic pseudocysts.
3. To distinguish solid and cystic lesions in the region of the pancreas.
4. In obstructive jaundice, to exclude a mass in the head of the pancreas.

Transducer and technique

A short focus, high resolution transducer of 3–5 MHz is advisable and the slope should be greater than for the liver at approximately 5–6 dB cm⁻¹ with a sensitivity of about 3–5 dB less than a liver scan.

Scanning planes

1. Longitidunal scans at 0·5 cm intervals near the midline with the patient supine and during quiet breathing are used to identify the major blood vessels in order to locate the pancreas. The body of the pancreas curves over the superior mesenteric artery which lies in a collection of high level echoes anterior to the aorta. The splenic vein lies behind the superior margin of the pancreas and the uncinate process in the angle of origin of the superior mesenteric artery from the aorta.
2. Oblique transverse scans at an angle of 30–40° to the spinal column with the patient supine during quiet breathing are then performed at 0·5 cm intervals from below the level of the costal margin to the epigastrium. The oblique transverse scans which are done with a compound motion should run along the long axis of the pancreas from the more caudally situated head of pancreas to the more cranial tail of pancreas lying at the splenic hilum. The superior margin of the body and tail of the pancreas lie in front of the splenic vein, and the head of the pancreas in front of the left renal vein as it enters the inferior vena cava.
3. Transverse axial scans with the patient supine, at 1 cm intervals between the umbilicus and epigastrium, are used to identify the body of the pancreas.
4. Prone longitudinal and oblique scans may be useful in identifying lesions in the region of the tail of the pancreas.
5. Erect scans with the patient sitting and after drinking 500 ml of water can show the body and the tail of the pancreas through the fluid filled stomach which acts as an acoustic window.

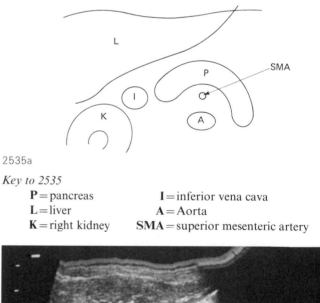

2535a

Key to 2535

P = pancreas	**I** = inferior vena cava
L = liver	**A** = Aorta
K = right kidney	**SMA** = superior mesenteric artery

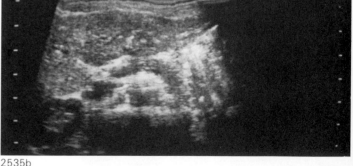

2535b

(**2535**) Normal pancreas lying in front of the superior mesenteric artery and aorta with the inferior vena cava to the right with the liver in front and the right kidney behind.

Normal appearances (2535, 2536, 2537, 2538)

The normal pancreas contains many small internal echoes with intense surrounding echoes due to mesenteric and retro-peritoneal adipose tissue. The central pancreatic duct may be seen outlined by brighter echoes of the wall.

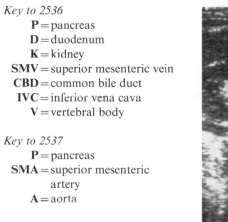

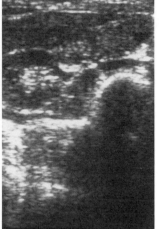

Key to 2536
- **P** = pancreas
- **D** = duodenum
- **K** = kidney
- **SMV** = superior mesenteric vein
- **CBD** = common bile duct
- **IVC** = inferior vena cava
- **V** = vertebral body

Key to 2537
- **P** = pancreas
- **SMA** = superior mesenteric artery
- **A** = aorta

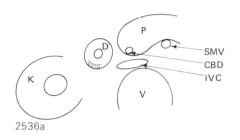

2536a

(2536) Normal head of pancreas.

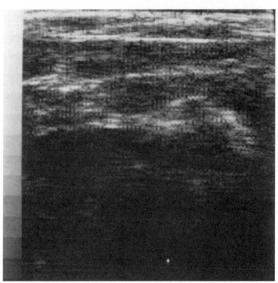

2536b

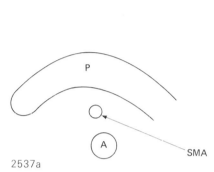

2537a

(2537) Pancreas shown on the real time scanner.

2537b

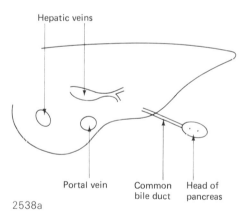

2538a

(2538) Sagittal oblique scan through the head of the pancreas.

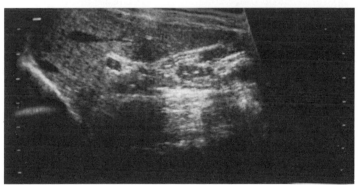

2538b

The aorta and inferior vena cava

Ultrasonography is an extremely valuable non-invasive method for examining the aorta to diagnose aneurysms, aortic dissections and thrombosis of the inferior vena cava.

Indications

1. For aneurysms of the aorta to distinguish lumen from surrounding thrombus.
2. For dissection of the aorta.
3. For patency of aortic prosthesis.
4. To diagnose thrombosis of the inferior vena cava.
5. To distinguish lymphadenopathy from an aneurysm.

Scanning planes and technique

A 1·5 MHz transducer is needed for obese patients but a 2·5–3 MHz transducer can be used in thinner subjects. While low sensitivity is required to show the wall of the aorta high sensitivity is needed for intraluminal thrombus.

1. Longitudinal scans are done with the patient supine on the 2/5 scale in full inspiration as a single pass from xiphisternum to pubis, starting in the midline. Half centimetre, para-sagittal scans on either side to cover the width of the aorta, will demonstrate any tortuosity. Scans further towards the right will show the inferior vena cava.
2. Oblique longitudinal scans along the line of the tortuous aorta can then be done at 0·5 cm intervals.
3. Transverse scans at right angles to the long axis of the aorta and with no transducer tilt, at 1 cm intervals as compound scans, will define the true calibre of the lumen and prevent superimposition of the aneurysm on the renal arteries.

Normal appearances (2539–2546)

The aorta is a sonolucent tube tapering from about 2·5 cm at the diaphragm to 1·5 cm at its bifurcation. The superior mesenteric artery forms a narrow sonolucent tube lying parallel and anterior to the middle part of aorta surrounded by intense echoes of the retroperitoneal adipose tissues. The left psoas muscle is visible behind the upper part of the aorta and the body of the pancreas is visible in front of the middle part of the aorta.

The inferior vena cava narrows as it traverses the liver and the fan-shaped confluent hepatic veins can be seen draining the liver to enter the inferior vena cava.

Para-aortic Lymph Nodes

Normal nodes are not distinguished on ultrasonography but lymphadenopathy produces scalloped mass lesions surrounding the aorta which are relatively free of echoes and can be recognised in both longitudinal and transverse scans.

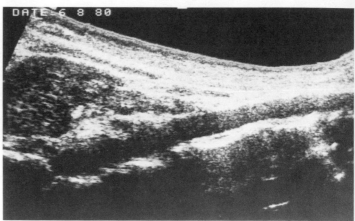

2539a

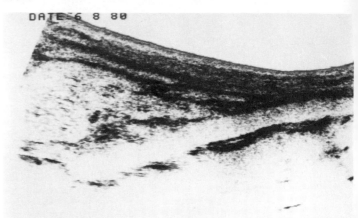

2539b

(2539) Aorta shown on longitudinal scan behind the left lobe of the liver on both (a) positive and (b) negative prints.

(2540) Aorta on longitudinal section showing origin of coeliac axis as well as the superior mesenteric artery lying in front of and parallel to the aorta.

(2541) Transverse section through the aorta, inferior vena cava, superior mesenteric artery and portal vein.

(2542) Longitudinal scan of aorta with superior mesenteric vein.

(2543) Large portal vein anterior to the inferior vena cava, lying in the hilum of the liver.

(2544) Real time scan through (a) aorta showing (b) superior mesenteric artery lying anterior to aorta.

(2545) Real time scanner M-scope recording of the mitral valve showing the difficulty in obtaining a clear recording because of the large size of the transducer.

(2546) Transverse oblique scan with cranial angulation showing confluence of portal veins, inferior vena cava and hepatic vein draining into it.

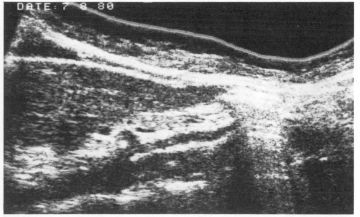

2540a

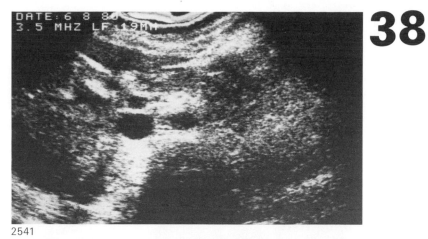

2541

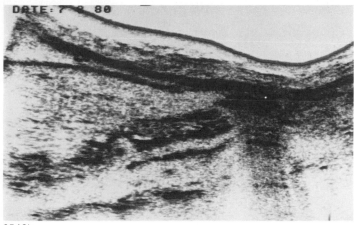

2540b

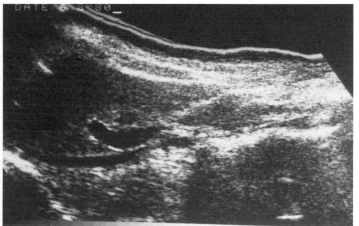

2542

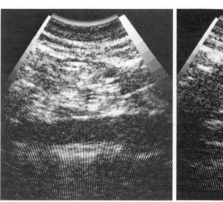

2543

2544a

2544b

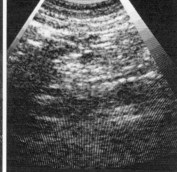

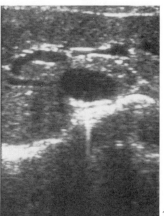

2546

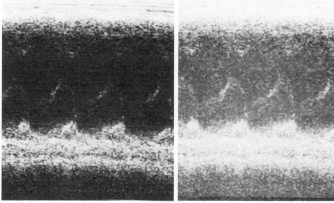

2545a

2545b

The Pelvis (non-obstetric)

Ultrasonography is recognised as the non-invasive method of choice in the pelvis and is particularly valuable in showing lesions of the uterus, ovaries and bladder, with the prostate being examined by a special rotating transducer from within the rectum.

Indications

1. Localisation of intra-uterine contraceptive device.
2. Uterine mass lesions—fibroids, or carcinoma of cervix or uterus.
3. Ovarian mass lesions—ovarian cyst or carcinoma.
4. Bladder carcinoma staging.
5. Lymphadenopathy
6. Ascites or intraperitoneal haemorrhage.

Scanning planes and technique

The pelvis is always examined with a full bladder which displaces the small intestine out of the pelvic cavity and acts as an acoustic window to the uterus, adnexae and ovaries. (2547)

Scanning of the pelvis should be 2/5 full size image, initially using a slope of 6 dB cm^{-1} with minimal suppression. The attenuation must be varied to produce a good grey scale range and the image centred on the screen by positioning the transducer midway between the symphysis pubis and fundus of the uterus.

1. Longitudinal scans starting in the midline are performed at 1 cm intervals on both sides of the midline. As the transducer reaches a few centimetre above the symphysis pubis it is rotated in an arc towards the feet.
2. Then transverse scans are always performed, starting above the level of the uterine fundus, at 1 cm intervals down to the pubis. The transducer should be tilted 10–20° towards the head using a compound motion.

Normal appearances

In the longitudinal scan the bladder appears as an echo-free area with the uterus lying behind it and in front of the sacrum. The uterus appears as a flattened, pear-shaped structure with a fine, uniform pattern of low level echoes, in continuity with the single line of cervical echoes. The cervix lies behind the junction of the superior and posterior walls of the bladder.

In transverse sections the bladder appears square with the cervix and uterus indenting its posterior wall, the ovaries are quite commonly shown on either side of the uterus as small, rounded areas of uniform low level echoes.

In the male the prostate indents the lower part of the posterior wall of the bladder and is seen if the transducer is tilted in a caudal direction on the transverse scans. The prostate is clearly visualised with a radial transducer positioned in the rectum.

852

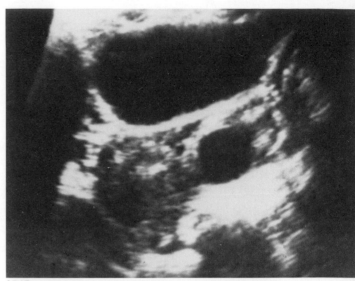

2547

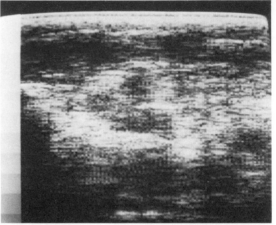

2548a

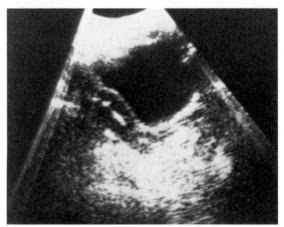

2548b

(2547) Transverse scan through the bladder with the uterus to the right and a sonolucent adnexal mass on the right shown to be a pelvic abscess.

(2548a) Complex mass arising out of the pelvis having the features of an ovarian carcinoma and proven at operation.

(2548b) Intra uterine contraceptive device (IUCD) within the uterus.

The Thorax

Cardiac Ultrasound

Non-invasive methods of cardiac imaging are now well established and in many clinical situations are replacing angio-cardiography especially for mitral valve disease. Many surgeons are now prepared to operate on the information obtained from ultrasonography without having recourse to more invasive procedures.

Cardiac ultrasound is particularly useful for assessing the mitral and aortic valves, pericardial effusion, chamber size and wall thickness of the left ventricle, cardiomyopathies and in some congenital heart lesions. The M-mode or time-position scan produces accurate measurements of valve movement and wall thickness, while real-time examinations using a sector scanner give a view of the spatial relationships of the heart.

Scanning planes and techniques

With the patient supine and the head-end of the bed raised 30°, the transducer is placed in the left 4th interspace close to the sternum. Directing the beam about 20° towards the head (2549A) shows the aortic valves, root of the aorta and left atrium. With the beam 10° towards the feet (2549B) the beam passes through the anterior wall of the right ventricle, the right ventricular cavity, the interventricular septum, the base of the left ventricular cavity and the posterior wall of the left ventricle. In this position the anterior and posterior mitral valve cusps are also in the ultrasound beam. With the beam directed 25° towards the feet (2549C) the beam traverses the ventricular walls, anterior right ventricle, interventricular septum, and the posterior left ventricular cavity in its maximum diameter.

The clearest real-time images are obtained with a sector scanner and modern equipment produces the corresponding M-mode or time-position scan by simply depressing a button on the keyboard. Images can also be obtained with a linear array transducer but because of its large size the ribs interfere with the image both on the sector scan and M-mode (2550).

Normal appearances

The normal appearances on the M-mode or time position scan are best shown diagrammatically for positions A, B, and C as in (2550).

In position A the main feature is the aortic valve, in B the mitral valve and in C the ventricular cavity.

To show the appearances of the corresponding real-time images, a recording is made on a video-cassette; still frame pictures being a rather poor representation of 'ultrasonic fluoroscopy' as shown by the real-time sector scanner. The movement of the mitral valve is particularly dramatic.

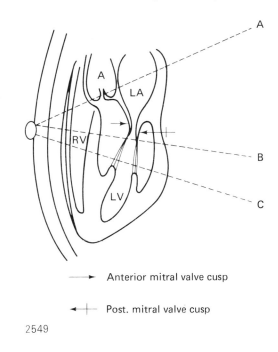

→ Anterior mitral valve cusp

←+ Post. mitral valve cusp

2549

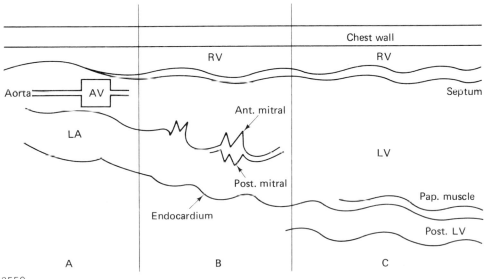

2550

The Brain

The adult cranium is far too reflective to allow brain imaging and for many years ultrasonography was used only to assess midline shift which proved of limited use and was completely superseded by computed tomography. It neonates a quite different situation prevails. The cranium is transonic and good anatomical detail of the ventricular system can be obtained for assessing ventricular size and intraventricular haemorrhage, and for diagnosing subdural haematomas. Furthermore, ultrasonography equipment can be portable and used without the infant being moved out of the incubator, no anaesthetic or even sedation being needed.

The Thyroid and Parathyroid glands

Glandular enlargement can be detected with ultrasonography and solid tumours can be distinguished from cysts.

Scanning planes and technique

With the patient supine a small waterbath is positioned on the anterior surface of the patient's neck using oil or gel to establish adequate transonic coupling between the waterbath and the patient's skin. Scanning is done at 0·5–1 cm intervals in the longitudinal and transverse axes.

Orbits

Ultrasonography is also used in the orbit but has largely been replaced by computed tomography because of the better anatomical definition. Ultrasonography is particularly valuable for occular lesions such as retinal detachment; the visualisation of the retrobulbar region with ultrasound cannot however match the detailed delimination possible with computed tomography which shows not only the intraorbital soft tissues but also the surrounding bone and adjacent structures such as the sinuses and brain.

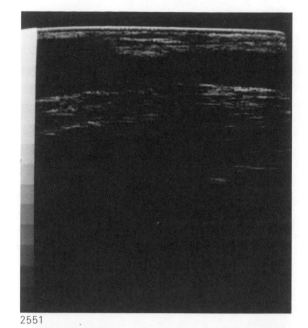

2551

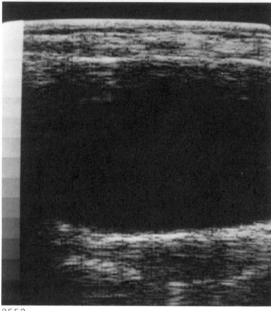

2552

(2551) Fibromuscular hyperplasia femoral artery on a real time scanner.

(2552) Right femoral aneurysm on a real time scanner.

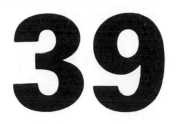

COMPUTED TOMOGRAPHY

COMPUTED TOMOGRAPHY

History

Unlike isotope scanning or ultrasonography, computed tomography (CT) emerged as a well developed diagnostic tool from the research laboratories. Oldendorf, a neurologist of Los Angeles, California, in 1961 described his experimental system for reconstructing the appearances of soft tissues by measuring 'radio density discontinuities' or, as they are now known, differences in tisue attentuation. Computer technology was poorly developed at the time and his ideas lay unrecognised till G. N. Hounsfield of EMI Laboratories at Hayes, Middlesex developed an experimental system in 1969.

The first pictures produced were of a brain specimen that had been fixed in formalin and of the torso of a pig in the region of the upper abdomen (2553). The initial results were sufficiently impressive to induce the Department of Health and Social Security (UK) to contribute financially to the project.

A functioning prototype was installed under the aegis of Dr James Ambrose at the Atkinson Morley Hospital in 1971. A year later when the first clinical results of brain scanning was reported, CT clearly had the potential for a major contribution in neuroradiology and since then air-encephalography has been almost entirely replaced and cerebral angiography cut to about 40 % of its previous level.

The first body CT device with a 20 second scanning time, which allows sections to be taken during suspended respiration, was installed by EMI at Northwick Park Hospital in 1974 with a grant from the Department of Health and Social Security. It was again immediately obvious that this new radiological method was highly successful, particularly for showing soft tissue masses in the abdomen in the diagnosis of lymphadenopathy, pancreatic tumours, liver metastases and abdominal abscesses. (2554, 2555, 2556)

General Principles

To obtain the readings required to reconstruct a picture of an axial section of anatomy, an X-ray tube and opposed photon detectors are required. The patient is scanned by a narrow beam of X-rays with both the collimated beam of X-rays being measured, and the intensity of the photons on the detectors being recorded.

The absorption of X-rays by the body can then be calculated along the beam paths where

$$\text{Absorption} = \text{Log} \frac{\text{Intensity of X-rays at source}}{\text{Intensity of X-rays at detectors}}$$

The readings from the detectors are converted into digital form and fed continuously into the micro-computer during each scan. In the body 180,000 simultaneous equations must be calculated to provide the tissue attenuation values in each cube of the section being scanned.

CT sections are usually 13 mm thick and in the body have a matrix of 320×320 pixels or picture elements while in the head the matrix is 180×180. In particular regions and for overcoming the partial volume effect, 5 mm and 2 mm sections are indicated. However with thinner sections increased radiation is needed to maintain the required spatial resolution.

(2553) The first body section (a pig's torso) done with computed tomography by Dr. G. N. Hounsfield at the EMI research laboratories, Hayes, Middlesex.

(2554) Mesenteric and para aortic lymph node masses in a case of non-Hodgkin's lymphoma.

(2555) Pancreatic carcinoma in the head of the pancreas adjacent to the duodenum. **D**=duodenum **L**=liver, **K**=kidney, **S**=spleen, **A**=aorta, **M**=mass (pancreatic carcinoma)

(2556) Subphrenic abscess displacing the liver, showing as a half-moon area of low tissue attenuation.

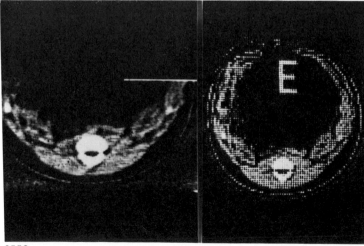

2553

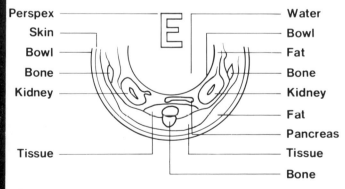

Perspex — Water
Skin — Bowl
Bowl — Fat
Bone — Bone
Kidney — Kidney
— Fat
— Pancreas
Tissue — Tissue
— Bone

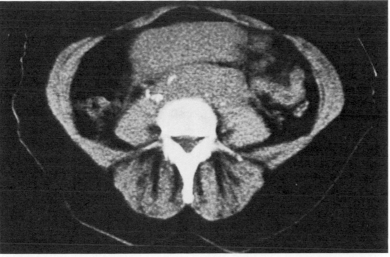

2554

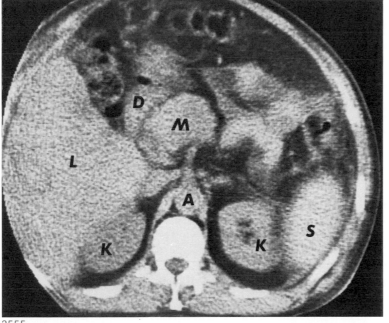

2555

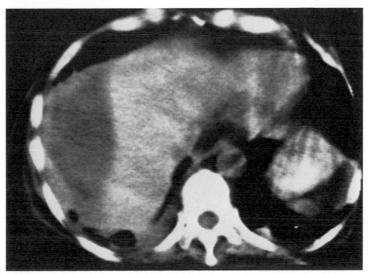

2556

The Apparatus

A CT scanning system consists of four major components: the scanning frame which obtains the readings, the processing unit for producing values of tissue attenuation in each section scanned, the viewing unit which presents the information as anatomical pictures, and a storage facility to retain the information for future display.

The Scanning Frame

The gantry or scanning frame incorporates the X-ray tube and detectors used to obtain the 300,000 readings taken through at least 180° to reconstruct each axial section. Because of the long exposure time the X-ray tube is oil-cooled with a fixed anode and the detectors are either crystal scintillation detectors or gas ionisation detectors. Sodium iodide is most commonly used for the crystal detectors but calcium fluoride and bismuth germinate are easier to handle although less efficient. Gas ionisation detectors usually contain Xenon or Xenon and Krypton.

Different scanner systems have been developed mainly to obtain faster scans. The original system, or first generation scanner, had a rotate/translate action with a parallel beam of X-rays. The second generation scanner uses a fan beam of X-rays with a rotate/translate action for the interlinked tube and detectors (2557). In the third generation system the interlinked tube and detectors rotate around the patient while in the fourth generation scanners the tube rotates and the detectors are stationery. The latest system has the tube outside the ring of stationery detectors (2558).

Rotate/Translate—first generation scanner

The mark I head scanner has a water-bath made of a latex cap around the aperture into which the head is inserted using collimated beams of parallel X-rays, two X-ray tubes and a bank of detectors to take two simultaneous, contiguous sections.

The interlinked X-ray tubes and detectors move across the head taking 160 readings for each traverse then rotate through 1° and move back again, rotating each time through a further 1° until 180° has been covered in 4.5 minutes. Thus 28,800 (160 × 180) readings are taken across the head from all angles in approximately a 1 cm thick slice with two adjacent slices being examined simultaneously.

The Mark I scanners had a long scanning time of 4.5 minutes.

Because of the waterbath only the head could be examined and not even the cervical spine or neck. However, the waterbath helped to obtain good fixation of the head to limit movements during the slow scan.

Rotate/Translate—second generation scanner

Non-movements scans of the head can be obtained by adequate fixation but in the body much faster scans were needed which could be completed during suspended respiration. Breathing movements cause movement artefacts whether in the chest or upper abdomen both on conventional radiographs and on CT. A scanning time below 20 seconds is obtained by using a 12° fan beam and rotating the interlinked X-ray tube and detectors through 10° after each traverse across the body. During each traverse 18,000 readings are taken and 300,000 for each section. Clearly the aperture between the X-ray tube and detectors needs to be larger for the body than for the head but different 'wedges' are available to examine larger or smaller areas. For head examinations and for children a 25 cm (10 in) 'wedge' or field size is used, for most adults a 32 cm (13 in) 'wedge' and for large individuals a 40 cm (16 ins) 'wedge'.

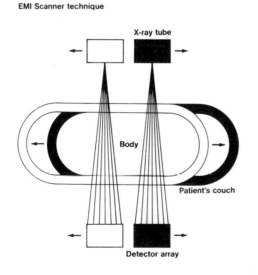

EMI Scanner technique

X-ray tube

Body

Patient's couch

Detector array

Movement of scanning frame

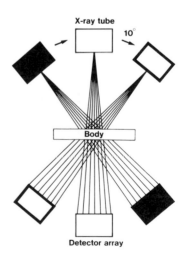

X-ray tube

10°

Body

Detector array

Scanning sequence

Rotate/Rotate—third generation scanner

The interlinked X-ray tube and detectors rotate around the patient to cover 360° although two or more rotations may be used for each scan. A wide fan beam of 35–50° is used and an arc of 20–50 detectors. Scan times down to 3 seconds are obtained with this system but it is prone to develop circular artefacts and the calibration cannot be checked once the patient is in position.

Rotating Tube/Fixed Detectors—fourth generation scanner

In this system the tube rotates around the patient and there are a large number of fixed detectors arranged in a circle, 1,000 or more being required to produce a high quality picture. Rapid scans of 1–2 seconds are possible and continuous calibration can be carried out during the scan.

Rotating Tube Outside Detector Ring/Fixed Detectors/Nutating action—fifth generation scanner

Both the third and fourth generation scanners have a short tube-detector distance. To increase this distance and use fewer detectors the X-ray tube rotates outside the ring of detectors and by using a nutating action the detectors nearest to the tube are moved away from the X-ray beam (2558).

Thus within the five year period since the introduction of the body scanner, the scanning frame has undergone a number of modifications mainly to reduce scanning times. By suitable modifications the rotate/translate system can operate at 12 seconds but is unlikely to produce scan times much below this figure. While the rotate systems are considerably faster, they are also considerably more expensive, bearing in mind that movement free scans can be obtained in more than 95% of patients with scan times of 14–15 seconds. The main indication for fast scans of 1–2 seconds is to show contrast filled blood vessels (angiotomography) and for very young children.

The slow scanners use oil-cooled fixed anode X-ray tubes but with faster scanners a rotating anode air-cooled X-ray tube is required for the higher output. A pulse mode is used as it simplifies the gating of the detectors. The 'wedges' are shaped bars of aluminium interposed between the X-ray tube and the patient which are used to compensate for different field sizes being scanned. In many machines these wedges are changed manually but corrections for field size on other manufacturers equipment can be done automatically.

The gantry housing the X-ray tube and detectors may be fixed, allowing only horizontal axial sections, or it may be tilted. Tilting the gantry is useful in head scans and in aligning vertebral bodies and their intervening disc spaces in the exact plane of the CT section.

The couch for the patient is positioned at right angles to the gantry (2559) and is now being made as a separate detachable unit on which the patient can be wheeled in and out of the examination room. The surface of the couch is usually hollowed out to fit the contours of the body but needs to be filled in to form a perfectly flat top when scans are being done for radiotherapy planning.

39

The couch top can be moved automatically either up and down to raise and lower the patient or horizontally to move the patient in and out of the scanner. The horizontal movement is usually controlled from the gantry and a digital read-out is provided to show the extent of the movement into the scanning aperture. In the most sophisticated equipment the table top can also be skewed to take oblique sections, and is used particularly for the pancreas.

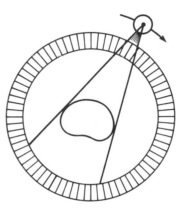

Stationary circular detector array with nutating sensor geometry

1,200 stationary detectors
Scan time 3 - 30 seconds

2558

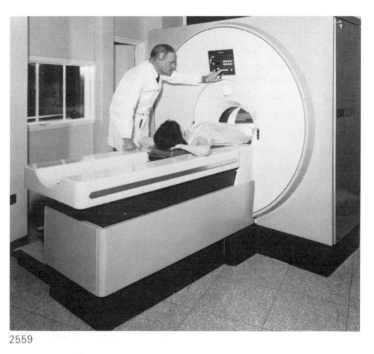

2559

(2557) Diagrammatic representation of the action of a second generation translate/rotate scanner with a fan beam of X-rays.

(2558) Diagrammatic representation of a fifth generation scanner with the X-ray tube outside the ring of detectors.

(2559) A computed tomography scanner showing the table and gantry.

Computed tomography

The Processing Unit
The processing unit consists of one or more mini-computers which start with the raw data received from the scanning gantry, such as the position of the scanning frame during a traverse, reference X-ray output, calibration information, and of course all the readings taken by the detectors. The first stage is to convert this raw data into edge readings or profiles which are then displayed as a picture on the cathode ray tube.

The profile readings are transformed into a picture by a complicated mathematical process called filtered back projection, or the convolutional method, which results in a file in the computer memory, known as a picture file, of 25,600 elements for a 160×160 picture or more than a 300,000 for a 320×320 picture. (2560)

Viewing
Viewing in most systems is by projecting a picture onto a television using recognised TV techniques. Each pixel or picture element represents a tissue attenuation or X-ray absorption value.

Tissue attenuation values have arbitrarily been divided either into 2000 Hounsfield (H) units or 1000 EMI (E) units, with air at -1000 H or -500 E units, water at 0, and a maximum of $+1000$ H units or $+500$ E units to encompass dense bone. Each section examined by CT can be viewed at different 'window' settings.

Window width and window level
The window settings used in viewing each section depend on the region of the body and the required spatial or contrast resolution. Window width refers to how many Hounsfield units are included in the picture and varies in steps of 200 or 100 from 800 down to 2. When 800 units are included the picture has a long grey scale with maximum spatial resolution, while with only 2 units shown there is no spatial resolution but maximum contrast resolution, the picture appearing as a bistable, black and white pictures (2561a, b). Thus when bone detail is required a wide window of 800 is used, for average soft tissue a window of 400–300, and when the liver or brain is being examined a window setting of 200–100.

The window level, on the other hand, is directly related to tissue attenuation values. When the values are low, as for lung, then a level of -800 to -600 is used, for soft tissues $0 - +40$; and for bone $+200 - +400$ (2562).

(2560) Print-out of tissue attenuation values (numbers) of a 1 cm axial section through the mid abdomen.

(2561) Varying appearances of CT section due to changing only the *window width* from 400 E units (800 H units) to 1 unit (2 H units). At wide window settings there is a long grey scale, good spatial resolution and poor contrast resolution. At narrow window settings there is poor grey scale with poor resolution and good contrast.

(2561b) Enlarged views taken from the independent viewing console (NC) by the use of a software programme showing how the appearances are changed by varying only the *window width* from 400–001 E units

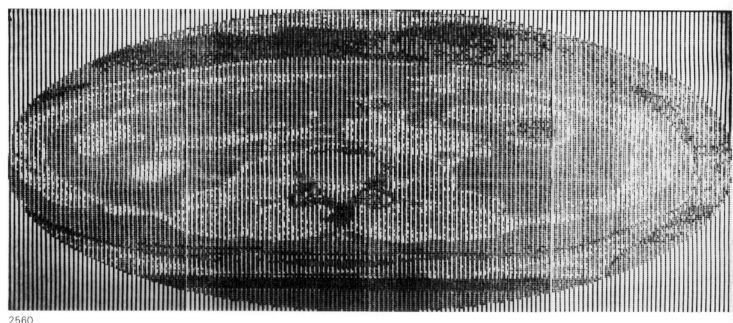

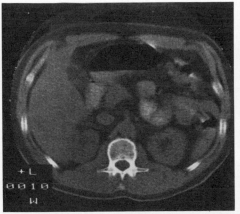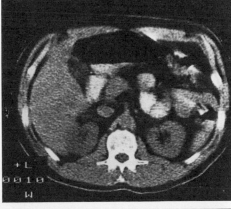

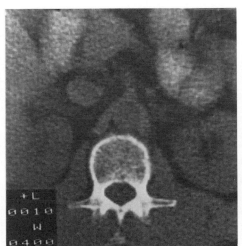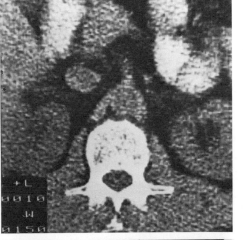

2561a

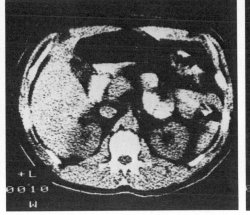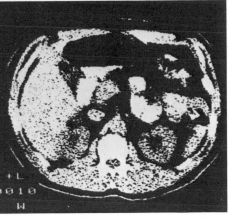

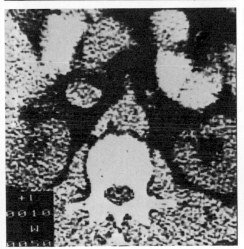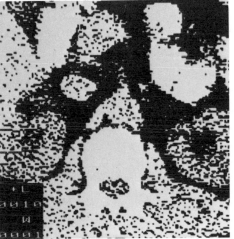

2561b

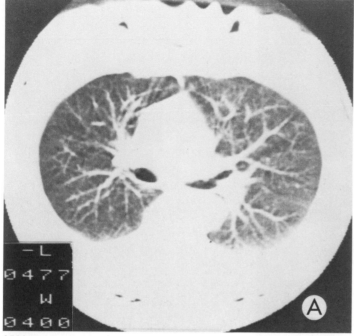

2562a

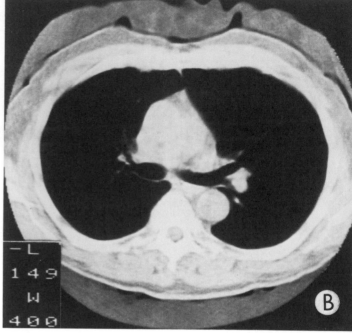

2562b

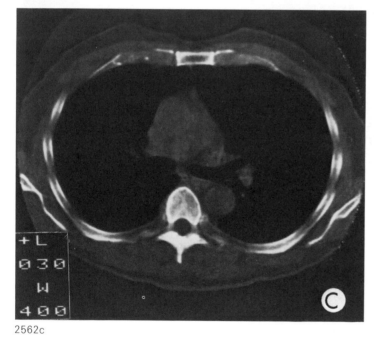

2562c

(2562a, b, c) Section through the thorax showing the effect of varying only the window levels from −477 which shows lungs to −149 showing soft tissues and +30 showing bone.

(2563) A software programme allows the measurement of tissue attenuation values in selected areas. In the supine position the anterior part of the lung has lower attenuation values than the posterior part due to gravity dependent lung perfusion.

(2564) Contrast enhanced ring lesion with surrounding oedema shown in axial sections.

(2565) Computer reconstructions into lateral and frontal sections.

Other viewing facilities

Various other possibilities in viewing include enlargement of any part of the section and showing a section between predetermined Hounsfield numbers. Thus, for instance, fat planes and lipoid tumours can be demonstrated by choosing only Hounsfield numbers between -80 and -20 while abscesses are shown with numbers between $+10$ and $+30$ H.

A small area of the picture can be examined with a variety of statistical modalities by using the 'region of interest' facility to allow tissue attenuation values to be determined in regions of various sizes and shapes (2563). Software programmes are available to view in frontal and coronal planes but require the original examination to be done with continuous or slightly overlapping sections (2564, 2565). There are also facilities available for computing distances, surface areas and volumes, thus making accurate measurements of organs and tumours possible.

Independent viewing console (IVC)

Initial viewing is at the console associated with the scanning gantry and is used for monitoring the examination, or for immediate diagnosis. For review or interrogation of the data, however, an independent viewing console away from the scanner is essential. The independent viewing console (IVC) allows detailed examination of the data, use of special software facilities, and the production of hard copy.

Data storage

The simplest method of storing pictures is on a hard copy whether on radiographic film, polaroid or bromide paper. There are now multiformat cameras which take from one to twelve pictures on a 25×30 cm (10×12 in) film. The advantages of bromide paper are that it contains very little silver and is relatively cheap, producing a print of excellent quality with a good grey scale.

Computer storage is initially on the main memory system disc and the new megabyte disc can hold 50–100 pictures which allows examination of the data directly from the disc on the independent viewing console where it can be transferred to magnetic tape or floppy disc. Otherwise the transfer of data is at the scanning console onto tapes or floppy discs with subsequent viewing on the IVC. Each magnetic tape must be provided with a directory in the form of a print-out from the computer, which contains the tape file numbers and patients identification.

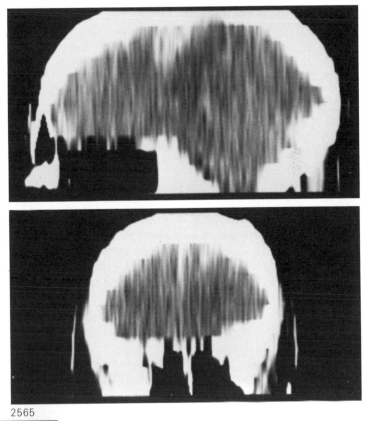

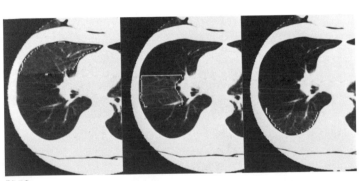

2563

2565

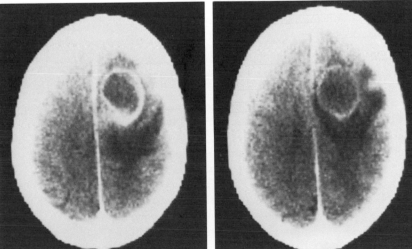

2564

General Comments

Although computed tomography is largely an automated process, neither the care of the equipment nor the management of a patient must be neglected. Computers require a dust-free environment, controlled for temperature and humidity, which is most easily obtained by housing the computer in a small separate air-conditioned room or cupboard.

The equipment is serviced at regular intervals by the manufacturing company, who provide a service contract, but regular checks by the technician or radiographer is also essential. The weekly and daily setting up procedures are listed in the hand book and the graticule alignment or tuning-fork tests are particularly important. If the graticule is out of alignment non-movement streak artefacts occur, particularly at tangents to dense areas such as the spine and pelvis.

Preparation for CT Examinations

There is a considerable variation in the preparation needed for CT examination of the various regions of the body, but irrespective of the clinical problem each patient should receive an explanation of the procedure and the nature of the apparatus. It is especially important to tell patients that they will be examined in a short tunnel and that the machine can be somewhat noisy. Occasional patients are claustrophobic and will need special reassurance. With these patients it may be necessary to carry out the examination in the prone position and it is also a good idea to have the patient inside the aperture starting at the furthest section and then move the patient out of the machine rather than into the machine.

Reassurance and explanation are at all times the basis of good management in radiography and particularly so with CT examinations. Correct preparation and good patient management result in scans of good diagnostic quality which is of course the whole purpose of the examination. The type of preparation depends not only on the region being examined but also on the equipment, and it is therefore important to understand the reason for the kind of preparation being advised.

There are two main reasons for patient preparation. The first is to overcome any movement artefacts, that can be produced by restless, uncooperative patients, from breathing and from bowel movements (2566). Quite clearly movements are more likely to occur with long scan times and will therefore be a particular problem with the 20 second scanner, but even with a 20 second scanner movement free scans can easily be obtained in the head, neck, pelvis and limbs. Conversely most movement artefacts can be easily overcome with 1–2 second scans.

The second major problem is to recognise bowel on abdominal scans. Although, by and large, fluid and solid structures have different attenuation values, small bowel is a notable exception and appears similar to solid organs. It is thus essential to label bowel with a contrast agent so as not to confuse it with mass lesions especially enlarged lymph nodes (2567). The only way of being quite sure that such a problem does not arise is to monitor each section noting whether the contrast medium is visible in the small bowel.

There is a very obvious difference in the quality of scans between obese and lean individuals. Where fat planes are well developed the organs are well demarcated from each other and can be clearly delineated (2568). But with absent fat planes, as in most children and in wasted patients, organ demarcation is absent, often resulting in difficult diagnostic problems (2569). It is particularly in these cases that labelling bowel with a contrast medium becomes essential and often also using intravenous contrast enhancement.

In summary therefore, patient preparation includes explanation and reassurance, taking cognisance of the type of scanning equipment, overcoming movements due to general patient movement, breathing and bowel movements, and adequately labelling bowel. CT produces much better results in obese subjects with well developed fat planes. However in certain circumstances unsuspected factors assume overriding importance, such as claustrophobia or severe backache, which do not allow the patient to lie in the scanner without mental or physical distress. These patients will of course present individual problems, irrespective of the area being examined.

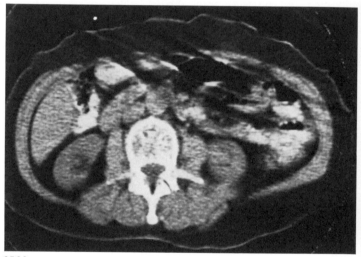

2566

(2566) Movement artefacts producing streaks across the anterior aspect of an abdominal section.

(2567) There is a loop of small bowel unfilled with contrast medium which mimics lymphadenopathy. (arrow)

(2568) Well demarcated abdominal organs in a patient with well developed fat planes.

(2569) With poorly developed fat planes particularly in (b) the internal organs are not easily distinguished from the mass (M) due to metastases from a Cushing's tumour of the adrenal. L=liver, K=kidney, S=spleen, C=colon.

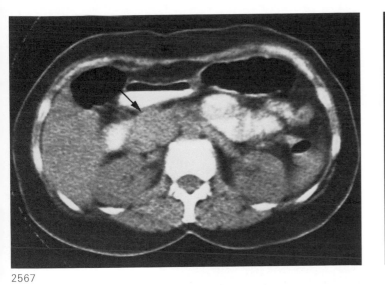
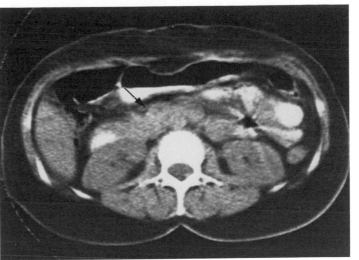

2567

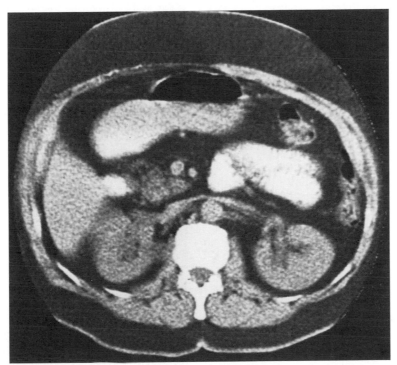

2568

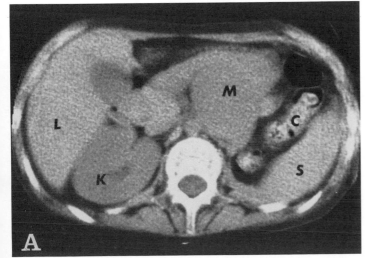
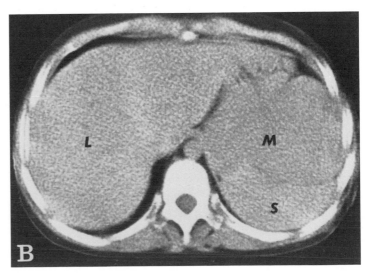

A

B

2569

Position of Patient

In the vast majority of cases scanning is performed with the patient supine. In special circumstances prone or decubitus scans need to be performed to elucidate particular problems, most commonly when small tumours are to be excluded, and particularly in examination of the pancreas. Prone or decubitus scans help to position the contrast medium adjacent to the suspicious area which may then clarify the diagnostic problem.

Contrast medium for stomach and small bowel

Computed tomography is an extremely sensitive method for discriminating between different attenuation values. Therefore very low concentrations of contrast medium usually suffice and conversely very high density substances produce streak artefacts. Until recently barium preparations have been quite unsuitable as there has been sedimentation in the bowel and concentration in the ileum which has resulted in the dense contrast causing artefacts. Consequently a weak solution of gastrografin came into a general use as the contrast medium of choice for labelling the stomach and small bowel for CT examinations.

Generally 300–400 ml of 2–3 % gastrografin, which is a tri-iodinated benzyl ring preparation, is given orally ½–1 hour before the examination and again 10 minutes before the abdominal scans actually start (2570, 2571). Ideally the whole of the small bowel and the stomach should contain the contrast medium so that the bowel is clearly labelled and cannot be mistaken for a tumour.

In some centres 20 mg of metaclopramide (Maxalon) is given orally as a hurrying agent just before the first dose of gastrografin to be sure to have the contrast in the distal ileum. This however will almost certainly empty the stomach completely of contrast, making the second dose imperative if the stomach and upper small bowel are to be visible. Recently a barium preparation from Australia has appeared on the market which claims to be an effective contrast agent for CT, but further trials are awaited.

Contrast for the colon

Gastrografin can also be given rectally, but not routinely. In selected cases the pelvic colon can be rapidly labelled in this way or the patient can be recalled after an interval when the gastrografin has reached the pelvic colon.

As a routine, oral calcium phosphate, 1 g three times per day starting 2 days before the examination, has been found to be an effective way of labelling the colon (2572). Calcium phosphate is inert, is not absorbed from the colon and produces no side effects.

Diet

In some centres a high residue diet, particularly including apples, is recommended. However with the large volume of gastrografin given, especially if preceded by metaclopramide, the gastrocolic reflex is likely to be activated, making the patient uncomfortable and provoking bowel movements. Other centres therefore recommend a low residue diet, to keep the colon relatively empty but hopefully labelled with calcium phosphate.

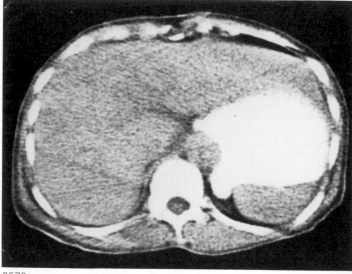

2570

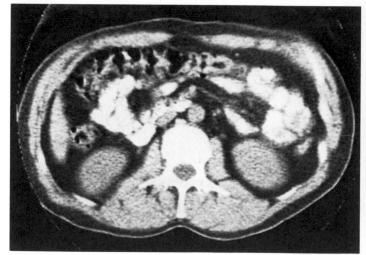

2571

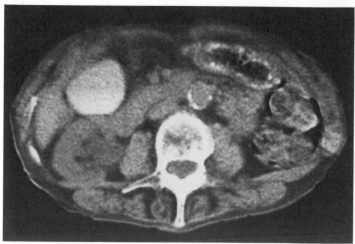

2572

Intravenous contrast enhancement

The use of intravenous contrast enhancement for CT of the brain and orbits is now well established and is often a routine procedure in suspected tumour cases (2573). The usual dose is about 40 g of iodine in a tri-iodinated benzyl ring compound given intravenously, such as 150 ml of meglumine diatrizoate (Conray '280') and may be given either as a bolus injection or drip infusion.

In body CT the use of intravenous contrast enhancement is considerably more complicated.

(a) For *malignant tumours* or inflammatory 'cysts' a regime similar to contrast enhancement in the brain is commonly used (2574).

(b) For the kidneys, ureters, or bladder half the dose is sufficient namely 15–20 g of iodine in a tri-iodinated benzyl ring compound (urographic type contrast agents). (2575)

(c) For vascular enhancement whether of the aorta, venae cavae, or portal venous system a quite different regime is needed. Rapid sequence, fast scans (angiotomography) are essential for a complete examination although a limited amount of information can be obtained with slow scanners. A bolus injection followed by an infusion maintains the concentration of contrast in the intravascular compartment showing the major vessels to best advantage and is applicable to the neck, thorax and abdomen. (2576)

(d) For the liver and pancreas, rapid sequence fast scans immediately following the usual dose of contrast for CT enhancement have been shown to be the most effective method of demonstrating metastases and vascular tumours. Fast scanners are thus essential for this type of examination. This is because in the liver and pancreas intravenous contrast agents achieve a higher concentration in normal tissue than in tumour within the first minute, thereby showing tumour as filling defects. Thereafter the concentrations equalise and the tumours become obscured.

New contrast agents for the liver and spleen may well be produced in the near future, which will overcome the problems associated with the urographic type water-soluble agents. These newer products are retained in the liver parenchyma for up to 48 hours and allow the ready visualisation of metastases.

(e) Biliary contrast agents such as iopanoic acid (Telepaque) and calcium ipodate (Solu-biloptin) have only been used with CT to a limited degree. The normal bile ducts and gall bladder are clearly shown but in clinical practice, this has few applications. (2577)

(f) Intrathecal metrizamide is used for demonstrating tumours of the spinal cord, small acoustic neuromas within the internal auditory meatuses and tumours at the base of the skull such as pituitary tumours encroaching on the basal cisterns. The contrast medium is injected by the lumbar or lateral cervical routes.

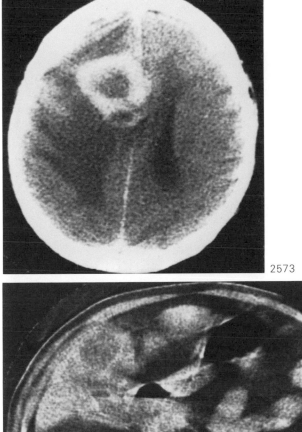

2573

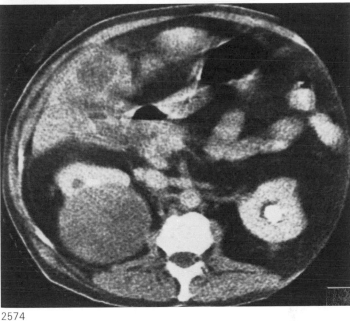

2574

(2570) Poorly developed fat planes. Without contrast medium in the stomach the liver would not be well delineated. There is a posterior prolongation of the fundus of the stomach between the aorta and spleen.

(2571) Contrast medium in the small intestine clearly distinguishes the bowel from the inferior vena cava and the aorta and eliminates the diagnosis of lymphadenopathy in this section.

(2572) The colon is easily identified because it contains calcium phosphate and the gall bladder is shown with calcium ipodate (Solu-biloptin)

(2573) Intravenous urographic agents are used for contrast enhancement of brain lesions such as this metastasis from a breast carcinoma.

(2574) Intravenous contrast enhancement of the kidneys in a right renal cystic kidney carcinoma.

867

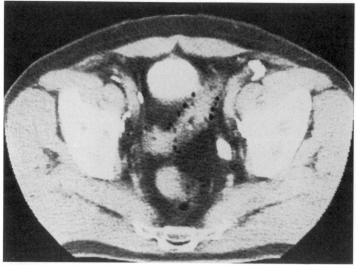

2575

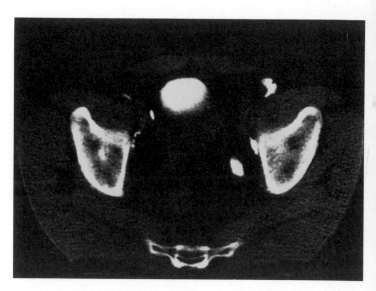

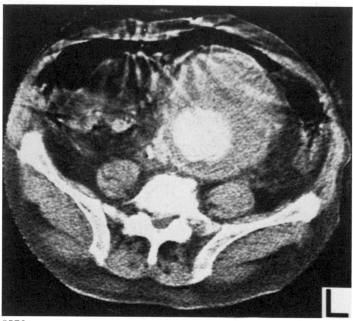

2576

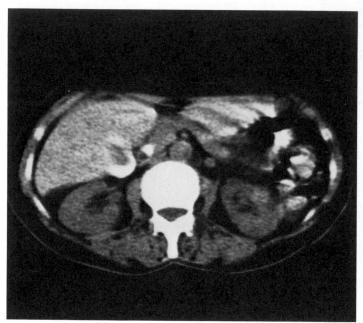

2577

(2575) Intravenous contrast enhancement of the bladder and right hydroureter.

(2576) Intravenous enhancement with a bolus injection and infusion showing the lumen with surrounding thrombus in an abdominal aneurysm.

(2577) Gall bladder and common bile duct shown after iopanoic acid (Telepaque), an oral cholecystographic contrast agent.

Preparation for Different Regions

There is considerable variation in the preparation required from one region to another. Little preparation is usually needed for head or thoracic scans, but it can be quite elaborate for the abdomen. The preparation may need to be modified for particular clinical problems or for urgent cases.

The Head and Neck

In larger children and adults little preparation besides explanation and reassurance is needed in examinations of the brain, orbits, face and neck. The most important aspects of these examinations are to obtain movement-free scans and the use of contrast enhancement.

Restless adults and infants will require sedation or even a general anaesthetic. The liaison between the scanning team, clinicians and anaesthetists is then all-important. With the development of ultrasonography for brain scanning of infants, there is now much less need for CT in this age group.

The Thorax

No specific preparation is required for CT examinations of the rib cage, pleura, lungs or mediastinum. With 18–20 second scans it is important to be sure the patient can maintain breath-holding during the actual scan. In doubtful cases deep rapid respiration, especially of oxygen, just prior to each scan, will allow breath holding for 18–20 seconds.

Some patients are not able to understand or carry out breath-holding without also pinching their noses to block the passage of air. If this type of patient holds his own nose, he can then also hold his breath for the required time.

Therefore, thorax scans can, by and large, be done without preparation provided the patient has had an adequate explanation, has been reassured and oxygen is available.

Contrast enhancement with urographic-type agents is frequently used in the mediastinum to delineate the major vessels, especially the aorta, and must be available for both a bolus injection and drip infusion.

Abdomen

The most complex preparation in CT is in examinations of the abdomen, but even within the abdomen there is considerable variation depending on the region or organ being examined and the nature of the suspected pathology.

Upper Abdomen

Liver, Spleen and Adrenal Glands

Most examinations in this region are carried out for intrahepatic tumours and abscesses, for subphrenic and subhepatic abscesses, and for suprarenal tumours. The major problem is in identifying the stomach (2578, 2579) and the fact that there may be a small prolongation of fundus between the aorta and left kidney, adjacent to the spine, which can resemble a tumour unless adequately filled with gastrografin. The rest of the stomach must also be identified, and especially its relationship to the tail of the pancreas. Gastrografin, 300–400 ml, must therefore be given orally to the patient about 10 minutes before scanning starts.

Contrast enhancement by intravenous urographic agents is frequently used in this region to identify the upper poles of the kidneys, adrenal tumours, and to show liver metastases and abscesses.

(2578) Water in the stomach resembling an upper abdominal subphrenic abscess or haemorrhage.

(2579) Contrast in the stomach clearly showing its position.

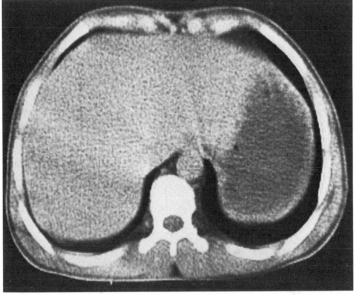

2578

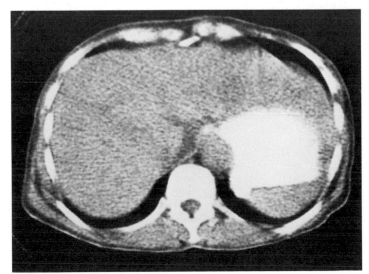

2579

The Pancreas

The preparation of the patient for examinations of the pancreas is somewhat more complex. The colon should be clearly marked and it is important to show the stomach, duodenum, and jejenum.

Calcium phosphate, 1 g three times a day for two days, and gastrografin, 300–400 ml 3–5% 10–15 minutes before the examination, are the important special features, but it is equally important to carefully observe each section done, to see that there is contrast in the bowel around the pancreas.

Intravenous urographic contrast may also be needed for contrast enhancement for angiotomography, but the main requirement is to stop all bowel movement with a myorelaxant when using the 18–20 second scanner.

Middle Abdomen

Lymphadenopathy, Aorta, Kidneys, Retroperitoneal Tumours

These patients require a full preparation with a low residue diet and calcium phosphate for 48 hours, metaclopramide on arrival in the department, 300–400 ml 2–3% gastrografin ½–1 hour before the examination and a further dose of gastrografin 10–15 minutes before the abdominal scans start. Close monitoring of the sections is essential to see that the bowel is adequately filled with contrast.

Intravenous contrast enhancement may also be necessary but the major problem is to stop all bowel movement with a myorelaxant. Glucagon is the myorelaxant of choice for CT scanning, although butyl-N-hyoscine bromide (Buscopan) is also used. The advantage of glucagon is that it produces no side-effects in the doses used for CT apart from the occasional case with nausea or slight diarrhoea at the end of the examination. Glucagon has a short action and therefore is given intravenously through an indwelling 'butterfly' needle, with topping up doses as is required. A loading dose of 0.25 mg is used initially and then 0.1 mg every 10–15 minutes depending on the bowel movement seen during the course of the examination.

The Pelvis

Bladder, Uterus, Ovaries, Colon and Bone

With most equipment, no worthwhile information can be obtained from the pelvis when metal hip prostheses are present, and this should be ascertained before the examination starts.

Pelvic examinations require a full preparation with low residue diet, calcium phosphate, metaclopramide and gastrografin. In addition, the bladder must be full, to displace small bowel from the pelvis (2580). It is therefore most important not to let the patient pass water till after the pelvis has been scanned. In cases where the rectum or sigmoid presents a problem in identification, the pelvic scans may be repeated after a delay of two hours, to fill the colon with the contrast given orally, or the patient may be given an enema of 300 ml of 2% gastrografin.

There is one other very important feature in CT examinations of the pelvis. Because of the surrounding bone and because this is a movement-free area when the bladder is well filled, high-photon or very slow scans are both necessary and possible. With rotate/translate systems, high definition scans which are movement-free can be obtained with a 60–70 second scan, and this is particularly indicated for patients with bladder carcinoma.

The urine in the bladder acts as an excellent negative contrast agent but should a positive contrast agent be needed, an intravenous dose of 30 ml of a 50% urographic contrast is sufficient.

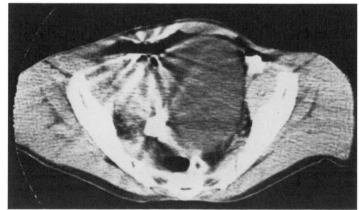

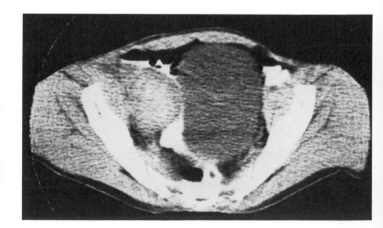

No preparation is needed to examine the limbs, although contrast enhancement by an intravenous urographic type contrast medium may be needed. (2581)

Preliminary Procedures

Before starting the CT examination a recent abdominal and chest film should be viewed. If such films taken within the last two weeks are not available, an abdominal and chest film should be done prior to giving the gastrografin. Not too infrequently an obvious abnormality or opacity is present on the abdominal or chest film which could otherwise present a problem. Certainly dense contrast medium in any quantity could produce unacceptable streak artefacts. It is also important to ascertain whether any calcifications are present on the abdominal film before being obscured by the gastrografin. Tumours treated with radiotherapy, and liposarcomas, for instance, may be partially calcified, and after gastrografin, this diagnostic feature could easily be misinterpreted.

(2580) Movement artefacts hiding a mass of lymph nodes but shown after bowel movements have been stopped with glucagon which is the myorelaxant of choice in CT apart from examination of the adrenals.

(2581) CT section through the thighs in case of haemangio-pericytoma. No preparation is needed but intravenous contrast enhancement may be required.

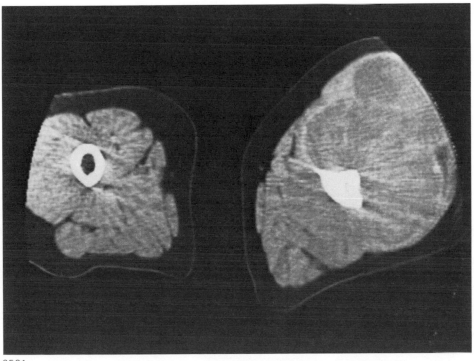

2581

Scanogram

CT examinations consist of axial sections and need to be localised to particular regions. The scanogram is used to decide where to take the sections and in reviewing the examination to know the level of the axial sections. Many of the latest models have an automatic scanogram device which moves the patient across the line of the stationary tube, and also shows the position of the scans which were taken (2582, 2583).

When this facility is not available a conventional scanogram with a slit beam diaphragm (2584) should be done before planning the CT examination. The patient lies supine on an X-ray table in the same position as on the CT scanner, using a long cassette with metal markers at fixed points on the body and skin marks to correspond. The positions for the fixed markers include the manubrio-sternal angle, xiphisternum, iliac crest and superior margin of the pubis. The exposure is made with a slit beam by moving the tube longitudinally down the body (2584).

The film is subsequently used to plan the examination with the axial sections to be taken marked on the film, and then becomes a record of the CT examination itself.

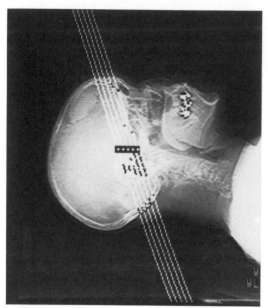

2582a

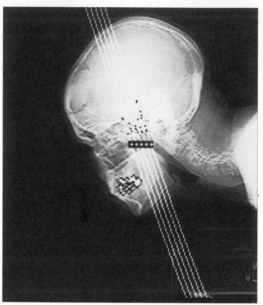

2582c

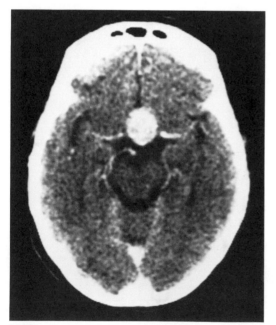

2582b

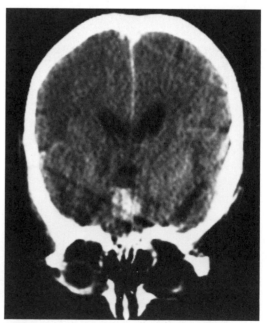

2582d

(2582a, b) Axial scan of pituitary tumour.

(2582c, d) Coronal scan of pituitary tumour.

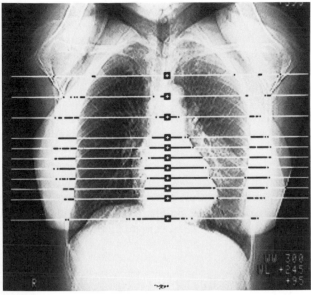

2583a

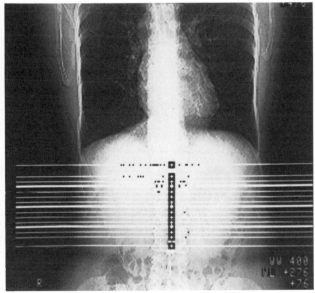

2583b

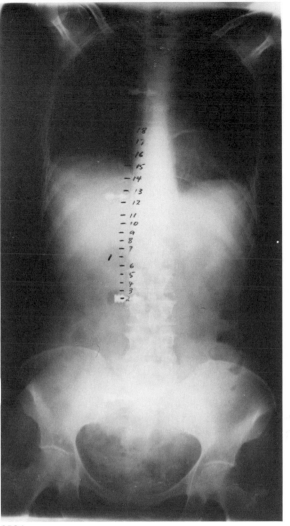

2584

(2582) Automatic scanogram prints showing positions of sections for an examination of the axial sections (a) and in the coronal plane (b).

(2583) Two automatic scanograms taken on the CT scanner; in (a) for a mediastinal cyst and in (b) for pancreatitis.

(2584) Scanogram done in the conventional way with a slit beam diaphragm and metal markers on the skin. The CT sections to be done are subsequently marked on the radiograph.

873

CT Scanning Technique
(Position of the patient and spacing between sections)

The Head, Face and Neck

CT scanning is almost invariably carried out with the patient supine although there are a number of important exceptions. The most notable exception in the head is for coronal sections which are most often done with the patient *prone* and the head extended, but in short-necked individuals coronal sections require a *supine* neck-extended position. A gantry tilt is extremely useful for coronal sections whether these are done supine or prone.

When the head and neck are being examined the patient enters the tunnel head first with the arms by the side of the body. The angulation of Reid's base line for the various regions of the brain has been considered previously (page 581), but in summary, most examinations are done with a 15–20° tilt; for the posterior fossa, a 25–30° tilt is used; and for the pituitary fossa and base of the brain a −10–0° tilt. The face and neck are done in true axial sections, with Reid's base line perpendicular to the table top for the face, but the chin tilted upwards by slight extension of head for the neck examination.

The major problem in the face and upper neck are metal fillings in teeth which on most equipment cause unacceptable streak artefacts. Should this be the case, then the head must be flexed or extended to move the teeth fillings out of the axial section. Teeth fillings are usually more of a hindrance in coronal sections of the head than in axial sections of the face and neck.

The sections through the head are usually contiguous 1 cm sections and through the face and neck, contiguous or at 1.5 cm intervals. The vocal cords require a fast scanner and 0.5 cm thick contiguous sections, while orbits can usually be examined quite adequately with slightly overlapping 1 cm sections. The major advantage of contiguous or slightly overlapping sections is that images in the coronal and sagittal sections can be reconstructed from the axial sections.

The patient must be told *not to swallow* during the examination of the neck as the movements associated with swallowing cause marked artefacts. This applies particularly to the slow scanners, but is applicable to all equipment.

Intravenous contrast enhancement is commonly used in the neck to show the jugular veins and carotid arteries, and for such tumours as the chemodectoma or carotid body tumour.

The Thorax

Although no preparation is needed for scanning the thorax there is a considerable variation in the position of the patient, the distance between sections and whether the examination is done in inspiration or not. For the thorax, the patient enters the aperture of the scanner feet first with the arms positioned above the head.

Anterior Mediastinum

The main clinical indication is for the detection or localisation of a tumour, particularly a thymoma, or lymphadenopathy.

■ The mediastinum is examined in deep inspiration to separate out the structures as far as possible (2585). The patient is supine, having entered the tunnel feet first, with the arms extended above the head. There is thus less tissue in the scan field, less chance of tangential artefacts from the upper humeri, and furthermore with many scanners the patient cannot fit into the scanner with the arms by the side of the chest.

■ One cm sections are done at 1–2 cm intervals depending on the clinical problem. In the search for small tumours the 1 cm sections must be contiguous, but to localise known tumours, diagnose lymphadenopathy, or distinguish fat, fluid or solid masses, sections at 2 cm intervals are adequate.

The Posterior Mediastinum

Most tumours or cysts in the posterior mediastinum are usually quite large and sections at 2–2.5 cm are adequate. The posterior mediastinum is usually examined in neutral respiration but it is most important to distinguish free or loculated effusions and pleural thickening by turning the patient into the prone or decubitus position and repeating the relevant sections. In the posterior mediastinum it is most important to also view with a wide window and at higher window levels to be sure there is no bone erosion or enlargement of the neural canal or intervertebral foramina.

The Aorta

The main indication for CT of the aorta is to show aortic aneurysms or dissection, and it requires contrast enhancement using a bolus injection followed by a drip infusion, and a fast scanner for rapid sequence sections at 2 cm intervals (angiotomography). The patient is in the normal position for thoracic scans, namely supine, feet in first, and the arms raised above the head.

The Lung Parenchyma

The conventional chest radiograph provides sufficient information for most pulmonary conditions but the detection of metastases is a relatively common situation where CT provides more detailed information because of the increased sensitivity of the system. Many more, and smaller, metastases are shown by CT than by conventional radiography, because metastases tend to be subpleural and peripheral in distribution (2586). Before a solitary metastasis is removed surgically, CT should be performed.

■ For the detection of metastases, 1 cm contiguous sections from the apices to the bases should be done, and the examination can then continue into the liver and suprarenals to exclude metastases in these regions as well.

When viewing these sections the bones must also be looked at using a wide window and high levels. (2587)

Most other conditions, such as sarcoidosis and tuberculosis, also show more disease on CT than conventional radiography, but this is almost always irrelevant to the management of the patient. One condition where CT has a role is in lung carcinoma, to see the presence or extent of mediastinal involvement.

■ One cm sections at 1·5 to 2 cm intervals through the lesion and draining lymph nodes are done, but to exclude metastases the examination is as previously described. For a bronchial carcinoma the section should be done in suspended deep inspiration to separate out the mediastinal structures.

The Pleura

CT is especially sensitive in showing minimal pleural disease and in demonstrating the extent of involvement of the thoracic wall and rib cage (2588). Pleural effusions or thickening are a not infrequent associated occurrence, and for a clearer view of the relevant area, or to distinguish effusions and thickening, the patient must be turned into the prone or decubitus position.

■ One cm sections at 2–3 cm intervals are usually sufficient for pleural disease. They can be taken in neutral suspended respiration with repeat sections prone or in the lateral decubitus position to distinguish between fluid and pleural thickening or to move the pleural effusion to uncover any underlying disease.

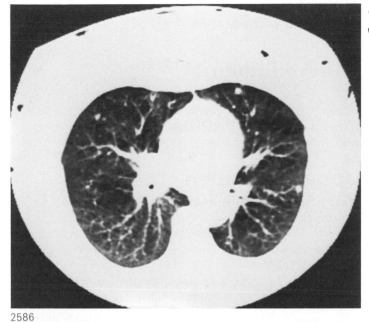

2586

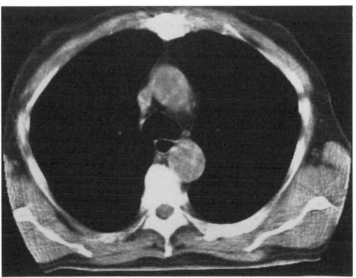

2585

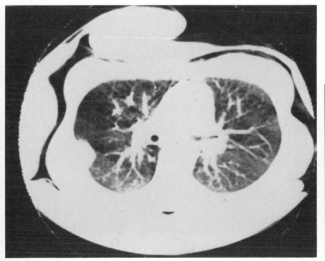

2588

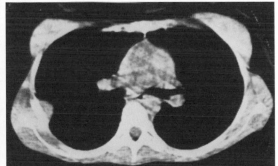

2587

(2585) Section through the thorax taken in deep inspiration to show the mediastinum.

(2586) Multiple small metastases not visible on the chest radiograph. Typically, metastases are peripheral and subpleural in distribution.

(2587) Bone metastases on thoracic sections which were unsuspected and only shown by viewing with wide window, high level settings for bone.

(2588) Pleural lymphoma bulging internally but not invading the underlying rib.

The Abdomen

CT now plays a major role in the diagnosis of intra-abdominal disease particularly in the detection of tumours, in the staging of malignancy, and in localising or diagnosing intraabdominal abscesses.

Upper Abdomen

Liver, Spleen, Subphrenic or Subhepatic Spaces

The type of pathology being sought in this region is usually quite large, particularly intrahepatic (2589) and subphrenic abscesses (2556).

■ Sections at 2·5–3 cm intervals will be adequate for diagnostic purposes but the area covered must be from above the diaphragm to below the level of the liver; an intrahepatic abscess can be in Reidel's lobe. The patient is in the usual CT position, supine with arms above the head, and there must be contrast in the stomach and upper small bowel.

If there is a suspicion of a subhepatic abscess, then prone and decubitus views will probably also be needed to distinguish it from fluid-containing bowel.

To detect liver metastases when the liver is not enlarged, adjacent section at 1 cm must be done, and preferably in rapid sequence within the first minute of a bolus of intravenous contrast medium.

The Adrenals

The search for endocrine tumours such as a pheochromocytoma or Cushing's tumour is an important indication for CT.

■ The patient is in the normal position, supine with arms extended at the shoulders, feet in first into the tunnel. Slightly overlapping or adjacent 1 cm sections are necessary, from the level of the diaphragm to below the level of the adrenals, and suspect sections will need to be repeated with intravenous contrast enhancement.

In extra-adrenal pheochromocytoma, preliminary localisation with biochemical assays from venous catheterisation will indicate the area to be scanned, which may be anywhere from the base of the brain to the pelvis. Adjacent 1 cm sections to cover the relevant area are required.

Glucagon is contraindicated in suprarenal CT for fear of producing a hypertensive crisis in a patient with pheochromocytoma.

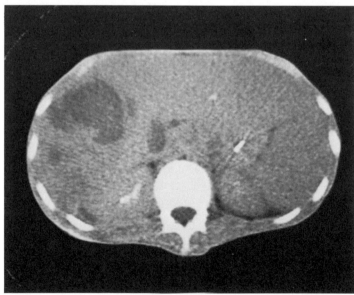

2589

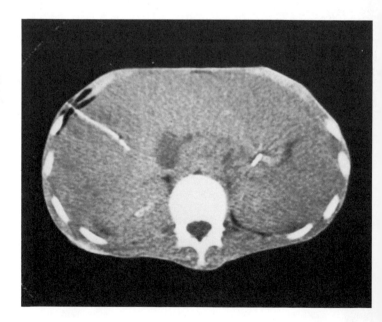

The Pancreas

CT examinations are usually carried out to identify a pancreatic carcinoma or pseudocyst of the pancreas (2590, 2591). It is essential to have gastrografin in the stomach, duodenum and jejunum to label the upper small bowel clearly, and with slow scanners it is imperative to stop all bowel movement with a myorelaxant, preferably glucagon. (2592)

■ For the pancreas, the patient is in the usual supine position, and adjacent 1 cm sections are done to cover the whole pancreas. The head of the pancreas is localised from a supine barium meal duodenal loop film, or from the gastrografin on the scanogram. The sections must start just below the level of the uncinate process of the head of the pancreas, moving cranially to cover the tail of the gland, requiring anything from 6 to 14 sections depending on the obliquity of the pancreas. Angiotomography is needed to diagnose very small tumours and suspect areas will need scans in the prone or decubitus position.

■ If a pseudocyst of the pancreas is detected, sections at 2–2·5 cm must be done from above to below the level of the pseudocyst as seen on the monitor during the scan.

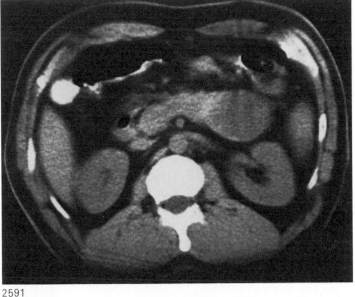

2591

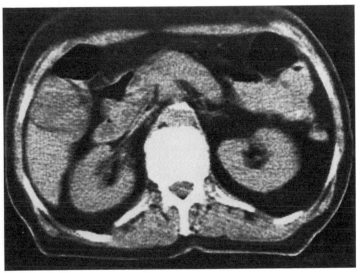

2590

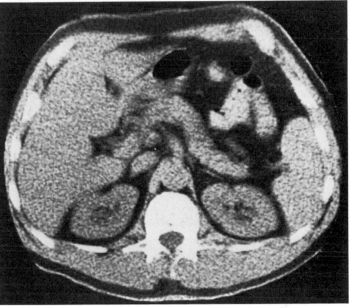

2592

(2589) Liver abscess delineated and subsequently a drain was inserted under CT control.

(2590) Small pancreatic carcinoma on the posterior aspect of the body of the pancreas.

(2591) Pseudocyst of the tail of the pancreas in case of chronic pancreatitis.

(2592) Normal pancreas lying in front of the superior mesenteric artery arising from the aorta.

Lymphadenopathy

The detection of enlarged lymph nodes (2593) in Hodgkin's and non-Hodgkin's lymphoma in the staging of the disease, is a major indication for CT, and has largely replaced lymphography.

A full preparation for the colon and small bowel is needed with careful monitoring during the examination. Any suspicious area without contrast-filled bowel clearly visible must be rescanned when the gastrografin has reached the area. A myorelaxant is essential with the slower scanners and for the pelvic sections the bladder must be full.

■ The patient is in the normal CT position, supine, feet in first into the scanner with arms above the head. One cm sections at 2·5–3 cm intervals are done, to cover the whole abdomen from just below the pubis to above the diaphragm. If there is any suspicion of intrathoracic disease further sections at 2–2·5 cm are taken to cover the thorax.

The sections through the diaphragm include two important lymph node regions, namely the pericardial and the retrocrural nodes (2594) and must therefore be included in the abdominal examination. The lymph node drainage from testicular tumours is to para-aortic nodes around the first and second lumbar vertebrae, but occasionally the lymph nodes of the pelvis are also involved. Metastases to the lung bases are also not infrequent, especially with teratoma of the testis.

■ One cm sections at 2 cm intervals from L5 to well above the level of the diaphragm will cover the major possible regions of spread of the disease, including para-aortic lymphadenopathy, liver and suprarenal metastases, and metastases to the lung bases. In some centres sections at 2·5 cm through the pelvis are recommended, and these must be done if there is any suspicion of spread of the disease.

■ For other malignant conditions infiltrating lymph nodes, such as melanoma, only the region of the relevant draining nodes is examined—usually the pelvis, with 1 cm sections at 1·5–2 cm intervals.

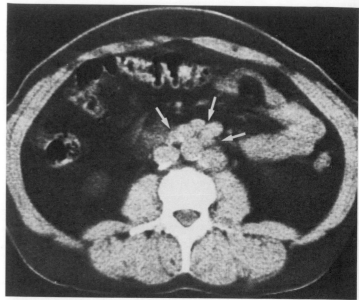

2593

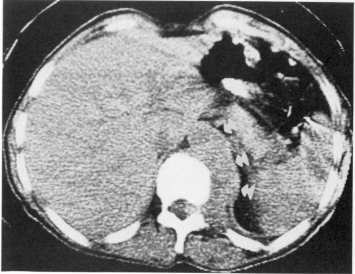

2594

(2593) Moderate para aortic lymphadenopathy (arrows) in a case of Hodgkin's disease.

(2594) Retrocrural nodes (arrows) due to lymphadenopathy from teratoma testis.

The Aorta and Inferior Vena Cava

For an effective CT examination of the aorta angiotomography is required, though limited but useful information can be obtained with a slow scanner. A bolus of contrast followed by a drip infuśon is given, the sections starting immediately the bolus injection has been completed. (2576)

■ One cm sections at 2 cm intervals are then done, from the diaphragm to the aortic bifurcation, in as rapid a sequence as possible.

For the inferior vena cava, a slow intravenous injection at the foot will show its full extent

■ One cm sections at 2 cm intervals from the pelvis to the diaphragm are done during the injection of contrast.

The Kidneys

The intravenous urogram remains the standard screening procedure to detect morphological abnormalities of the kidney. Patients coming for CT scan will therefore have supine films of the region to localise the position of the kidneys, which is then marked on the scanogram. The main indications for CT include distinguishing tumours from cysts, (2595) detecting perinephric haemorrhage or abscess, and seeing whether a mass lesion arises in the kidney or in adjacent structures. Not infrequently unsuspected hydronephrosis, due to obstruction of the ureter by enlarged paravertebral lymph nodes, is detected in examining patients with abdominal malignancy.

■ One cm sections at 1·5–2 cm intervals are done from just above to just below the kidneys and repeat sections after intravenous contrast enhancement will be needed to elucidate 'mass' effects which are not obviously a cyst. Rapid sequence angiotomography is valuable for showing involvement of the renal vein and inferior vena cava by tumour thrombus.

Retroperitoneal Sarcoma

There is no effective method at present other than CT of clearly defining the position and extent of retroperitoneal sarcomas (2596). These are usually large tumours and may contain calcium. A recent plain film of the abdomen is essential before the CT examination starts, and for artefact-free scans a full preparation is required, delineating small bowel and preventing bowel movements with a myorelaxant.

■ One cm sections 2·5–3 cm intervals from above to below the level of the mass must be taken. Intravenous contrast enhancement does not usually contribute any significant extra information within the tumour, but clearly defines the kidneys and ureters in relationship to the retroperitoneal sarcoma which frequently encroaches on the abdominal cavity.

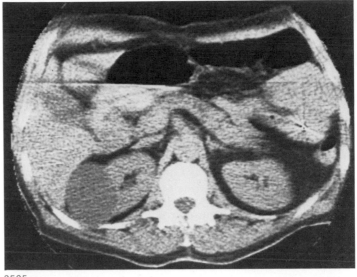

2595

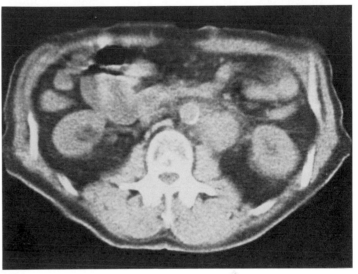

2596

(2595) Cyst of the right kidney adjacent to the liver.

(2596) Retroperitoneal sarcoma lying between the aorta and the left kidney and anterior to the psoas.

The Pelvis

The main indications for CT of the pelvis are the delineation of mass lesions, whether due to tumour or abscess, including carcinoma of the bladder, cervix and ovary and recurrent carcinoma of the colon. Bone tumours and their soft tissue component are also clearly shown by CT. Lymphadenopathy has been previously considered (p. 878).

A full preparation is essential for pelvic examinations. The bladder must be well filled and a myorelaxant must be used both to stop any bowel movements and relax the bladder. (2597)

■ The pelvis is examined with 1 cm sections done contiguously from the pubis to the sacrum. If a mass is uncovered, sections at 2–2·5 cm intervals must be done till the whole of the mass has been shown, as well as the region of the draining para-aortic lymph nodes. For an ovarian carcinoma the draining lymph nodes are in the region of first and second lumbar vertebrae at the hila of the kidneys. If contrast medium is needed to delineate the bladder, an intravenous injection of 20–30 ml of 50% urographic agent is sufficient and scanning starts 15 minutes later.

Staging of malignancy

A knowledge of both the extent of the disease and the total bulk of the tumour is required for the accurate staging of malignancy. This would in theory require total body scanning, which is clearly impractical as a routine. CT is used, by and large, only when there is evidence that the primary tumour is no longer confined and the examination is directed to areas where metastases are known to occur. The most extensive examinations are for lymphoma patients when frequently both the abdomen and thorax are scanned at 2–2·5 cm intervals. (2598)

■ For abdominal malignancies the para-aortic nodes, liver, adrenals, and lung bases must be covered, and for most intrathoracic tumours the lungs, liver, adrenals, and upper abdominal nodes, with sections at 2 cm intervals. When viewing, the bones must be included with wide window and high level settings.

Body CT examinations in malignancy are particularly indicated when serum tumour markers such as carcinoembryonic antigen (CEA) are positive.

Radiotherapy

Scanning for radiotherapy planning is a major indication for computed tomography. The tumour mass will invariably have been delineated at a previous CT examination and therefore no special preparation is necessary.

The patient must lie on the scanner table in exactly the same position as will be needed on the radiotherapy couch, which is usually supine but may be prone. The main variations from diagnostic CT are that the scanner top must be quite flat, with the hollows of the scanner table top filled in, and the scan is done in quiet breathing. The patient must be positioned

accurately with skin markers to correspond exactly to the position on the radiotherapy table.

For the face and neck, positioning is simplified by scanning the patient in the plastic radiotherapy shell which produces a reproducible position from radiotherapy couch to scanner table. The skin must be accurately marked to show the positions of the relevant scans.

■ One cm sections are done at 2·0–2·5 cm from above to below the level of the tumour, with the patient in the exact position to be assumed on the radiotherapy couch and during quiet breathing. Skin positioning marks must remain on for the radiotherapy sessions.

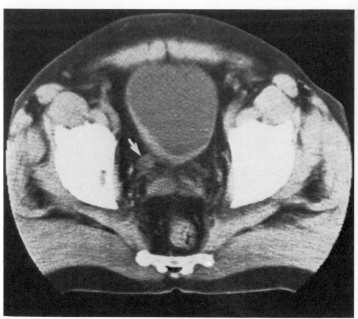

2597

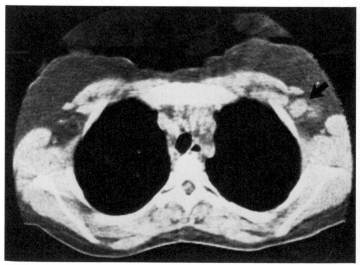

2598

Tumour and abscess localisation

For cytology and aspiration

The CT service should be organised in such a way as to undertake the aspiration and drainage of abscesses and fine needle aspiration cytology under CT control.

The examination is performed in the normal way and then a localising section is done over the relevant area and the skin marked at the level of the axial section. The section is viewed and the depth of the lesion and angle of the needle estimated. Using local anaesthetic, a small needle is positioned to correspond with the entry and angulation of the aspirating needle and the same section scanned to check on the position of the needle. The traverse of the table must be accurately calculated so that the needle can be sited in the exact position for scanning and aspiration (2599).

The needle or catheter is then inserted to the required position and depth, and cytology or aspiration and drainage as indicated is carried out. For cytology a check scan for localisation of the needle tip is advised before the aspiration.

Following abscess aspiration the pus must be sent for microbiology, and cytology slides should be correctly prepared after tumour fine needle aspiration. Follow-up scans at 10 days and one month will be needed after abscess drainage.

Radiation dose

Normally the radiation received by a patient during a CT examination is about the equivalent of a plain film examination of the abdomen and certainly considerably less than an intravenous urogram or barium meal, but the rationale of CT radiation dosage must be appreciated. Provided there are no adjacent, repeat, or overlapping sections, the radiation dose for one section is the same as the whole examination because each section scanned is irradiated with a narrow beam of X-rays; the radiation dose is therefore not summated. However, with adjacent sections there is an increase of about 50% due to scatter.

With a rotate/translate scanner the skin dose on the tube side is about 3 rads and about 0·5 rads at the opposite side with 1 cm sections, but to maintain spatial resolution the dose needs to be greatly increased for 5 mm and 2 mm sections.

The region that causes most concern is the lens of the eye, particularly for thin section examinations of the pituitary fossa. The eyes must be away from the rotating side of the tube which should be under the table and not over it as in the early CT scanners. If the tube rotates over the table, these thin section examinations in the region of the orbit must be done with the patient prone and face down.

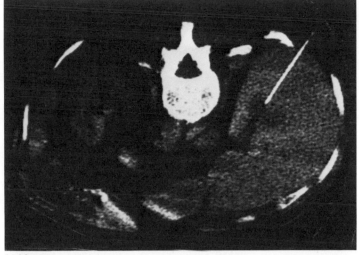
2599a

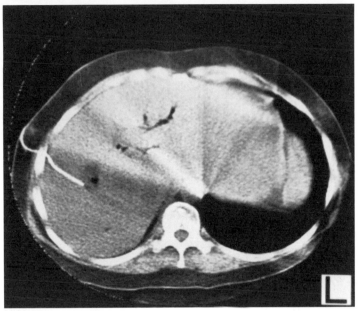
2599b

(2597) Thickened bladder wall due to carcinoma causing a right hydroureter (arrow).

(2598) Mediastinal and left axillary lymphadenopathy (arrow) in a case of lymphoma.

(2599a) Needle in the liver shown on CT section to localise the tip of the needle in an abscess.

(2599b) Catheter inserted into small liver abscess with CT control.

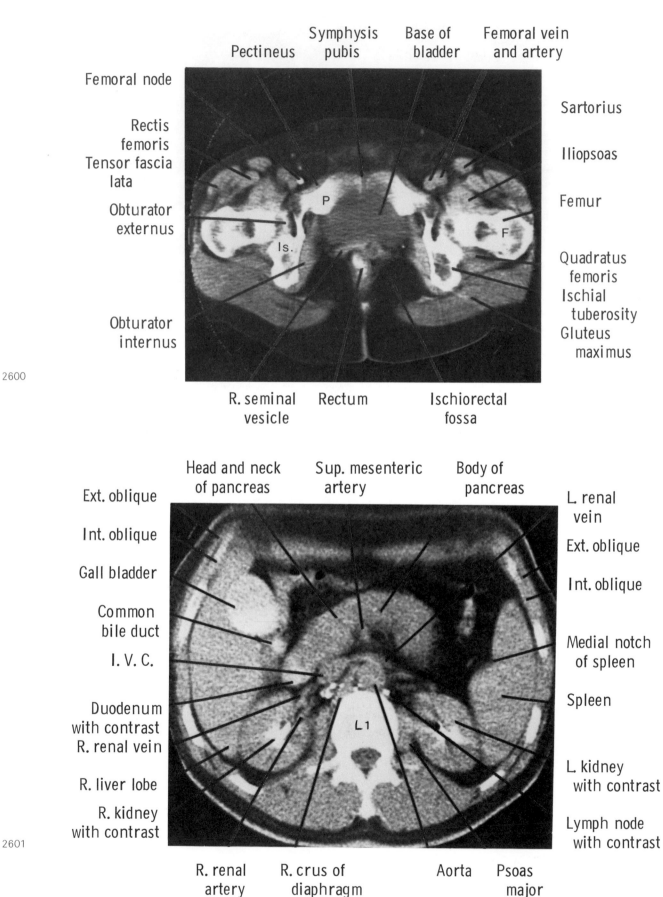

Pectineus · Symphysis pubis · Base of bladder · Femoral vein and artery

Femoral node

Rectis femoris
Tensor fascia lata

Obturator externus

Obturator internus

Sartorius

Iliopsoas

Femur

Quadratus femoris
Ischial tuberosity
Gluteus maximus

P

Is.

F

2600

R. seminal vesicle · Rectum · Ischiorectal fossa

Head and neck of pancreas · Sup. mesenteric artery · Body of pancreas

Ext. oblique

Int. oblique

Gall bladder

Common bile duct

I. V. C.

Duodenum with contrast
R. renal vein

R. liver lobe

R. kidney with contrast

L. renal vein

Ext. oblique

Int. oblique

Medial notch of spleen

Spleen

L. kidney with contrast

Lymph node with contrast

L1

2601

R. renal artery · R. crus of diaphragm · Aorta · Psoas major

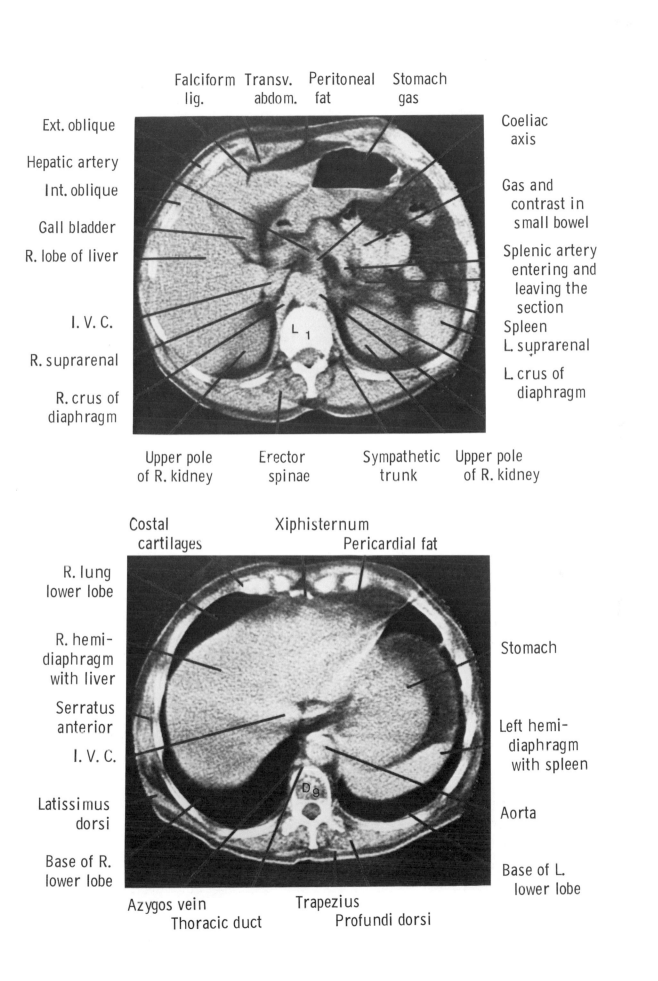

Falciform lig.
Transv. abdom.
Peritoneal fat
Stomach gas
Ext. oblique
Hepatic artery
Int. oblique
Gall bladder
R. lobe of liver
I. V. C.
R. suprarenal
R. crus of diaphragm
Coeliac axis
Gas and contrast in small bowel
Splenic artery entering and leaving the section
Spleen
L. suprarenal
L. crus of diaphragm
Upper pole of R. kidney
Erector spinae
Sympathetic trunk
Upper pole of R. kidney

L 1

2602

Costal cartilages
Xiphisternum
Pericardial fat
R. lung lower lobe
R. hemi-diaphragm with liver
Serratus anterior
I. V. C.
Latissimus dorsi
Base of R. lower lobe
Stomach
Left hemi-diaphragm with spleen
Aorta
Base of L. lower lobe
Azygos vein
Thoracic duct
Trapezius
Profundi dorsi

D 9

2603

Machine Management

There are four main aspects of managing computed tomography equipment.

    a)   The 'switching on' procedure
    b)   entering patient data
    c)   selecting radiographic factors
    d)   patient positioning and scanning

A.   'Switching on' procedure

1.   With equipment from some manufacturers such as the Phillips tomoscan '300' the mains isolator is left on continually to keep the detector bank at a uniform working temperature to maintain the stability of the CT numbers. Otherwise the main isolator must first be switched on before proceeding.

2.   Switch on the main switch of the Operator's Viewing Console (OVC).

3.   The system including the 80 megabyte disc is then run up for 1 minute.

4.   The computer core memory (96K) is brought into operation by the 'bootstrap' procedure by pressing the appropriate buttons on the front panel of the computer.

5.   The date and time is typed into the Visual Display Unit (VDU) and equipment is ready for 'Tube warm up' procedure consisting of 7 exposures over a 10 minute period.

6.   Magnetic tape is loaded and the system is ready for patient scanning which starts with the positioning of the patient.

B.   Entering patient data

The Operators Viewing Console (OVC) has both a computer keyboard as well as single function buttons for more rapid manipulations.

    Press 'Patient data' button and enter:—
        Patient's name
        Patient's identification (hospital number)
        Date of birth
        Sex
        Free comment up to 40 digits usually takes 1 minute.

C.   Selecting radiographic factors

    (i)   Field of view
    (ii)   Slice thickness—varies from 3 to 12 mm, with a choice of 13 calibration files.
    (iii)   Slice 'pitch'—distance between sections
    (iv)   Scan times—210°—2·8 seconds
                   360° fast—4·2 seconds
                   360° slow—8·4 seconds

N.B. 210° produces 300 profiles
      360° fast produces 600 profiles
      360° slow produces 1200 profiles

D. Patient positioning and scanning

1.   Select patient orientation e.g. feet first, supine. A light beam is used for positioning the table and after pressing the appropriate button on the table the patient is automatically moved into the scan plane.

2.   The scanogram on the Operators Viewing Console (OVC) is selected with a single function button and the gantry is automatically adjusted to the scanogram or vertical position.

3.   An exposure is made which moves the patient on the table with the tube pulsing every 1·5 mm for a length of 35 cm giving an instant reconstruction as shown on the Visual Display Unit (VDU).

4.   The 'Select—slice' button is pressed and a light pen is used to select the level at which the scan is to be started.

5.   Press 'Go-to-scan-plane' button on scanning table and the patient is automatically moved to the scanning level selected which is accurate to within 1 mm.

6.   Table movement is selected from either 'table inward' or 'table outward' button and the machine is ready for scanning.

7.   The next scan is selected and the table moves automatically to the next position.

8.   Scanning times on fast scanners range from 3·8 seconds with interim reconstruction times of about 10 seconds and final reconstructions at 20 seconds.

9.   The images are automatically filed onto tape but can also be filed on floppy-discs or photographed on a free standing camera.

10.   There may be a delay between scans for tube cooling. With low photon dose there is no waiting time, for medium dose 30 seconds cooling time and with high photon dose 1 minute tube cooling time.

Low	dose 120 Kv 150 mA—skin dose	1 rad
Medium dose 120 Kv 350 mA—skin dose		1·5–2 rad
High	dose 120 Kv 450 mA—skin dose	3 rad

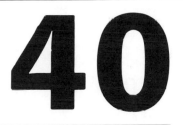

NUCLEAR MAGNETIC RESONANCE IMAGING (ZEUGMATOGRAPHY)

40 SECTION 40

NUCLEAR MAGNETIC RESONANCE (NMR) IMAGING (ZEUGMATOGRAPHY)

Introduction

Isotope scanning, ultrasonography and computed tomography are mature clinical tools but nuclear magnetic resonance scanning has only just reached the stage of clinical evaluation. There is at present a very limited number of centres with apparatus for examining patients and then only brain and extremity scans can be done. Nevertheless, the potential of this method in tumour diagnosis is considerable and inherently has many advantages. It is completely safe at diagnostic energies, has no radiation effect, the equipment has no moving parts, scans can be acquired in any desired plane and bone or gas does not degrade the image. NMR is thus likely to be a major scanning modality in the future.

History

In chemistry and physics NMR has been a well established technique for analysis of dynamics and structure of various compounds for the last 30 years but it was only after Lauterbur in 1973 showed how projections could be reconstructed using NMR signals that investigation began of this scanning modality. The next important development came when Hinshaw in 1974 produced three-dimensional image reconstruction by a system known as 'spin-mapping' and subsequently made even faster picture times possible by simultaneously scanning complete lines of each plane to produce a two-dimensional view. The Nottingham team were thus able, by 1978, to produce images of the human wrist and guinea pig skull. The first head scans bearing a striking similarity to CT were produced by Moore and Holland in 1979.

Principles of NMR Scanning

Water is universally present in body tissue and the hydrogen nucleus or proton is particularly favourable for NMR scanning. Protons have two fundamental properties which are relevant to NMR; spin and a small magnetic moment. Protons thus behave as small spinning magnets and when placed in a magnetic field, their magnetic moment μ tends to turn in a direction parallel to the field (2604). But because of the spin the protons respond to this force like a gyroscope, with their axes precessing about the direction of the magnetic field (B) (2605).

The frequency (v) of the precession is proportional to the force or couple (c) (2606), as propounded in the theorem of Larmor, and therefore to the magnetic field (B)

i.e. $v = cB$

where c depends on the gyromagnetic properties of the nucleus. For protons in a magnetic field (B) of one tesla, the frequency (v) is 42·6 MHz. In practice this is the order of short wave frequency used in NMR scanning.

If a coil is now wound around a volume of protons (water), subjecting it to a radio frequency (rf) current at the Larmor frequency v in the previous equation, then the resonant short pulse can be arranged to turn the magnetisation through 90°. This is called a 90° pulse.

The protons now precess at 90° around the magnetic field (B) at the same frequency v and induce a minute current (electromotive force, emf) in the coil which, when amplified, can be displayed on an oscilloscope. This signal is called a free induction decay (FID) and lasts for some seconds. The time constant of this decay is the *transverse relaxation time* or T_2.

If a resonant radio frequency of twice the previous length is applied through the coil, the magnetisation of protons will be rotated through 180°, and at the end of the pulse lies in the opposite direction to the original magnetic field. The return of the protons to their original position is exponential and is known as the *spin—lattice relaxation time or T_1*.

For pure water T_1 and T_2 are equal being several seconds, and for cellular water several tenths of a second. For malignant tissue the values for T_1 and T_2 are about twice as long as for normal tissue.

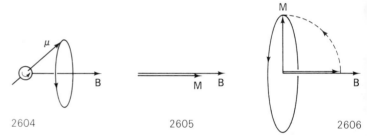

2604   2605   2606

Methods of NMR Imaging

To produce NMR images not only must there be a magnetic field but the object must also be subjected to a small magnetic gradient so that the protons along the line of the increasing gradient will show progressively increasing NMR frequencies. A proton NMR spectrum can therefore be shown which will be a linear profile of proton density within the field gradient. Thus a tube of water in such a field with a gradient across it will produce a linear profile as shown in (2607).

To produce a two-dimensional display, as is required for scanning images, either the field gradient must be moved progressively around the subject or the subject must be rotated within the field gradient. Many linear profiles can then be

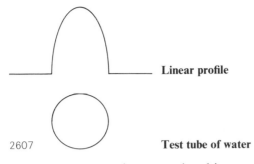

Linear profile

2607 **Test tube of water**

reconstructed by computer to produce a sectional image. The first NMR images of Lauterbur in 1973 used this projection reconstruction method.

It is interesting to note that the spatial resolution of the images is not dependent on the wave length of the radiation, which is of the order of 10 metres, but on the gradient of the magnetic field. The magnetic field on which the spatial resolution depends is coupled to the electromotive force of the protons in the object, hence the term zeugmatography from the Greek *zeugma* meaning 'that which joins together'.

There are a number of methods for acquiring signals given off by the protons after being subjected to the resonating magnetic field. While the original approach used by Lauterbur allowed small test tubes to be scanned, it is too cumbersome to be used for image reconstruction for anatomical sections, especially in clinical practice. However if a time-dependence is applied to the gradients during measurements the required computation becomes possible. The method first successfully applied by Hinshaw is known as 'spin-mapping'.

In 'spin-mapping' the object is in a uniform magnetic field with three field gradients applied at right angles to each other and modulated at different low frequencies. Because each alternating gradient has a plane in which the field is constant—the null plane—the point where the three planes meet will be a null point or point where the field is constant. The recorded NMR signals taken through a low pass filter will then come from the region of the null point. By moving this point across the body at successive intervals a cross-sectional image can be obtained, and this overcomes the necessity for reconstructing the point of origin of the NMR signal.

The multiple sensitive point method produces images much more quickly by acquiring signals from a whole line of tissue simultaneously rather than from individual points. It is also possible to collect data simultaneously from a whole pre-selected two dimensional section. Each method has advantages and disadvantages. At present Moore and Holland have pioneered a NMR head scanner by collecting data along pre-selected lines in a particular plane.

The NMR signals can also be detected in two distinct ways, either being continuous with the system in a steady state of excitation or pulsed with a reduced sensitivity below the T_1 time between radio frequency pulses.

There are thus a number of different combinations possible to produce an NMR scanner. There is no firm method that will finally prove to be the most successful.

For practical clinical purposes an air-cored magnet with a central gap of about 40 cm in diameter is needed, having a uniform field to at least 1 part in 10^4, and up to 1 part in 10^6 for some NMR techniques. Because the thickness of tissue gives rise to attenuation and phase shift of the radio frequency signal in the body, to keep artefacts to a minimum the NMR operating frequency is kept below 10 MHz for whole body imaging and 20 MHz for the head. This gives an upper limit of the field strength for body of 0·23 T (tesla) for the body and 0·46 T for the head.

Super-conducting solenoids of the size required for body imaging would be too expensive, and therefore air cored magnets with a complex Helmholz geometry have been adopted, which consist of two large central coils with two smaller diameter coils outside these. It is also an advantage to use a system which is particularly insensitive to field non-uniformity, and this can be achieved if the field gradient used to form a projection is strong (0.6 m T cm^{-1}) compared with the main field non-uniformity.

If this system is used, the equipment requires no exhaustive protection against stray magnetic fields and can be placed in a normal hospital environment. However, photo-multipliers, cathode-ray tubes as used in image intensifiers, Gamma cameras and ultrasound scanners must be at least 6 m from the centre of the magnet. Watches and similar scientific equipment must be kept away from the magnet, which will disturb their function, and the magnet must be protected, preferably by a large wire cage, so that no loose iron objects will 'fly' towards the magnet when in operation. The force and speed with which nuts, bolts and spanners in the vicinity of the magnet will travel towards its centre could be lethal for a patient lying within the air-core during an examination.

The computation requirements are virtually identical to those of X-ray CT systems. The Fourier transform functions, back projection and system controls can be handled by a small mini-computer, but for faster processing, as is currently practiced with X-ray CT, dedicated hardware processors are needed.

Present Status of NMR Equipment

There are no machines being used for regular day-to-day examinations of patients in hospital practice, although equipment is on the point of being installed in some hospitals. Brain scans of normal volunteers show a remarkable similarity to CT scans but with significant differences due to the nature of the physical characteristics of the wave energy being used. For instance, with X-ray CT bone produces marked attenuation, whereas with NMR no signals originate from bone nor for that matter from within normal blood vessels with active movement. Already the best NMR images of brain are superior to those of routine CT brain scans, but take 1–2 minutes to produce. NMR images of the human abdomen or thorax suitable for clinical use have now been produced, and could well be available shortly in hospital practice.

40 Nuclear Magnetic Resonance

Advantage of NMR Imaging

NMR imaging uses non-ionising electromagnetic radiation and at the radio frequencies required to produce images in humans, appears to be without detectable hazard. Scanning can be achieved in any plane simply by switching the orthogonal x, y and z co-ordinates. Thus axial, coronal and sagittal sections can be produced directly (without reconstruction programmes as is required for X-ray CT). Adjacent sections, whether in axial, coronal or sagittal planes, can be done by electrical switching without moving the patient.

The anatomical images are likely to be as good as those taken with X-ray CT, and could therefore be substituted in the vast majority of clinical conditions, but with the added advantage of the possibility of greater tissue characterisation than is possible at present. Work on NMR to date indicates quite strongly that the relaxation time (especially T_1) is significantly increased for biopsy samples of cancerous tissue. If malignancy can be diagnosed with certainty *in situ*, diagnostic imaging will indubitably make an even greater impact in medical management, than that already achieved with nuclear medicine, ultrasonography and X-ray computed tomography.

Other diagnostic possibilities include imaging of blood vessels and the determination of blood flow. Non-contrast angiography will then be possible, with the added advantage of non-invasive blood flow determinations and visualisation of thrombus.

Further in the future NMR imaging with other nuclei including carbon, sodium and phosphorous may become possible, leading to biochemical analysis *in situ* in a variety of normal and pathological states. Moreover, NMR 'contrast' agents may be developed to give yet more useful clinical information.

NMR imaging equipment contains no moving parts and is unlikely to be more expensive then X-ray CT and possibly considerably less so.

Disadvantages of NMR Imaging

At present the scanning times for acquiring data for NMR images of the abdomen and thorax are too long to produce images free of movement artefacts, and clearly this problem must be overcome before body imaging is accepted in clinical practice.

The possibility of a serious accident from metal objects flying into the air core of the magnet while a patient is in position will need stringent precautions. The effects on patients with epilepsy are still to be determined, and scanning cardiac patients having pace-makers could well be contraindicated.

The non-visualisation of bone has both advantages and disadvantages. There is the possibility of imaging bone marrow for haemopoietic diagnoses but scanning metabolic or diffuse bone disease is likely to be non-informative.

To compete effectively with the other imaging modalities, NMR must ultimately either yield new but relevant information, or be cheaper, if it is to make a clinical impact. The non-ionising nature of the electro-magnetic radiation used in NMR could well be an overriding consideration in the future.

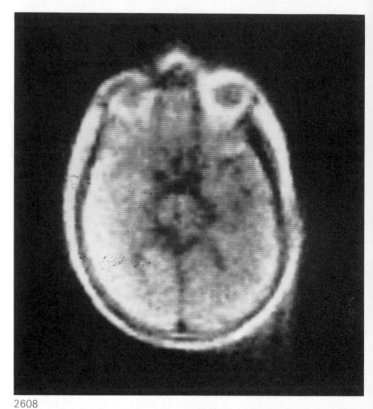

2608

2609

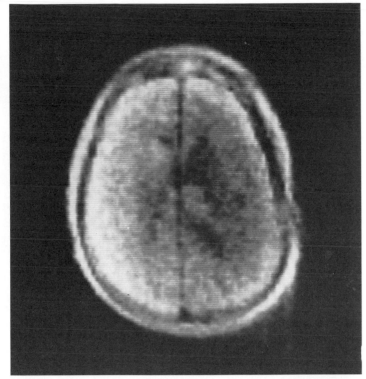

2610

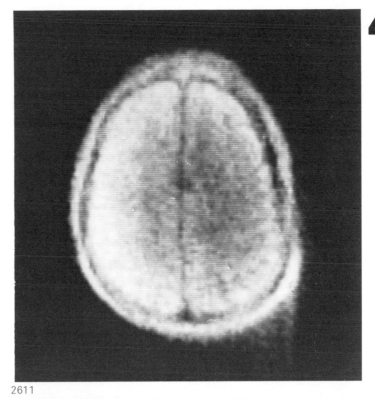

2611

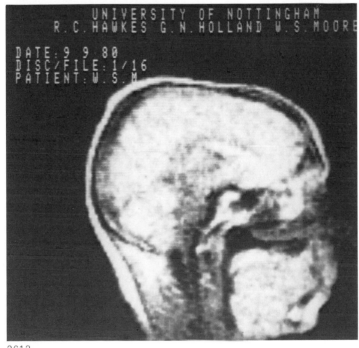

2612

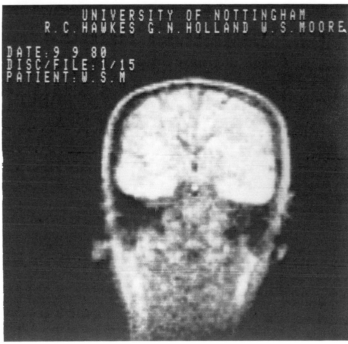

2613

(2608) NMR scan in the axial plane through the base of the brain showing the orbits and midbrain. The bone appears black as it produces no signals while the orbital and subcutaneous fatty tissue are intensely white. Blood vessels also appear black.

(2609) Section taken just above the orbits showing blood vessels but with this particular system the ventricles are not clearly visible.

(2610, 2611) The midline and brain tissue immediately under the bone are clearly visible but not the ventricles.

(2612) Sagittal section through the head and face in the midline showing cerebrum, cerebellum, midbrain and spinal cord. The picture is produced by the direct acquisition of data and not by reconstruction from axial sections.

(2613) Sagittal section through the mastoid air cells, ear lobes and posterior nasopharynx showing the cerebral hemispheres.

Figures by kind permission of Dr. W. S. Moore, G. W. Holland and R. C. Hawkes of the Department of Physics at the University of Nottingham, England.
This research work is currently being supported by G.E.C. Medical Equipment Limited, England.

EFFECTS OF RADIATION AND RADIATION PROTECTION METHODS IN DIAGNOSTIC RADIOLOGY

THE EFFECTS OF RADIATION, AND RADIATION PROTECTION METHODS IN DIAGNOSTIC RADIOLOGY

Introduction

There are both benefits and hazards associated with ionising radiation, which is still essential for diagnosis in a large number of clinical situations. In the last decade, many technical developments have been introduced which obviate or curtail the use of X-rays, including image intensification, rare earth screens and fibreoptic endoscopy. The greatest saving in radiation has, however, come with the introduction of ultrasonography in obstetrics and gynaecology. Though less spectacular, automatic exposures with iontomat devices prevent unnecessary repeat examinations and the almost universal introduction of the ten-day rule protects the very early pregnancy from ionising radiation when the fetus is most vulnerable.

At the other extreme of modern technology, computed tomography can extract the maximum diagnostic information when ionising radiation is used. If nuclear magnetic resonance scanning, which also requires computers, fulfills its expectations, there will be a further decrease in the indications for ionising radiation in medical diagnosis.

Nuclear medicine presents special problems in radiation protection because of the mobility of the isotope both before and after the examination. Radiopharmaceuticals are well controlled in the laboratory and in transit to the scanning room, but disposing of the isotopes that will be excreted from the patient following examination, such as contaminated urine and faeces, needs special attention, as does the 'radioactive' patient.

Radiation protection thus continues to be an important aspect of the policies and functions of a radiology department, which must also conform to national and international codes of practice, the most recent being a recommendation from the Council of European Directives.

The dose of radiation is given in rems, rads and roentgens (r). The rem, or 'rad-equivalent-man', takes into account the biological effects produced by different types of radiation following the same dose measured in rads. However, there is little difference between rems, rads and roentgens in the effects of X-rays on soft tissues. These units are defined on pp. 898–9.

Ionising radiation produces both somatic effects (those experienced directly by the individual) and genetic effects (those passed on to later generations) and each is considered in some detail.

Somatic effects of radiation

Only relatively large doses of radiation can produce serious effects and should never be encountered in diagnostic radiography.

High doses of radiation to the whole body, such as those received by the victims of the atomic bombs in Japan in 1945, produce an acute illness within a few hours of exposure, with subsequent death in many instances. A dose of 500r produces this illness in all cases and about 50% die. Small parts of the body can tolerate much higher doses of radiation. 500r to an area of skin received during radiotherapy only produces a reddening and loss of hair. 4000r or more may be given in radiotherapy, when the skin becomes very sensitive and prone to infection, and at this stage is covered with dilated blood vessels.

Apart from the above effects, which appear soon after exposure, doses of radiation can cause leukaemia and many forms of cancer at a later date. Leukaemia, which may appear as much as 10 years after exposure is uncommon, and even after exposure to large doses of radiation the likelihood of suffering from it is still small. Cancer can occur more than 50 years after exposure, so that individuals exposed in later life will die from other causes before any radiation-induced cancer has had time to appear.

Some parts of the body are more sensitive to radiation than others, particularly the blood forming organs, the lens of the eye and the reproductive organs. A whole-body dose as low as 25r can produce a temporary change in the blood count. 200r to the eye can cause cataract formation and with 750r will occur in most cases. Doses to the gonads of 200r will produce temporary sterility and 300r to 600r may cause permanent sterility.

It seems relevant here to quote from the 1956 report of the Medical Research Council, 'The Hazards to Man of Nuclear and Allied Radiations': 'Under modern conditions of occupational exposure, for example, among radiologists and radiographers, there is no evidence of any impairment of fertility. Furthermore there is no suggestion that female radiographers suffer from radiation-induced menstrual disturbances which might be accompanied by diminished fertility.'

Miscarriage and stillbirth can be caused by high doses of radiation to pregnant women, such as those received during radiotherapy or by the population of Hiroshima in 1945 and there is also evidence to show that irradiation of the fetus at an early stage can cause developmental abnormalities. Hence the rigid application of the 'ten-day rule'. All women of child-bearing age must be radiographed only in the first ten days of the menstrual cycle, unless there are overriding urgent medical indications or adequate contraceptive precautions have been taken.

Genetic effects of radiation

The nucleus of all cells of the body contain a number of chromosomes in which there are a large number of genes that determine the hereditary nature of each individual. The genes and chromosomes in each cell of the body are identical, half being inherited from each parent, apart from the sperm or ovum which contain only half the genes and chromosomes of the body cells. Thus it is that on average a particular gene is passed on to half of one's children, to a quarter of one's grandchildren, to an eighth of one's great grandchildren, until after a large number of generations it will be spread widely in the population.

Genes occasionally undergo a sudden change into a different

form and is known as a mutation. If this happens in a sperm or egg cell, the gene will be passed on to later generations in its changed form. Mutations normally occur at a low rate caused, among other things, by natural background radiation coming from cosmic rays and small amounts of radioactivity in our bodies and in the surroundings. Many mutations produce harmful effects on the population, often severe including mental defects, mental illness, blindness and neonatal deaths, stillbirths and congenital malformations. Their existing levels are due to the natural mutation rate to which mankind has always been subjected. However, any additional radiation to the reproductive organs from the time of one's own conception until the conception of one's child, increases the mutation rate and therefore the occurrence of these harmful genetic effects in later generations.

The additional dose of radiation to double the natural mutation rate has been estinated to be between 30r and 80r to the reproductive organs up to the age of 30 years, this age being taken as the average age of reproduction. As background radiation in this country contributes only about 3r in 30 years it must account for less than 10% of natural mutations. The genetic effect has been shown to be negligible if a relatively small group of prospective parents receives this 'doubling' dose or even somewhat more; but if the average dose throughout the population were as high as this, then all genetic effects would eventually be doubled.

A nuclear disaster, whether by an industrial accident or war, would increase the average radiation dose to the survivors and hence to the world population to greater than the doubling dose, to maim and stultify large numbers in subsequent generations through genetic effects.

Permissible doses of radiation

In view of the harmful genetic effects produced by relatively small doses of radiation to the whole population, it is obviously necessary that rules should be made to ensure that such effects are kept within acceptable limits. Today, when radiation is widely used in diagnosis and treatment of disease and in industry, a balance must be found between the advantage of using radiation in certain circumstances and the possible risks. A report of the International Commission on Radiological Protection published in 1960 gives a number of recommendations on maximum permissible levels of radiation, in addition to background radiation, to different groups of people, based on the most up-to-date information. Table 1, page 899 summarizes these recommendations. It was decided that a dose of 5 rems to the gonads up to the age of 30, averaged throughout the population, would produce a genetic effect small enough to be acceptable, and that a small group of radiation workers could be allowed to receive 60 rems to the gonads between the ages of 18 and 30 years. The average dose of 5 rems is somewhat less than twice the normal background radiation and 60 rems is roughly equal to the doubling dose. In order to limit the average gonad dose in the population to 5 rems it is obvious that members of the general public must have a maximum permissible dose in 30 years of less than 5 rems. It is emphasized in the recommendations that these are all *maximum* doses and that every effort should be made to keep all doses to the minimum possible. It will be seen in Table 1 that radiation workers are permitted to receive somewhat larger doses of radiation to some parts of the body other than the gonads. This is because no genetic effect is produced except when the gonads are irradiated, and any somatic effects to the other parts of the body will not in general be produced by such low doses.

The maximum permissible doses laid down in these recommendations do not include radiation doses received from medical exposure. The International Commission recommends that, '... the genetic dose to the whole population from all sources additional to natural background radiation should not exceed 5 rems (per 30 years) plus the lowest practicable contribution from medical exposure'.

Responsibility for dose reduction in diagnostic radiology

All medical workers therefore carry a grave responsibility, particularly those in diagnostic imaging, for any additional genetic effects produced in the population through ionising radiation. Because of the importance of reducing radiation radiographers must know, in some detail, how to minimise the dose to other medical personnel, to patients and to themselves.

Protection for the radiologist and the radiographer

All diagnostic X-ray departments should conform with requirements laid down in the Ministry of Health's 'Code of Practice for the Protection of Persons Exposed to Ionizing Radiations'. This involves radiation protection to walls, floors, ceilings and doors to shield persons in adjacent rooms, the use of modern equipment with adequate protection around the X-ray tube apart from the main beam and protection for the radiologist during fluoroscopy. Protective body aprons and gloves should always be available for use during fluoroscopy.

In addition to these protective measures, there are a number of ways in which radiographers can actively help to keep radiation to a minimum to themselves and to fellow workers.

(1) To always remember the 'inverse square law' and keep as far as possible away from all sources of radiation, whether primary or scattered and to *never* stand in the primary beam. If a child or unsteady patient needs to be supported this should be done by an accompanying parent or person not concerned with the X-ray department who should be provided with protective clothing and positioned so as to avoid the primary beam.

(2) To always use the smallest possible X-ray beam which minimizes radiation to the radiographer. The main source of scattered radiation is the area of the patient directly within the X-ray beam and is approximately proportional to the size of the area. In a small room it is essential to provide a protective screen with a lead glass window to reduce the scatter to the radiographer.

(3) Never to remain in the X-ray room unnecessarily during exposures.

(4) During erect fluroscopy to stand, whenever possible, behind the radiologist where protection is provided by the lead glass of the screen and by the apron suspended from it. During horizontal screening, the radiographer must always wear a lead apron to protect the body.

(5) To make regular inspections, every 3 months of all protective gloves and aprons to detect any splitting or holes. Aprons can be inspected simply by screening, but the easiest way to inspect gloves is to lay them on a double-wrapped film and expose to X-rays sufficient to penetrate them slightly, using the highest kilovoltage available. Examples of such radiographs of gloves are reproduced by Osborn (1956).

(6) Every radiation worker is required by the 'Code of Practice' to wear either a film badge or a pocket ionization chamber which is normally worn outside any protective clothing, usually on the lapel or in the breast pocket, thus giving an indication of the dose received by unprotected parts of the body. The radiographer should co-operate in wearing these badges or ionization chambers and in returning them at the required time for dose assessment. A continuous personal record can then be kept of every worker's dose. Investigation into any dose higher than normal may point to improvements needed in general technique or may be an early indication of faulty equipment.

Protection of the patient

The use of up-to-date equipment and accessories helps to reduce radiation to the patient. Recommendations in this connection have been made in 'The Code of Practice', in the report 'Radiological Hazards to Patients' and by the International Commission on Radiological Protection. These recommendations include the use of light beam localizers, accurate timing devices and aluminium filters. A permanent total filter of 2 mm aluminium should be fitted to all radiological equipment. An unfiltered X-ray beam contains a wide range of photon energies and the very soft components will be absorbed in the superficial layers of the patient and will not reach the film. An aluminium filter will absorb these soft rays thus reducing the skin dose to the patient and making little or no difference to the film dose.

No patient must be radiated unnecessarily and therefore it must be ascertained whether the relevant information can be obtained from films previously taken, possibly at another hospital, or by some completely different method. Fluoroscopy should not be used when the same information can be obtained by radiography as doses are invariably less for radiography.

In view of the importance of minimizing radiation to the fetus, the pelvis should not be radiographed during pregnancy unless this is absolutely necessary. It should be remembered that any woman of child-bearing age could be in the early stage of pregnancy, and to avoid this possibility radiographic examinations of the pelvis would be best undertaken during the first 10 days of the menstrual cycle.

In considering the role of the radiographer in minimizing radiation to the patient the most important factor is good radiographic technique which will produce good radiographs, and reduce irradiation of the patient to the minimum especially the gonads. In this, the following points are of importance:

(1) Always position the patient accurately using immobilizing devices when necessary and practicable. If the exposure has to be repeated, the radiation to the patient is doubled.

(2) Always use the smallest possible field sizes. If the edges of the beam show as a margin on the film one can be sure that an excessive field size was not used and ideally, should become the general practice. The use of a circular cone to cover a rectangular film exposes more of the patient than necessary or otherwise wastes the corners of the film, so it is obviously preferable to have an adjustable rectangular aperture fitted with a light beam localizer which assists the accurate positioning of the beam.

(3) When possible direct the beam away from the gonads, for example, when radiographing the upper limb with the patient in the sitting position.

(4) Gonad shields should be used where the gonads are likely to be in the primary beam, unless they interfere with the examination itself. Shields of 0·5 mm lead equivalent will reduce the gonad dose to about 5% of the unshielded dose, most of which is due to radiation scattered from the rest of the beam. A number of different devices for protecting the gonads have been designed in recent years some of which are positioned on the patient and others attached to the cone or light beam diaphragm.

(5) The fastest possible film screen combinations should be used for the required diagnostic information. With rare earth screens there is no longer the inevitable graininess associated with high speed screen film combinations and perfectly acceptable results can be obtained with 20–25% of previous exposures. The lower exposures prolong the life of equipment, especially the X-ray tube and allows lower output units to produce very short time exposures, overcoming movement blurring.

(6) The longest practicable focus–film distance should be used. For a given film dose the skin dose is less for a long than for a short focus–film distance and the diagram illustrates two situations: in the first, the focus–skin distance is 23 cm (9 ins) and the focus–film distance 46 cm (18 ins), in the second, the distances are increased to 68 cm (27 ins) and 90 cm (36 ins)

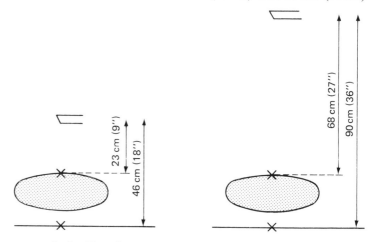

respectively. For the same tube exposure in the two examples the film dose in the second example will be a quarter, and the skin dose one-ninth of those in the first example. If, therefore the tube exposure in the second example is four times that of the first, the film dose will be equal, but the skin dose will be reduced to four-ninths or less than half.

(7) The kilovoltage used should be neither too low nor too high.* Soft X-rays are readily absorbed by the body and

* As there is some confusion in the use of the terms 'soft' and 'hard' in describing radiation *versus* its photographic effect—high kilovoltage, therefore hard radiation, produces a flat effect in the radiograph; conversely, low kilovoltage, therefore soft radiation, produces a steep contrasty radiograph.

therefore, to give the required film dose, a large dose must be given to the patient. On the other hand, if a very high kilovoltage is used, the penetrating power will be increased so much that the X-rays will tend to pass through the film as well as the patient. Also, scatter outside the beam is greater for high kilovoltage than for low kilovoltage radiation, so that if the gonads are out of the main beam they will receive a smaller dose at the appropriate lower kilovoltage. Thus, for minimum gonad doses the use of 70–110 kVp is recommended.

(8) A check on the alignment of the light and X-ray beams of all light beam localizers should be made periodically and can easily be done with a large double-wrapped film. Using a field somewhat smaller than the film, small strips of metal should be laid along the four edges of the light beam to mark their positions on the film. An exposure sufficient to penetrate the metal and leave a clear outline of the X-ray field will show any discrepancy between the two fields. Correct alignment can make all the difference between the gonads being in or out of the beam, especially in chest radiography where the focus–film distance is considerable.

Estimation of skin dose from nomogram

Where an extensive radiological examination is contemplated it is advisable to keep a careful account of the skin dose from the beginning. A quick indication of skin dose received by the patient and how it varies with an added filter, kilovoltage and focus–*skin* distance can be obtained by referring to the nomogram on the next page, constructed by measuring the output of a number of X-ray sets and taking the largest, a ward-mobile machine, as the 'standard'. The actual dose from other sets may be somewhat less but will not in general be less than half the value estimated from the nomogram, Osborn (1956 and 1963). It is thus possible to get a reasonable estimate of skin dose.

To use the nomogram, a straight line is required, and this can conveniently be either a length of black thread stretched taut, or a fine black line ruled on celluloid. This line should be laid over the chart so as to cross the top and bottom scales at values corresponding to a specified exposure. The bottom horizontal scale represents kilovolts peak (kVp); the line should cross this scale at a position determined by the lower row of figures if *no* external filter is used, or by the upper row of figures if a 2 mm aluminium filter is used. (For undercouch work, the couch top may legitimately be regarded as a filter for the purpose of estimating radiation exposure, and this applies also to a vertical stand with the tube in the screening position). The top horizontal scale represents the focus–*skin* distance (FSD) *not* the focus–*film* distance (FFD) and it is scaled in centimetres as well as in inches for convenience.

When the line is correctly adjusted on the two outer scales, the point at which it crosses the middle horizontal scale should be observed, and the numerical value noted. This indicates the dose delivered in milliroentgens (mr) per milliampere-second (mAS), from which the total surface dose for any other value of milliampere-seconds can easily be calculated.

Example 1. A patient was radiographed at 90 kVp, 12 mAS, 2 mm aluminium filter at a focus–*skin* distance of 50 cm. From the nomogram is read the value of 38 mr per mAS, but the tube exposure was 12 mAS and therefore the dose was $38 \times 12 = 456$ mr. (N.B. With no added filter the dose would have been $95 \times 12 = 1140$ mr. This is two-and-a-half times the skin dose with 2 mm aluminium filter).

Example 2. A patient is screened at 85 kVp, 3 mA, 2 mm aluminium filter, at a focus–*skin* distance of 30 cm. How long is permitted for a maximum skin dose of 20 r (20,000 mr)? The nomogram value corresponding to the above conditions is 92 mr/mAS; hence for 20,000 mr we have $20,000/92 = 217 \cdot 4$ mAS. At 3 mA, this would give an exposure time of $72 \cdot 5$ seconds.

Existing levels of genetic doses in Great Britain

In 1957 to 1958 a survey was made of genetic doses to the population of Great Britain, resulting from diagnostic and therapeutic radiology. A Committee was set up under the chairmanship of Lord Adrian and the results obtained are recorded in the Committee's Second Report 'Radiological Hazards to Patients'.

Table 2 on page 899 is taken from the report and gives the mean gonad doses received in different diagnostic examinations. It was calculated that doses from all diagnostic examinations in Great Britain are equivalent to an average gonad dose (ie genetic dose) of 14·1 mr per year to each person in the population. A similar calculation for genetic dose from radiotherapy gave a figure of 5·2 mr per year to each person.

Table 3 on page 900 shows the genetic dose per person from the different sources of radiation to which the population is exposed. These figures are derived from those in the Second Report of the Medical Research Council on radiation hazards (1960). The last column gives the genetic doses received in a generation of 30 years showing that this amounts to 0·08 rad above background plus 0·579 rad from medical exposure. This should be compared with the recommended maximum value of 5 rems above background plus the lowest practicable contribution from medical exposure. The first figure is obviously well below the acceptable level, but the contributions from medical exposure can be reduced considerably by the adoption of all possible protection measures.

A detailed analysis of the results obtained in the Adrian Committee survey has shown that the genetic dose from diagnostic radiology is as high as 14·1 mr to each person per year mainly because some hospitals do not take sufficient care to use low dose techniques. For example, it was found that in the chest examinations of the survey the ovaries of 51 % of the adult females were in the X-ray beam as was also the scrotum of 10 % of the adult males, for which there is no justification. It was shown that, if the techniques of the 10 % of hospitals giving the largest doses were brought up to the average standard of all the others, the figure of 14·1 mr to each person per year would be reduced to about 10 mr. If all techniques were as satisfactory as that in the 25 % of hospitals giving the lowest doses, then the genetic dose could be reduced to 2 mr to each person per year. With improvements also in techniques in the treatment of non-malignant disease by radiotherapy, it is estimated that the total genetic dose to each person per year from diagnostic and therapeutic radiology could be reduced from 19·3 mr to about 6 mr.

The importance of technique in reducing radiation hazards should not now need to be emphasized. Radiographers must realize that they are in control of a potentially hazardous machine and it is their duty to use it with the utmost care. Only then are they making their maximum contribution to the well-being of patients by helping to diagnose disease in the present population with the minimum hazard to future generations.

Radiation Precautions After Nuclear Medicine Examination

Radiation precautions for isotopes are especially important when patients return to the ward or go home after a nuclear medicine examination. Radiographers must understand the basic principles associated with patients who 'contain' radioactivity to limit exposure to ionising radiation to as low a level as possible.

No appreciable hazard exists to hospital personnel from ionising radiation within a patient unless a large amount of radioactive material has been given, which does not occur with diagnostic nuclear medicine. There is no risk of radiation to nurses or family from being close to such patients, but when a patient contains therapeutic radioactivity special precautions are necessary. However, all body fluids and excreta of patients who have received radionuclides are considered to be radioactive and special precautions must be taken.

1. Direct contact with the patient's blood, faeces, urine, vomitus or other body fluid must be avoided. Rubber gloves must be worn to handle all such materials.
2. If clothes or bedclothes become contaminated by such body fluids, the radiology or nuclear medicine department must be informed and the contaminated materials saved for monitoring.
3. Similarly if a dressing covering the site of injection of Gold-198 becomes contaminated, notify the nuclear medicine department.
4. If patients have received large amounts of iodine-131 they should not bath for at least 24 hours thereafter. Otherwise simple precautions such as wearing rubber gloves and washing hands after bathing patients should be taken.
5. Bedpans must only be handled with rubber gloves and thoroughly flushed before returning to general use. Bedpans used by patients having had large amounts of iodine-131 should be flushed out thoroughly and the same bedpan retained for that patient during his hospital stay.
6. If there is any spill of radioactivity, mop up immediately, saving all material including the mop used and notify the nuclear medicine department immediately.
7. If needles, capsules or seeds of radioactivity being used for treatment become dislodged, they should only be handled with forceps or tongs and never be touched directly. Notify nuclear medicine department immediately.
8. If a patient containing more than 5 mCi of radioactivity dies, notify the nuclear medicine department and if a patient containing needles, capsules or seeds of radioactivity dies, the physics section of the radiotherapy department must be notified immediately.

Each hospital will have its own set of detailed rules for radioactivity precautions which must be rigidly observed, and if there is any doubt about precautions to be taken in specific circumstances, the physics or nuclear medicine department must be consulted.

There should be no limitations to visitors of patients containing radioactivity unless precautions to the contrary are shown and usually pertains only to encapsulated radioactivity within a patient.

Proposals for the Directive by the Council of European Communities presents the basic measures for protection of persons undergoing medical examination or treatment. Unfortunately the final Directive is not available at present, only draft proposals of the first seven articles summarising the responsibilities of the member of states.

References

Ardran, G. M. and Kempt, F. H. (1957). Protection of the male gonads in diagnostic procedures. *British Journal of Radiology*, **30** (353) 271–3.

Abram, E., Wilkinson, D. M. and Hodson, C. J. (1958). Gonadal protection from X radiation for the female. *British Journal of Radiology*, **31** (366) 335–6.

Whitehead, G. and Griffiths J. T. (1961). The Leicester gonad protector: a device to afford localised protection from diagnostic X-irradiation. *British Journal of Radiology* **34**, 135–6.

Kendig, T. A. (1960). Reduction of fetal irradiation in pelvimetry. *Radiology*, **75**, 608–11.

Osborn, S. B. (1956). In: Hazards to man of nuclear and allied radiation. *Medical Research Council* (HMSO), Cmd. 9780.

Osborn, S. B. (1963). Variations in the radiation dose received by the patient in diagnostic radiology. *British Journal of Radiology*, **36**, 230–4.

NOMOGRAM FOR ESTIMATING THE SURFACE
RADIATION EXPOSURE TO THE PATIENT

FOCUS-SKIN DISTANCE

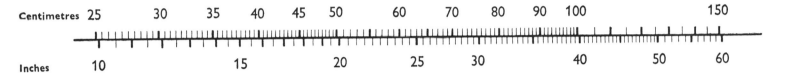

Centimetres 25   30   35   40   45   50   60   70   80   90   100   150

Inches   10   15   20   25   30   40   50   60

MILLIRÖNTGENS PER MILLIAMPERE-SECOND

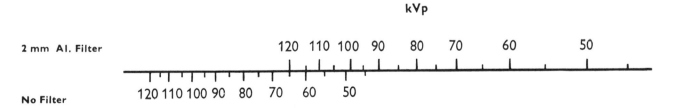

500 400 300   200   100 80 60 50 40   30   20   10 8   6 5 4   3   2   1

kVp

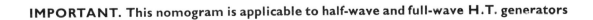

2 mm Al. Filter   120 110 100 90   80   70   60   50

No Filter   120 110 100 90 80   70   60   50

IMPORTANT. This nomogram is applicable to half-wave and full-wave **H.T.** generators

Definitions of terms

Absorbed dose of any ionizing radiation: amount of energy imparted to matter by ionizing particles per unit mass of irradiated material at the place of interest. Expressed ideally in rads but for X and gamma rays of quantum energy up to 3 MeV, the roentgen (r) may be used.

Collimation. In radiology; the limiting of a beam of radiation to the required dimensions.

Computer. Electronic equipment which performs calculations and stores data. The calculations performed include simple functions, intergration, differentiation and simultaneous equations. Computers may be *analogue*, *digital* or *hybrid* (*mixed digital analogue*).

Analogue operates with continuously varying amplitudes such as pictures or graphs whereas *digital* operates on units.

Cosmic rays. Ionizing rays entering the earth's atmosphere from unidentified extra-terrestrial space and resulting in the presence of photons, electrons, neutrons, protons, mesons, etc., by collision with atoms in the atmosphere.

Detectors. These are a part of the circuit capable of extracting a signal by reacting to electromagnetic radiation.

Gantry. This is the supporting frame which houses the X-ray tube and detectors of a computed tomography machine.

Half-value layer (HVL). The thickness of a specified absorbing material which, when introduced into the path of an X-ray beam, reduced the dose-rate to half its original value.

Hertz (Hz). This is the unit of frequency indicating the number of cycles per second. In ultrasonography, the frequency is indicated in megahertz (mHz) or millions of cycles per second.

Ionizing radiation. Electromagnetic radiation (X-ray or gamma-ray photons or quanta), or corpuscular radiation (alpha-particles, beta-particles, electrons, protons, neutrons, and heavy particles) capable of producing ions.

Lead equivalent. The thickness of lead affording the same protection under specified conditions of irradiation as the material in question. The lead equivalent of a substance, such as lead glass or lead rubber, which attenuates the radiation essentially by its lead content, is largely independent of the quality of the radiation. The lead equivalent of all other protective materials and also building material for protective walls (concrete, brick, etc.) and barium protective glass shows a dependence on the quality of the radiation.

Lead glass (protective glass). Glass, containing a high proportion of lead compounds, which absorbs radiation passing through it. Used as a transparent protective material.

Lead rubber. Rubber containing a high proportion of lead compounds. It is used as a flexible protective material.

Nutation. (adjective—Nutating) A particular type of rotation with a periodic variation of the inclination of the axis of rotation (similar to the oscillation of the earth's polar axis which occurs about every nineteen years).

Quantum. The smallest quantity of energy in the form of a bundle or packet of waves of electromagnetic radiation which can be associated with a given phenomenon. (Electromagnetic radiation sometimes appears to consist of waves and at other times of particles. Such particles may be regarded as bundles of waves.)

Quantum energy. Energy contained in a quantum of radiation and proportional to the frequency of the radiation waves. (The energy E of a quantum of radiation of frequency f if hf where h is Planck's constant.)

Photon. A quantum of light or electromagnetic radiation which is equal to Planck's constant (h) multiplied by frequency (v) in Hz.

Piezo-electric effect. The process of conversion of electrical energy to a mechanical effect such as to produce sound waves and vice versa the conversion of mechanical effects by, for example, sound waves into electrical energy. A property which is possessed by crystals such as quartz and barium titanate.

Precess. The effect shown by a gyroscope such as a spinning top when a force is applied to it in such a way as to change the direction of its rotation, similar to a spinning top as it begins to slow down with the long axis inclining towards the horizontal.

Rad. Unit of absorbed dose. It is 100 ergs per gramme. Millirad (mrad): 1/1,000 rad.

Radiation (*as applied to X-rays*):

1. Primary radiation: radiation coming directly from the target of the X-ray tube. Except for the useful beam, the bulk of this radiation is absorbed in the tube housing.
2. Secondary radiation: radiation, other than the primary radiation, emitted by any matter irradiated with X-rays. Often loosely called scattered radiation.
3. Scattered radiation: radiation which during passage through a substance has been deviated in direction. It may also have been modified by an increase in wavelength (Compton effect). It is one form of secondary radiation.
4. Stray radiation: radiation not serving any useful purpose. It includes secondary radiation and any radiation, other than the useful beam, coming from within the X-ray tube and tube housing (such as stem radiation). This is the radiation against which special protective measures have to be taken.
5. Useful beam: that part of the primary radiation which passes through the aperture, cone or other device for collimating the X-ray beam.

Relative Biological Effectiveness (RBE). Ratio of the dose (expressed in rads) of 200 to 250 kV X-rays to the dose (in rads) of any type of ionizing radiation which produces the same biological effect. Most of the clinical evidence on the effects of ionizing radiations has been obtained with 200 to 250 kV X-rays. Accordingly, this is used as the base line, being given a biological effectiveness of unity.

Rem (Rad-Equivalent-Man). Quantity of any ionizing radiation such that the energy imparted to a biological system per gramme of living matter by the ionizing particles present in the locus of interest, has the same biological effectiveness as 1 rad of 200 to 250 kV X-rays. Millirem (mrem): 1/1,000 rem.

Roentgen (r). Unit of dose of X and gamma rays, but not other ionizing radiation, Defined as below:

'The Roentgen shall be the quantity of X or gamma radiation such that the associated corpuscular emission per 0·001293 gramme of air produces, in air, ions carrying 1 electrostatic unit of quantity of electricity of either sign.' (It becomes increasingly difficult to measure the dose in roentgens as the quantum energy of X or gamma radiation approaches very high values. The unit may, however, be used for most practical purposes for quantum energies up to 3 MeV.)

Milliroentgen (mr):   1/1,000 r.
Microroentgen (μr):   1/1,000,000 r.

X-ray tube housing. An enclosure which covers the tube and sometimes also other portions of the X-ray equipment (transformer) and which limits the major portion of radiation emitted from the tube to the useful beam.

TABLE 1
SUMMARY OF RECOMMENDATIONS OF ICRP FOR MAXIMUM PERMISSIBLE DOSES OF RADIATION, EXCLUDING MEDICAL EXPOSURE

	Maximum Permissible Dose in rems			
	in 13 weeks	in 1 year	up to age N years	up to 30 years
A. Radiation Workers				
(i) Gonads, blood-forming organs, lens of the eye.	3	5	5 (N–18)	60
(ii) Skin and thyroid gland.	8	30		
(iii) Hands, forearms, feet, ankles.	20	75		
(iv) All other organs and tissues.	4	15		
B. Non-radiation Workers who work near or may occasionally enter areas where radiation is used				
i) Gonads, blood-forming organs, lens of eye and all internal organs.		1·5	1·5 (N–18)	18
(ii) Skin and thyroid gland.		3		
C. Some members of the public, for example those living in the neighbourhood of radiation areas. (Including children and pregnant women)				
All tissues.		0·5	0·5N	15
D. Average gonad dose per head of population				5
E. Therefore all other members of the population (to maintain average of 5 rem)				less than 5

TABLE 2
MEAN GONAD DOSE PER EXAMINATION IN MILLIROENTGENS

	Type of Examination	Male	Female	Fetus
1.	Chest, heart, lung (excluding mass miniature radiography)	2·75	5·4	5·5
2.	Barium meal	44	333	448
3.	Abdomen	105	183	281
4.	Abdomen obstetric	—	367	723
5.	Intravenous Pyelography	765	585	843
6.	Pelvimetry	—	745	885
7.	Pelvis, lumbar spine, lumbo-sacral joint	370	392	536
8.	Hip, upper femur	740	102	154

TABLE 3
APPROXIMATE GENETIC DOSES TO THE POPULATION OF GREAT BRITAIN IN 1957–1960

Source of Radiation	Genetic Dose per Person	
	in millirads per year	in rads per 30 years
Natural Background	100	3
Medical Exposure:		
Diagnostic Radiology	14·1	0·423
Therapeutic Radiology	5·2	0·156
Total	19·3	0·579
Other Sources:		
Fall-out	1·2	0·035
Miscellaneous	Less than 1	Less than 0·03
Occupational exposure	0·5	0·015
Total Less than	2·7	Less than 0·08

WORKING METRIC EQUIVALENTS OF DIMENSIONS AND QUANTITIES

SUPPLEMENT TWO

WORKING METRIC EQUIVALENTS OF DIMENSIONS AND QUANTITIES

LINEAR

Inches		Centimetres
$\frac{1}{8}$	=	0·32
$\frac{1}{4}$	=	0·64
$\frac{1}{2}$	=	1·3
$\frac{3}{4}$	=	1·9
1	=	2·5
$1\frac{1}{4}$	=	3·2
$1\frac{1}{2}$	=	3·8
$1\frac{3}{4}$	=	4·4
2	=	5·1
$2\frac{1}{4}$	=	5·7
$2\frac{1}{2}$	=	6·3
$2\frac{3}{4}$	=	7·0
3	=	7·6
$3\frac{1}{2}$	=	8·9
4	=	10
$4\frac{1}{2}$	=	12
5	=	13
$5\frac{1}{2}$	=	14
6	=	15
$6\frac{1}{2}$	=	17
7	=	18
$7\frac{1}{2}$	=	19
8	=	20
$8\frac{1}{2}$	=	22
9	=	23
$9\frac{1}{2}$	=	24
10	=	25
11	=	28
12 (1 foot)	=	30
13	=	33
14	=	36
15	=	38
16	=	41
17	=	42
18	=	46
19	=	48
20	=	51
22	=	56
24 (2 feet)	=	61
26	=	66

LINEAR

Inches		Centimetres
28	=	71
30	=	76
32	=	81
34	=	86
$35\frac{1}{2}$	=	90
36 (3 feet)	=	91
38	=	97
$39\frac{3}{8}$	=	100 (1 metre)

Inches		Metres
40	=	1·02
42	=	1·07
44	=	1·12
46	=	1·17
48 (4 feet)	=	1·22
$49\frac{1}{2}$	=	1·25
50	=	1·27
54	=	1·37
56	=	1·42
59	=	1·50
60 (5 feet)	=	1·52
66	=	1·68
72 (6 feet)	=	1·83
79	=	2·0
84 (7 feet)	=	2·13
96 (8 feet)	=	2·44

Centimetres		Inches
1·0	=	0·4
2·0	=	0·8
2·5	=	1·0
3·0	=	1·2
4·0	=	1·6
5·0	=	2·0
6·0	=	2·4
7·0	=	2·8
8·0	=	3·2
9·0	=	3·6

To convert centimetres to inches multiply by 0·4
To convert inches to centimetres divide by 0·4

WEIGHT

Pounds avoirdupois		Kilograms
1	=	0·4536
5	=	2·268
10	=	4·536
20	=	9·072
30	=	13·608
50	=	22·680
80	=	36·288
100	=	45·360
125	=	56·7
140	=	63·5
146	=	66·2
150	=	68·0
157	=	71·2
160	=	72·6
168	=	76·2
200	=	90·7

Kilograms		Pounds avoirdupois
1	=	2·2046 = 35·27 oz.
2	=	4·4092
3	=	6·6138
4	=	8·8184
5	=	11·0230
6	=	13·2276
7	=	15·4322
8	=	17·6368
9	=	19·8414
10	=	22·0460
15	=	33·069
20	=	44·092
25	=	55·115
30	=	66·138
35	=	77·161
40	=	88·184
45	=	99·207
50	=	110·230
55	=	121·253
60	=	132·276
65	=	143·299
70	=	154·322
75	=	165·345
80	=	176·368
85	=	187·391
90	=	198·414
95	=	209·437
100	=	220·460

FLUID

Millilitres		Ounces	Minims
	=		16·9
2	=		33·8
3	=		50·7
4	=		67·6
5	=		84·5
6	=		101
7	=		118
8	=		138
9	=		152
10	=		169
20	=		338
30	=	1	27
40	=	1	196
50	=	1	365
60	=	2	54
70	=	2	223
80	=	2	391
90	=	3	80
100	=	3	249
200	=	7	19
300	=	10	268
400	=	14	37
500	=	17	287
600	=	21	56
700	=	24	305
800	=	28	75
900	=	31	324
1,000	=	35	94
(1 litre)			

35·2 ounces = 100 ml = 1 litre = 0·220 gal.
  1 gal. = 4·56 litres.

Drams		Fluid ounces		Millilitres
1	=	$\frac{1}{8}$	=	3·55
2	=	$\frac{1}{4}$	=	7·10
4	=	$\frac{1}{2}$	=	14·20
8	=	1	=	28·40
		2	=	57·00
		4	=	114·00
		8	=	228·00
		12	=	342·00
		16	=	456·00
			=	(1 USA pint)
		20	=	568·20
			=	(1 British pint)

TEMPERATURE CONVERSION CHART

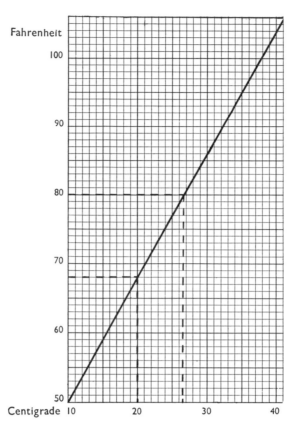

Radiographic film is available in the following centimetre and inch sizes:

cm		inches	
13 × 18	24 × 30	$4\frac{3}{4} \times 6\frac{1}{2}$	10 × 15
15 × 30	30 × 40	$6\frac{1}{2} \times 8\frac{1}{2}$	12 × 15
15 × 40	35·6 × 35·6	8 × 10	7 × 17
18 × 24	35·6 × 43·2	6 × 12	14 × 14
20 × 40		10 × 12	14 × 17

Roll film $\begin{cases} 30 \text{ cm} \times 15 \text{ metres} \\ 30 \text{ cm} \times 25 \text{ metres} \end{cases}$

TABLE OF CONTRAST MEDIA
(See Section 35)

Angiography

(Aortography)

1. Triiodinated benzoic acid		
Derivatives	*Trade name*	
Diatrizoate	Hypaque	Sodium or Meglumine salts
	Urografin	
Iodamine	Uromiro	
Iothalamate	Conray	
Metrizoate	Triosil	
2. Ioxaglate	Hexabrix	
3. Metrizamide	Amipaque	

Examination	*Quantity ml*	%	*Approx. g. Iodine per 100 ml*	*Preferred contrast agent*
Aortography	20–40	60	28	
Brachial arteriography	10–15	60	28	Meglumine salts Ioxaglate
Cardioangiography	40–50	70–80	40	
Coronary arteriography	5–6	60	28	Ioxaglate Metrizamide
Cerebral arteriography	6–8	60	28	Ioxaglate Metrizamide Meglumine salts
Femoral arteriography				
Bilateral	20–40	60	28	Meglumine salts Ioxaglate
Unilateral	15–20	60	28	
Selective Visceral arteriography				
Coeliac axis	40	60	28	Meglumine salts
Hepatic	30	60	28	
Inferior mesenteric	20	60	28	
Pancreatic	10–20	60	28	
Renal	10	60	28	Ioxaglate
Splenoportography	50	60	28	
Venography	50–70	60	28	Meglumine salts Ioxaglate

Biliary System
Cholecystography
(oral)

Dirivatives	*Trade name*	*Dose*
Iopanoic acid	Telepaque	2g
Ipodate	Biloptin	2g
Calcium Ipodate	Solu-bioptin	3g

Examination	*Contrast agent*	*Trade name*	*%*	*Quantity*
Cholangiography (intravenous)				
	Iodipamide	Biligrafin	30	30 ml
		Biligrafin 'forte'	50	20 ml in 250 ml normal saline
	Ioglycamine	Biligram		20 ml
Cholangiography (operative)				
	Iothalamate	Conray		
	Iodamide	Uromiro		
	Metrizoate	Triosil	25	5–20 ml
	Diatrizoate	Hypaque / Urografin		
Cholangiography (percutaneous transhepatic)				
	Iothalamate	Conray		
	Iodamide	Uromiro		
	Metrizoate	Triosil	45	10–50 ml
	Diatrizoate	Hypaque / Urografin		
Endoscopic Retrograde Cholangiopancreatography				
	Metrizamide	Amipaque	60	2–3 ml (in pancreatic duct)
	Ioxaglate	Hexabrix		5–10 ml (in common bile duct)
	Meglumine salts			

Central Nervous System
Myelography with Metrizamide

	Quantity in ml	*Amipaque %*	*Approx. g. Iodine/100 ml*	
Lumbar Region	10–15	35	17	
Dorsal Region	12–15	40	20	
	10–12	50	25	Metrizamide-Amipaque
Cervical Region	7–10	50	25	
Ventriculography	3–5	50	25	
Myelography	Ethyl iodophenyl Myodil undecylate 6–9			

Dacrocystography

Meglumine salts		1–2 ml	60%	
Ioxaglate	Hexabrix	1–2 ml	60%	

Gastro-intestinal System

Barium sulphate

	Contrast agent	% w/v
Liquids	Baritop Micropaque	100 and 120
Powder	Baritop	100–130
	Barosperse } made	100
	Barytgen } up	100–130
	EPI-C } to	
	E-Z }	170

Triiodinated benzoic acid derivatives

Gastrografin
Gastroconray

Examination		Quantity	% w/v
Oesophagus	Liquid	50–100 ml	100
	Powder made up to	50–100 ml	100
Stomach			
single contrast	Liquid	200–300 ml	80
	Powder made up to		80
Double contrast	Liquid	150–200 ml	100–120
	Powder	150–200 ml	120–170
Small bowel	Liquid	300–600 ml	100
follow through	Powder (Barosperse)	300–600 ml	100
Small bowel enema	Liquid	600–1,000 ml	15–20
Colon			
single contrast	Liquid	300–600 ml	80
	Powder	300–600 ml	
double contrast	Liquid	300 ml	120–130
	Powder	300 ml	120–130
Grastrografin		50–100 ml	
Gastroconray		50–100 ml	

Genito-urinary System

Urography (intravenous)

	Contrast agent	Trade name	Quantity	% w/v	Dose
	Diatrizoate	Urografin } Hypaque }			
	Iodamide	Uromiro }			
	Iothalamate	Conray }	40–70 ml	60–70	15–30 g
	Metrizoate	Triosil }			
Urography (high dose)	Methyl glucamine		100 ml	60–70	40 g
Urography (infusion)			250 ml	25–30	20 g
Antegrade Pyelography			10–40 ml	25	3–4 g
Retrograde Pyelography			5–10 ml	25	1–2 g
Cystography			200–300 ml	25	20–30 g
Cysto-urethrography	Methyl glucamine		200–300 ml	25	20–30 g
Hystero-salpengography	Methyl glucamine Ioxaglate		5–10 ml	60–65	4–8 g
Urethrography	Methyl glucamine		100 ml	25	15–20 g

Locomotor System
Arthrography

	Contrast Agent	Trade name	Dose
	Metrizamide	Amipaque	5–10 ml
	Ioxaglate	Hexabrix	5–10 ml
	Mythyl glucamine salts		5–10 ml
Discography			
	Metrizamide	Amipaque	1–2 ml
	Ioxaglate	Hexabrix	1–2 ml
	Methyl glucamine salts		1–2 ml
Lymphography			
	Ultra-fluid	Lipiodol	up to 7 ml (per leg) up to 5 ml (per arm)

Respiratory System
Bronchography

	Dose	
Dionosil Aqueous	6–10 ml	⎫
Dionosil oily	6–10 ml	⎬ per lung
Hytrast	6–10 ml	⎭

		Quantity	% w/v
Sialography	Methyl glucamine salts	1–2 ml	60
Sinography	Triiodinated benzoic acid derivatives	5–30 ml	60

INDEX